Intensive Care Therapeutics

INTENSIVE CARE
THERAPEUTICS

edited by

JOSEPH M. CIVETTA, M.D.

Professor of Surgery, Anesthesiology,
  Medicine, and Pathology
University of Miami School of Medicine
Director, Surgical Intensive Care Unit
University of Miami/Jackson Memorial
  Medical Center
Miami, Florida

APPLETON-CENTURY-CROFTS / New York

Copyright © 1980 by APPLETON-CENTURY-CROFTS
A Publishing Division of Prentice-Hall, Inc.

Cover photograph copyright © 1980 by Robert Goldstein.

80 81 82 83 84 / 10 9 8 7 6 5 4 3 2 1

Prentice-Hall International, Inc., London
Prentice-Hall of Australia, Pty. Ltd., Sydney
Prentice-Hall of India Private Limited, New Delhi
Prentice-Hall of Japan, Inc., Tokyo
Prentice-Hall of Southeast Asia (Pte.) Ltd., Singapore
Whitehall Books Ltd., Wellington, New Zealand

Library of Congress Cataloging in Publication Data
Main entry under title:

Intensive care therapeutics.

    Bibliography: p.
    Includes index.
    1. Chemotherapy. 2. Critical care medicine.
I. Civetta, Joseph M. [DNLM: 1. Critical care.
2. Intensive care units. WX218 I106]
RM263.I48   615'.58   79–20772
ISBN 0–8385–4305–7

Cover design: Janet Konig
Line drawings in Chapters 1, 2, and 6 by Hal Keith

PRINTED IN THE UNITED STATES OF AMERICA

CONTRIBUTORS

Clyde H. Beck, Jr., M.D.
Clinical Professor of Medicine
University of California—San Diego
School of Medicine
La Jolla, California

D. David Glass, M.D.
Associate Professor of Surgery
Dartmouth Medical School
Director, Intensive Care Unit
Mary Hitchcock Memorial Hospital
Hanover, New Hampshire

Alan S. Livingstone, M.D.
Assistant Professor of Surgery
University of Miami School of Medicine
Staff Surgeon
Veterans Administration Hospital
Miami, Florida

D. Stewart MacIntyre, Jr., M.D.
Assistant Professor of Medicine
University of Miami School of Medicine
Director, Infection Control
University of Miami/Jackson Memorial Medical Center
Miami, Florida

George H. Rodman, Jr., M.D.
Assistant Professor of Surgery and Anesthesiology
University of Miami School of Medicine
Chief, Trauma Unit
Associate Director, Surgical Intensive Care Unit
University of Miami/Jackson Memorial Medical Center
Miami, Florida

CONTENTS

PREFACE

In a world in which the medical professional is bombarded by books, journals, articles, tapes, conferences, presentations, continuing education, and other types of communication, why should we compound the issue by creating yet another amalgam of ideas? Our answer, and perhaps our justification, is that, although the existence of intensive care is an incontrovertible fact, its growth seems to have come as a surprise to most educators. The curricula of medical schools, nursing diploma and degree programs, respiratory therapy courses, and other paramedical educational programs seem to include intensive care exposure only as a tantalizing afterthought. House officer rotations in certain subspecialties attempt to remedy this, but continuing education courses in intensive care only underscore the fact that this gap exists. Moreover, we feel that intensive care offers a unique application of the basic sciences, physiology, and pharmacology. These subjects are the determinants of medical practice in the intensive care unit. This handbook offers a succinct and understandable presentation of applied science to be utilized not only in quiet study but in the heat of the battle as well. While pharmacokinetics, molecular structure, and other important drug properties must of necessity be omitted to comply with these goals, this appears to be justifiable, since such information in the text might actually interfere with rapid acquisition of the practical knowledge that is necessary in a crisis.

Our approach has been a basic one. We hope you will read the text, refer to the summaries in acute situations, and then reread the text and use the references when the acute situation has been resolved.

The organization of this text involves a somewhat different approach to medical information. Usually, information is separated into basic sciences and clinical medicine and further subdivided into subspecialties of medicine, surgery, neurology, pediatrics, psychiatry, and the like. Realistically, none of these classification systems is all encompassing, and significant overlaps are tolerated without comment. For instance, urology and gynecology contain both the medical and surgical aspects of those particular subspecialties. In the case of the pediatrician or gerontologist, the only claim to specificity is the age of the patient. Intensive care cuts across the spectrum of human illness in a different dimension. We "intensivists" have concentrated our attention on a particular point of the patient's illness rather than on a chronologic definition or subspecialty differentiation.

The organization of this text has been guided by the need to resolve a particular issue: Is intensive care a specialty sufficiently differentiated to justify the investment of our time and money? This issue, of course, involves the definition of a specialty. Is there a specific core of knowledge? Does one require an expertise not otherwise available and does this specific experience create an individual of special talents? In our parochial view, the answer to each of these questions is yes!

While it is common to hear protestations that "all clinicians are intensivists by trade," the unique perspective that one obtains from the daily experience of the intensive care unit would suggest that this belief is more apparent than real. It was the gradual realization of the unique perspective of the full-time intensivist that prompted the decision to create this text. The types of drugs, routes of administration, dosages, problems treated, intercurrent problems, drug interactions, host resistance, therapeutic efficacy, and specific drug selection in intensive care are truly unique. Our own efforts at amassing this body of information proved so tedious, so changeable, and yet so vital that we elected to create yet another reference, which we sincerely hope will not provide an additional bookend support, briefcase stabilizer, or library adornment, but rather will quickly become dog-eared and discarded only when its contained knowledge is truly yours.

OBJECTIVES

The determiners of educational programs now require one to crystallize what is to be achieved from an exercise. Perhaps it is useful to suggest what we hope this volume will offer. To this purpose we can describe a certain set of desired objectives.

1. Structural and pharmacologic principles, while important, seem to be less than easily categorized according to pharmacologic effects both in terms of physiology and differential diagnosis and in terms of a proposed therapeutic schema for common intensive care problems. Whether one considers hypotension, seizures, agitation, or the like, it is perfectly obvious that these might have diverse etiologies including sepsis, hypoxia, neurologic manifestations, and so on. The interrelationships are clear and important: What steps must be taken and in what order? From another viewpoint, there are certain pharmacologic and pharmacodynamic aspects of intensive care that are not clearly differentiated in standard treatises of disease or of drug usage. Thus, the dissecting-out of the specific intensive care subset

of pharmacologic agents is difficult when one approaches the standard multi-thousand-page internal medicine or pharmacologic text.

2. The physiologic orientation attempted is intended to provide a basic framework to understand current medications and to allow similar understanding of newer agents, newer indications, and whatever updating becomes the standard of the future.

3. Of course, specific knowledge is stressed: routes of administration, dosages, modifications because of drug interactions, and drug indications not commonly understood in the general population. Finally, specific pharmacologic properties of importance to the critically ill patient will be stressed since they might be unappreciated or unimportant in ambulatory and/or routine hospital in-patient usage. For instance, the introduction of cimetidine as an H_2 antagonist has extremely important applications to treat stress gastrointestinal bleeding either as a primary diagnosis or as a disastrous intensive care complication.

4. The intensive care experience often represents the entire hospital exposure to certain disease states. Although a gastroenterologist regards diseases of the entire digestive system as his domain, intensive care complications involving the G.I. tract come only to his attention when the intensivist informs him of their existence. Thus, there is a peculiar concentration of multiple subsystem complications. One might then infer that the therapeutic response to various pharmacologic and other therapeutic manipulations might be best known not by the traditionalist, but by those individuals—intensivists—who observe all treated cases. In amassing concentrated experience in disastrous complications, the intensivist has had to develop pragmatic and immediate solutions to common problems. Such knowledge is not necessarily found in more standard volumes, and a major goal of this text is to disperse this information in a form more readily useful to the intensivist.

5. Problem solving in the intensive care unit is a way of life. It requires a multidisciplinary approach and an exposure to real situations. One cannot be content with an understanding of textbook and/or laboratory pharmacologic effects. We must learn to interpret the individual patient's response which, of course, is colored by co-existing disease, previous therapy, age, and the multitude of other factors that uniquely determine the condition of a particular patient at the time treated. These problems can be construed in a priority-oriented structure. Real situations can be true emergencies in which therapy may often precede diagnosis. An urgent situation may permit diagnosis to proceed ahead of therapeutic intervention, but the distinction is of minor importance in terms of the time involved. There are two other classes of intensive care problems relevant to pharmacologic interventions: potential problems, such as metabolic encephalopathy or stress G.I. bleeding, in the prolonged critically ill state and the creation of iatrogenic problems. The highest incidence of side-effects of any particular

mode of therapy is often found in the intensive care unit because the patient's physiologic reserve is exhausted. The daily experience is the creation of the "worse possible case." In other words, if there is a limited but potential nephrotoxic effect of a particular antibiotic, its emergence as a clinical problem is most likely in the situation in which patients with underlying renal disease are subjected to hypovolemia and other nephrotoxic insults. Should concomitant antibiotic therapy be deemed necessary, one might predict that the incidence of clinically important nephrotoxicity would be enhanced.

Problem solving cannot be considered to follow some "cookbook" recipe. A reasonable approach based on physiologic principles and experience is the most that we can hope to offer.

6. Finally, the physiologic interpretation of the critically ill state requires a certain understanding of apparatus and technique. Should we attempt to include all aspects of critical illness, we, too, could create a 2000-page tome. The information that is crucial to the understanding of methodology will be presented, and by the adequate referencing of the text we hope to provide an opportunity for the investigation of those areas that cannot be covered in minute detail.

PERSPECTIVE

The intensive care unit is an area of polypharmacology. A multitude of interventions to treat and/or prevent established conditions may or may not be appropriate. We hope to create a physiologic and pharmacologic data base for the interpretation of commonly advocated regimens. To achieve this, we have compiled the relevant data in a systematized format and have defined pharmacologic interventions in terms of the physiologic symptoms commonly observed in the intensive care unit.

This text, then, attempts a global approach to a specific area. It is a beginning, not an end; it is clinical, not lab-oriented. But most of all, it is hoped that it may provide a ready and effective reference source for the individual who is in the front line, who faces problems requiring immediate solution, and who perhaps silently wishes, at that particular moment, that he was not!

Although this volume is structured according to certain types of physiologic systems, it is probably fair to state that no pure case ever existed in an intensive care unit. Therefore, while emphasis rests on a particular system in an individual section, we hope to reemphasize the multidisciplinary aspects of critical illness by examining specific problems in each chapter.

Can all of these goals be accomplished? If some of the crisis orientation and history associated with intensive care can be removed and a logical approach to sudden and devastating complications can be initiated, then we would judge this effort and perspective to have been worthwhile.

Intensive Care Therapeutics

ONE

General Use
Medications

Alan Livingstone

ANALGESICS

Analgesics are defined as agents that alleviate pain without causing loss of consciousness, and it is readily apparent that many patients in a surgical intensive care unit will require this type of medication. While it has been observed that people do not die of pain, the elimination of needless suffering is a desirable goal which should be obtained as expeditiously as circumstances allow. There are, of course, times when the administration of narcotic analgesics is contraindicated, such as in a patient with an unstable cardiovascular system, a person with head trauma, or during the preoperative evaluation of an acute abdomen. However, once the clinical picture has stabilized or cleared, pain should be relieved with drugs such as morphine. The further advantage of narcotic analgesics in the intensive care unit setting is that they also provide sedation. There are now over 20 narcotics available, but when the drugs are administered in equianalgesic doses, the differences in major side effects are not significant. The familiarity with just a few of these preparations will serve most clinical situations (Table 1-1).

TABLE 1-1
Representative Narcotic Agonists and Antagonists
Used Parenterally

Drug	Dose (mg)	Dose Interval (hr)
Opium alkaloids and opiates		
Morphine	10	4
Heroin	3	3–4
Hydromorphone (Dilaudid)	2	4
Codeine	120	4–5
Synthetics		
Meperidine (Demerol)	100	3–4
Anileridine (Leritine)	25	3–4
Methadone (Dolophine)	7.5–10	4
Pentazocine (Talwin)	30	4
Narcotic antagonists		
Naloxone (Narcan)	0.4–0.8 (I.V.)	p.r.n.
Nalorphine (Nalline)	5–10 (I.V.)	—
Levallorphan (Lorfan)	1 (I.V.)	—

MORPHINE—THE PROTOTYPE NARCOTIC

Analgesia and Anxiolysis Since the isolation of morphine from opium in 1807, it has become the standard against which other narcotic analgesics must be compared. Morphine is known to relieve pain primarily by acting on the central nervous system, modifying the central reception and interpretation of pain. While anesthetics achieve analgesia by putting the patient completely to sleep, morphine accomplishes this end without significant loss of consciousness. However, there is often some drowsiness, mental clouding, and physical inactivity.[1] In larger doses there is increased sedation and sleep may occur. The sites of morphine-induced analgesia are summarized in Goodman and Gilman's general reference volume[2] by Jaffe and Martin,[3] but the exact mechanisms by which it exerts its effects remain unknown. The recent discovery of enkephalins and endorphins is beginning to give us a better understanding of the pharmacophysiologic activity of narcotics.

Several years ago, binding sites for opiates were discovered on the cell membranes of neurons in areas of the central nervous system known to be important in pain perception. From a teleologic viewpoint, this suggested that these receptors must ordinarily bind some endogenous substance or substances, very likely involved in the modulation of pain appreciation, and because of similar stereochemistry, opiates cross-react with these binding sites. Research designed to answer these questions has resulted in the discovery of a number of peptides in the pituitary and brain with narcotic-like activity.[4] Hughes et al. have identified in pig brains two pentapeptides, Leu-enkephalin and Met-enkephalin.[5] Ling[3] has isolated from the pig pituitary several larger polypeptides named endorphins, comprised of between 16 and 30 amino acids. Interestingly, the endorphins all contain the whole pentapeptide sequence of Met-enkephalin.[6] In turn, the amino acid sequences of the endorphins make up a portion of the molecular structure of β-lipotrophin, a substance that has been extracted from the pituitary gland but previously had no known function. This has led to the suggestion that β-lipotrophin may be the prohormone for Met-enkephalin and all the endorphins (Table 1-2).[5]

The full spectrum of activity of these substances has not yet been elucidated. Early in vitro studies indicate that β-endorphin is 5 to 10

TABLE 1-2
Is β-Lipotrophin a Prohormone?

Degradation: Amino Acid Sequence	Polypeptide
61–65	Met-enkephalin
61–76	α-Endorphin
61–96	β-Endorphin
61–77	γ-Endorphin
61–87	δ-Endorphin

From Guillemin R: N. Engl J Med 296:226, 1977

times more potent than morphine, and the enkephalins and α- and γ-endorphins, on a molar basis, are about as active as morphine. In laboratory animals, each of the endorphins has unique effects.[4] For example, α-endorphin produces transient analgesia mostly of the head and neck, and has a tranquilizing effect on the animal. Administration of β-endorphin results in a catatonic syndrome in association with total body analgesia. In contrast, γ-endorphin has no narcotic effect, but produces agitation and even violence in animals. The exact roles that enkephalins and endorphins normally play in humans is not known, but continued research into their actions will undoubtedly help us understand the mechanisms involved in the production of analgesia by morphine and other narcotics.

While the narcotic activity of morphine is its most important clinical attribute, that aspect of morphine that produces sedation and anxiolysis should not be underestimated. This can be an extremely valuable side effect in the very ill patient who is being constantly monitored and manipulated in the intensive care unit.

Other Central Nervous System Actions Morphine directly depresses the respiratory center. All opioids have this effect and, in equianalgesic doses, the amount of respiratory depression produced is similar with all these agents. In therapeutic doses, morphine decreases the rate of breathing, tidal volume, and consequently, the minute volume of respiration.[7] Further, it suppresses the normal responsiveness of the brain stem to hypercapnia but not to hypoxia. Consequently, oxygen should be administered with care to the patient medicated with morphine, particularly to those patients in the immediate postoperative period when they have not fully awakened from the effects of the anesthesia. These effects on respiration must be considered when a patient is on a respirator, and it may be necessary to adjust the tidal volume, rate of respiration, and the inspired oxygen concentration.

A characteristic effect of morphine is that of pupillary constriction. In a traumatized patient, morphine makes it difficult to gauge the response of the pupils to light as miosis occurs even in total darkness. However, it does not totally abolish the ability of the pupil to dilate, and with expanding intracranial pressure and cerebral ischemia, mydriasis still occurs.

Morphine directly stimulates the chemoreceptor trigger zone of the medulla, often producing nausea and vomiting. This can be minimized by keeping the patient recumbent, and by the concomitant administration of an appropriate phenothiazine. Once again, these side effects are approximately equal among the various narcotics when they are given in equianalgesic doses.

Cardiovascular System Effects In patients who have decreased intravascular volume, or who are bleeding actively, morphine should be used with caution because of the problem of hypotension. This is at least in part due to peripheral vasodilatation, a property that may be of some value in postoperative vascular and cardiac surgery patients. Since most patients in an I.C.U. are in the supine position, morphine has little effect on the pulse rate or on the blood pressure. However, orthostatic hypotension may occur if the patient's position is suddenly changed.

The normal heart is minimally affected by morphine, but in patients with coronary artery disease, it may produce a decrease in the left ventricular end-diastolic pressure, cardiac index, and cardiac work. Thus, the time-honored use of morphine to treat congestive heart failure has a physiologic basis, as well as the desirable effect of reducing anxiety. Not all narcotics have this salutory effect. Pentazocine, for example, increases cardiac work by 22 percent, making it a less desirable drug for patients with myocardial disease.[8]

Other Effects   The actions of morphine on the gastrointestinal tract combine to produce constipation. The tone in the pylorus, ileocecal valve, and anal sphincter is increased. The tone in the antrum of the stomach, small bowel, and colon is raised but propulsive contractions are markedly diminished. The resultant effect of these forces is marked prolongation in transit time through the G.I. tract.

Morphine has fairly widespread activity on other smooth muscle as well, producing increased tone in the ureters, detrusor muscle of the urinary bladder, and vesical sphincter. This may induce urinary retention, particularly in patients with benign prostatic hypertrophy. Morphine also markedly increases biliary tract pressures, occasionally to the point of producing colic. This may even be associated with elevated serum amylase and lipase. Not all analgesics have the same effect on common duct pressures, and Economou and Ward-McQuaid have shown that the increases may be less after the use of drugs such as meperidine.[9] Meperidine may, therefore, be a better drug to use in patients with suspected biliary tract disease, pancreatitis, or after choledochotomy (Table 1-3).

Routes of Administration and Metabolism   Morphine, as well as most of the other narcotics, is well absorbed from the G.I. tract, after subcutane-

TABLE 1-3
Important Narcotic Actions

Effects	Side Effects
Analgesia	Respiratory depression
Anxiolysis	Miosis
Sedation	Nausea
Cough suppression	Delayed emptying of G.I. tract, bladder, biliary tree
Vasodilation	Vasodilation

ous or intramuscular injection, and, of course, instantaneously after intravenous injection. The maximum effect after oral ingestion is considerably less than after parenteral injection. The most certain route of administration, particularly in a patient who may have erratic absorption from the tissues (such as patients with unstable cardiovascular systems, or cold patients in the immediate postoperative period), is by intravenous injection, where the use of the drug can be closely titrated to achieve the desired effect. However, it must be noted that even after intravenous injection of morphine, maximum analgesia is not evident for approximately 20 minutes because of the relatively slow rate of penetration of the drug into the brain. In the postoperative, intubated patient suffering from pain and apprehension, the I.V. route is ideal. Not only is unpredictable absorption avoided, but the total dose of narcotic administered can be reduced. A dosage of 1 to 3 mg I.V. is often sufficient to allay pain and anxiety, and provide adequate sedation to facilitate ventilation of the patient.

The narcotics are detoxified predominantly in the liver.[10] Morphine is conjugated with glutamic acids and then excreted in the urine. Because of the metabolic pathways, all narcotics are relatively contraindicated in patients with hepatic insufficiency of any cause. (For drug dosages, see Table 1-1).

SYNTHETIC ANALGESICS

The actions of most of these drugs are very similar to those of morphine and, in equianalgesic doses, the sedation, respiratory depression, and cardiovascular effects are comparable to those of morphine. The activity of meperidine (Demerol) is essentially the same as morphine; however, it has a decreased incidence of constipation and urinary retention. In pancreatitis and biliary tract problems, meperidine is probably a better drug than morphine because it does not increase the bile duct pressure or cause spasm of the sphincter of Oddi. There have been claims that, because of the metabolic pathways involved in the elimination of meperidine, it might be a safer drug than morphine to use in patients with hepatic insufficiency. Since meperidine, as with morphine, is metabolized predominantly in the liver, it should be used cautiously, if at all, in patients with severe liver disease.[10] This general rule should be applied to all narcotics.

Fentanyl (Sublimaze) is used extensively as an intravenous anesthetic, often in combination with droperidol in a preparation marketed as Innovar. This analgesic, which is about 80 times as potent as morphine, can produce profound respiratory depression. Although this is usually of short duration, it can be readily reversed by a narcotic antagonist, if necessary.

Methadone is mentioned only as a reminder that drug addicts may be on an oral maintenance program of this analgesic agent. In the postoperative period or during a serious illness, these patients need parenteral narcotic replacement to prevent an acute withdrawal syndrome. Maintenance methadone, with supplemental morphine in small amounts, can be simultaneously administered to provide any necessary pain relief. These patients may be extremely manipulative and the staff may be uncomfortable in dealing with their demands for medication. Personal feelings of reluctance to administer narcotics to an addict after surgery can interfere with the primary goal of alleviating suffering. Rehabilitation of a drug addict is a chronic problem that cannot be addressed in the convalescent period. However, incorporation of social service and other non-I.C.U. personnel can help alleviate the feelings of inadequacy that the manipulative patient is more than willing to engender.

SUMMARY OF THERAPEUTIC INDICATIONS AND PRECAUTIONS

Narcotics are most commonly used for the treatment of severe pain and occasionally for control of severe diarrhea or nonproductive coughing. They should be used cautiously, if at all, in patients with hypovolemia, cardiovascular instability, or hypoadrenalism because of the danger of hypotension. In fulminant ulcerative colitis, they may precipitate toxic megacolon. Narcotics should not be administered before a definitive diagnosis has been made in the case of an acute abdomen and a decision is made regarding therapy. They are contraindicated in head injuries and other situations where there is cerebral edema because the narcotics will exacerbate any increase in intracranial pressure, produce respiratory depression, mental clouding, miosis, and vomiting, making it difficult, if not impossible, to thoroughly evaluate these patients. In patients with hepatic insufficiency, narcotics can induce hepatic coma. Severe, chronic obstructive lung disease and asthma are relative contraindications for their use since they can induce histamine release and provoke bronchospasm. Meperidine is probably preferred over morphine in patients with pancreatitis, biliary tract disease, and benign prostatic hypertrophy. The respiratory depressant and hypotensive effects of narcotics may be potentiated by the simultaneous administration of phenothiazines and related drugs (Table 1-4).

The value of titrated, small doses of morphine in congestive heart failure or in postoperative, respirator-dependent patients has been discussed. Large doses of narcotics have been used for general anesthesia, e.g., 1 to 5 mg of morphine per kilogram of body weight. After surgery, these patients need ventilatory support for up to 24 hours because of the induced respiratory depression. Recently, some anesthesiologists have preferred to use fentanyl instead of morphine because of its shorter half-life, giving supplemental doses as necessary when the pulse rate or blood pressure increases.

TABLE 1-4
Clinical Indications for Narcotics

Situation	Indicated Drug
Analgesia ± sedation	Morphine
Biliary tract surgery	Meperidine
Pancreatitis	Meperidine
Benign prostate hypertrophy	Meperidine
Narcotic reversal	Naloxone

NARCOTIC ANTAGONISTS

These drugs compete with narcotics for receptor sites, blocking or reversing the effects of the narcotics. The most widely known drugs in this category are naloxone (Narcan), nalorphine (Nalline), and levallorphan (Lorfan). Naloxone is essentially a pure narcotic antagonist and is the drug of choice in all situations where the reversal of a narcotic effect is necessary. The action of naloxone is evident almost immediately after administration, rapidly reversing narcotic induced respiratory depression. The dosage is 0.4 to 0.8 mg I.V. and can be repeated when necessary. Nalorphine and levallorphan are not only narcotic antagonists but also partial agonists. They, in themselves, in large doses, can produce respiratory depression. Therefore, these two drugs are indicated only when naloxone is unavailable.

Reversal of narcotics must always be carefully monitored since the half-life of the antagonist may be shorter than that of the agonist. This can result in late recurrence of the narcotic depression state.

SEDATIVES AND TRANQUILIZERS

In the last several decades, there has been an amazing—and probably unnecessary—proliferation of drugs useful in the allaying of anxiety and production of sleep. Although these drugs do have some different indications and effects, the knowledge of several is more than sufficient in most clinical situations. The terminology in this field is often confusing and some drugs can be properly assigned to different classes according to dosages used. Conventionally, sedatives are drugs that produce a calming effect. Many diverse drugs may have this effect although they are classified in other groups (for example, narcotic analgesics and antihistamines). Hypnotics are drugs that induce sleep. Tranquilizers are agents that act on the emotional state, quieting or calming the patient without affecting clarity or consciousness. Major tranquilizers reduce psychotic symptoms, and minor tranquilizers are useful in the treatment of anxiety, tension, or psychoneurosis.

BENZODIAZEPINES (VALIUM, LIBRIUM, SERAX, DALMANE)

Twenty years ago this new class of compounds was discovered and, since that time, they have been established as the drugs of choice in most clinical situations for patients with anxiety or insomnia requiring drug treatment.[11] There has, again, been an unnecessary development of a large number of drugs in this category and this has been referred to as the "benzodiazepine bonanza."[12] There are few major differences between the individual benzodiazepines currently available; thus, familiarity with just a few will suffice.[13] The most commonly used drugs in this case are chlordiazepoxide (Librium), diazepam (Valium), oxazepam (Serax), and flurazepam (Dalmane).

Effects The predominant effect of the benzodiazepines is on the central nervous system (Table 1-5). In low doses they relieve anxiety, but as the dosage increases, the sedative effect becomes more apparent, and when the dosage is large enough, they produce sleep. Flurazepam has been approved for the treatment of insomnia while diazepam has not, but diazepam is probably just as effective as a hypnotic if the dose is sufficient. This is of particular importance in the I.C.U. since diazepam, and not flurazepam, can be administered parenterally. Unlike other hypnotics, such as the barbiturates, REM sleep does not appear to be affected by flurazepam, and there is little development of tolerance when it is taken daily for several weeks.

Given rapidly, intravenous diazepam can produce a transient respiratory arrest. Consequently, when this route is employed, respiratory support must be available. When used in the usual oral doses, there

TABLE 1-5
Actions of Benzodiazepines

Drug	Predominant Effects
Chlordiazepoxide (Librium)	Anxiolysis and sedation
Diazepam (Valium)	Anxiolysis, sedation, and control of status epilepticus
Oxazepam (Serax)	Anxiolysis and sedation
Flurazepam (Dalmane)	Hypnosis

In large enough doses, all the benzodiazepines will produce sleep.

are very few significant side effects of the benzodiazepines. Even very large oral overdoses seen in suicide attempts are seldom lethal. The care of such a patient is symptomatic and supportive, and although he may sleep for several days, respiratory and cardiovascular suppression are minimal.

Diazepam is often prescribed as a skeletal muscle relaxant. The predominant clinical effect is probably centrally mediated with reduction of anxiety and production of a relaxed state, rather than a direct effect on skeletal muscle.

The clinical usefulness of diazepam in status epilepticus will be discussed in the section on anticonvulsants (page 21).

Routes of Administration and Metabolism Parenteral administration of drugs produces a more rapid and predictable onset of action. Consequently, in the I.C.U., diazepam and chlordiazepoxide are the benzodiazepines most commonly used because, unlike oxazepam and flurazepam, they can be given parenterally. When the I.V. route is selected, the rate of administration should not exceed 5 mg/min of benzodiazepine to prevent respiratory depression. These drugs can all be given orally and, as mentioned, chlordiazepoxide can also be given intravenously or intramuscularly. Diazepam is interesting in that it is well absorbed after oral ingestion and, of course, has an immediate effect intravenously; however, it is poorly absorbed after intramuscular injection and should not be given by this route if a rapid, predictable effect is critical. At present, oxazepam and flurazepam are only available in oral preparations.

The benzodiazepines are metabolized by the liver, sometimes to active intermediate metabolites, but eventually the derivatives are excreted predominantly in the urine. Oxazepam has a shorter half-life than the other benzodiazepines with a simple one-step elimination pathway, and appears to have fewer cumulative effects.[13] It has been suggested that oxazepam may be the sedative of choice in liver failure, but it must be remembered that all drugs should be used cautiously, if at all, in this clinical setting. Usual dosages are listed in Table 1-6.

TABLE 1-6
Usual Dosages of Benzodiazepines

Drug	Usual Dosage
Chlordiazepoxide (Librium)	10 mg t.i.d.
Diazepam (Valium)	5 mg t.i.d.
Oxazepam (Serax)	10–20 mg t.i.d.
Flurazepam (Dalmane)	15–30 mg q.h.s.

Summary of Therapeutic Indications and Precautions   The relief of anxiety and insomnia are the most common indications for these drugs. These actions may be particularly useful in critically ill patients. In the intensive care unit, not only are the surroundings ominous and the threat of illness real, but the environment necessary to produce physiologic stability tends equally to ignore psychologic realities. Therefore, anxiolysis and production of an appropriate sleep should be conscious goals. The muscle relaxing, sedative, and amnesic properties of intravenous diazepam facilitate the performance of cardioversion and endoscopy. Chlordiazepoxide and diazepam are also important drugs in the treatment of alcohol withdrawal syndromes including delirium tremens. It may be necessary to use very large doses in this situation, e.g., 200 to 400 mg per day of chlordiazepoxide, or 100 to 200 mg per day of diazepam. The dosage must be titrated carefully depending upon the response of the patient.

It has clearly been demonstrated that tolerance to and physical dependence on benzodiazepines can occur. Withdrawal symptoms may become apparent with stoppage after chronic use, but this is rare when usual clinical dosages have been employed. The suicide potential with this class of drugs is extremely low even when very large amounts are taken orally. They have few interactions with other drugs except for an additive effect with other CNS depressants including alcohol. Except by rapid intravenous administration, they have minimal effects on the respiratory or cardiovascular systems.

SEDATIVE ANTIHISTAMINES

Many antihistamines have pronounced sedative activity, and several of these are commonly employed in the postoperative period. Drugs such as hydroxyzine (Vistaril) and promethazine (Phenergan) are often used in combination with a narcotic analgesic for their antianxiety and antiemetic properties, as well as in an effort to reduce the required dose of narcotic. The dose of hydroxyzine in this setting is 50 mg I.M. and that of promethazine is 25 mg I.M. They have no advantage over the benzodiazepines in terms of the quality and quantity of sedation induced. These drugs are discussed in greater detail in the section on antihistamines.

THE BARBITURATES

The barbiturates have been used extensively for 75 years. Benzodiazepines can now be considered to have replaced them for producing sedation and hypnosis except in certain selected situations. The ultrashort acting barbiturates such as thiopental are still used extensively as intravenous anesthetics. Certain of the barbiturates, particularly pheno-

TABLE 1-7
Barbiturate Uses

Effect	Representative Drugs and Usual Doses
Sedation and anxiolysis	Phenobarbital, 15 mg P.O. or I.M. q.i.d. (benzodiazepines preferred)
Hypnosis	Phenobarbital or pentobarbital (Nembutal), 100 mg P.O. or I.M. q.h.s. (benzodiazepines preferred)
Anesthesia	Thiopental, 150–300 mg I.V.
Status epilepticus	Phenobarbital, 150–400 mg I.V. (Valium is drug of choice)
Chronic seizure control	Phenobarbital, 100 mg P.O. b.i.d.
Cerebral resuscitation	Thiopental, up to 30 mg/kg I.V.

barbital, are important in the emergency control of convulsions and the chronic treatment of epilepsy states. These specific indications will be discussed in the section on anticonvulsants. A potential new application for barbiturates has been recently described. Experimental and clinical studies indicate that barbiturates may be useful in cerebral resuscitation after focal[14] and global[15] brain ischemia. The tentative results of an uncontrolled clinical trial using thiopental after cardiac arrest suggest that barbiturates may have a brain damage-ameliorating effect.[16] The current uses of barbiturates are listed in Table 1-7.

Since many authorities now advise against prescribing barbiturates for production of simple sedation and hypnosis,[11] discussion in this section will be brief. The reasons for this disenchantment with the barbiturates are manifold. When used as hypnotics, tolerance develops rapidly, confusional states are not uncommon, REM sleep is eliminated, and hangover the following day can occur.[17] The potential for suicide and/or abuse is substantial and documented. Unlike the benzodiazepines, overdosage of barbiturates produces severe respiratory depression and often is lethal. Not only can the use of barbiturates by themselves have serious consequences, but they also can produce important drug interactions secondary to their ability to induce liver microsomal enzymes that metabolize other drugs.* This sometimes necessitates an adjustment in dosages when other drugs are administered concurrently with barbiturates.[17] Further, the rapid cessation of barbiturate usage in the chronic user can produce a severe withdrawal syndrome consisting of insomnia, agitation, nausea, vomiting, delirium, and even grand mal seizures.

The ultrashort-acting and short-acting barbiturates, such as thiopental and pentobarbital are metabolized predominantly by the liver. The inactivated metabolites are conjugated with glucuronic acid and ex-

* See Table 1-11, page 24.

creted in the urine. Phenobarbital, a long-acting barbiturate, is metabolized partially by the liver, but about one-third of it is excreted unchanged in the urine. Therefore, in patients with renal failure, the dosage of phenobarbital should be reduced or eliminated. Similarly, the use of all barbiturates should be curtailed in patients with liver disease and completely avoided in patients with liver failure. In compensated cirrhotics, if a mild sedative is necessary, small doses of oxazepam can be used.

Barbiturate Poisoning   In the I.C.U., patients are rarely medicated with barbiturates but the recognition and treatment of barbiturate overdosage is still a significant problem (Figure 1-1). The clinical picture reflects the ingestion of excessive amounts of a sedative. The patient may be drowsy or in unresponsive coma, respiratory depression and hypothermia may develop, and shock, renal failure, and death can ensue. Current management of these overdoses is mostly supportive, and has reduced the mortality rate to below 2 percent.[17,18,19] If the patient is deeply comatose with respiratory failure, he should be intubated and if necessary—as determined by an increased PCO_2—mechanically ventilated. Hypotension, which is usually secondary to peripheral vasodilatation and occasionally myocardial depression, should be corrected with crystalloid infusion and dopamine if necessary. A Swan-Ganz catheter will aid in

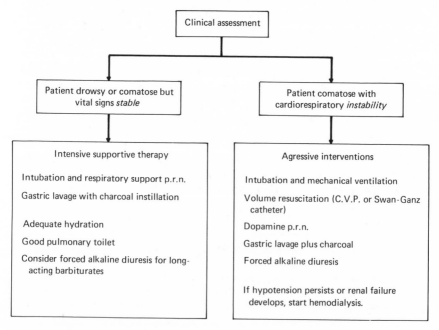

Fig. 1-1.   Management principles for barbiturate poisoning.

the diagnostic process. Volume deficiency or decreased cardiac output in these cases require data, not conjecture. If pulmonary artery occlusive pressure (PAO or wedge) is low (< 12 to 15 mm Hg), crystalloid infusion is indicated. Myocardial depression can be corrected with $CaCl_2$, digoxin, or dopamine (see Chapter 4). An attempt is usually made to prevent absorption of further drug from the gastrointestinal tract if the poisoning can be reasonably suspected to be of recent origin. In the comatose patient, gastric lavage with instillation of activated charcoal is safer and more efficacious. Endotracheal intubation is always an expeditious prophylactic measure. Blood is usually drawn for toxicology, but in general, the levels correlate only partially with depth of coma or survival.[18] The major benefit of toxicology is to confirm the presence of barbiturates and occasionally to identify other drugs that may have been simultaneously ingested. Many authorities recommend forced diuresis and alkalinization of the urine to increase barbiturate elimination, but there is little in the way of prospective evidence to show that this improves survival. In fact, overly vigorous hydration may result in electrolyte imbalances, pulmonary edema, and death unless adequate cardiovascular monitoring is also employed.[19] Forced alkaline diuresis is of greatest benefit in long-acting barbiturates, e.g., phenobarbital, and has modest effect on the excretion of short- and intermediate-acting barbiturates such as pentobarbital. When this therapeutic modality is employed, a diuresis of 8 to 20 liters per day with a urine pH close to 8 is optimal. Of course, the patient must be carefully monitored to prevent pulmonary edema or severe metabolic alkalosis. If PAO is maintained in the 13 to 17 torr range, the risk of inducing pulmonary edema is minimal. In severe poisoning where the patient's vital signs cannot be maintained with adequate hydration and vasopressors are required, or if renal failure occurs, peritoneal dialysis and particularly hemodialysis should be used. Exchange transfusions and passage of blood through ion exchange resins or charcoal have been used in desperate situations. Analeptics are no longer used. With intensive supportive therapy, death from hypotension, respiratory failure, pneumonia, and renal failure can be prevented in most patients.

PHENOTHIAZINES

The phenothiazines used to be classified as major tranquilizers, but perhaps it would be more appropriate to label them as antipsychotic agents. While some of them, such as chlorpromazine, do produce sedation initially, tolerance develops rapidly to this sedative action and the side effects of the phenothiazines are so significant that they should not be used for sedation or relief of anxiety alone. Some phenothiazines have pronounced antiemetic and antihistaminic effects but, in general, these drugs are of greater interest to the psychiatrist than to the intensivist.

Accordingly, they will only be briefly reviewed. However, they retain a major utility for treating that specific entity—intensive care psychosis. The phenothiazines can be subdivided into three groups depending on the side chain in their molecular structure (important because this markedly alters the clinical activity and side effects). The first group, which has an aliphatic side chain, includes chlorpromazine (Thorazine). The second includes thioridazine (Mellaril) and has a piperidine side chain. The third group includes perphenazine (Trilafon) and trifluoperazine (Stelazine) and has a piperazine side chain (Table 1-8).

TABLE 1-8
Antipsychotic Agents

Drug	Usual Daily Dosage (mg)	Acute Psychosis I.M. Dosage q 4–6 hr (mg)
Phenothiazines		
Aliphatic		
Chlorpromazine (Thorazine)	200–800	25–50
Piperidine		
Thioridazine (Mellaril)	200–800	—
Piperazine		
Trifluoperazine (Stelazine)	4–20	1–2
Perphenazine (Trilafon)	8–32	5–10
Butyrophenones		
Haloperidol (Haldol)	2–10	2–5

Effects   While it is clear that the phenothiazines are extremely effective as antipsychotic agents, the exact manner in which this activity is accomplished is not fully understood. They unfortunately have severe side effects that cannot be totally separated from the antipsychotic action of the drug. Sedation can occur with initial treatment, particularly with the aliphatic phenothiazines. Even a few milligrams intravenously will produce postural hypotension in a person who has not previously received chlorpromazine. This complex effect is secondary to α-adrenergic blockade, inhibition of centrally mediated pressor reflexes, and perhaps myocardial depression. Fortunately, tolerance develops rapidly to the hypotension and sedation, but not to the antipsychotic action. Therefore, the very large doses that are sometimes required for chronic control of psychosis are not limited by these undesirable side effects. In contrast, severe extrapyramidal symptoms including a parkinsonian syndrome and akathisia occur more commonly with the piperazine group. These usually respond readily to anticholinergic, anti-Parkinson drugs such as benztropine. A rare but severe neurologic syndrome that may be permanent and unresponsive to drug therapy is tardive dyskinesia.[11] Other known side effects are related to the anticholinergic activity of these drugs and include urinary retention, dry mouth, and blurred vision. Photosensitivity, skin rashes, and cholestatic jaundice can occur. Agranulocytosis has also developed and has been a fatal complication. These side effects are almost exclusively confined to the psychiatric patient and not when used in the I.C.U.

A number of phenothiazines are good antiemetics, and promethazine (Phenergan) is used extensively for this action. Promethazine has almost no antipsychotic effect and is classified in the section on antihistamines.

Haloperidol   Haloperidol (Haldol) is a butyrophenone useful in the treatment of psychosis. Although structurally unrelated to the phenothiazines, it does have similar effects and side effects as the piperazine phenothiazines.[20] It does not usually cause hypotension, but has a high incidence of extrapyramidal side effects. Cholestatic jaundice is unusual. Currently, it is widely advocated to treat the perceptual disorders seen in the I.C.U.—the I.C.U. psychosis spectrum.

Therapeutic Indications and Precautions of the Phenothiazines   Phenothiazines and haloperidol should be used in the acute treatment of psychotic disorders in the I.C.U. They have modest usefulness as antiemetics, but in general should not be used for sedation or the treatment of simple anxiety states.

In the intensive care unit setting, these drugs will be employed in two main situations. The first is in the management of an "I.C.U. psychosis." In fact, a number of psychiatric syndromes in the critically ill patient have now been characterized.[21,22] These range from acute fear, anxiety, and agitated depression, to an acute schizophreniform reaction with thought disorder and delusions, or delirium with its impairment of cognitive functions. Often these states will respond to reassurances and explanations by the intensive care staff, making the patient understand what is happening to him, and keeping him oriented to time and place. A benzodiazepine, e.g., diazepam in as low a dose as 2 to 5 mg I.V. every 4 to 6 hours, will often assist in controlling fear, anxiety, and agitation. Occasionally, it will be necessary to treat an acute schizophreniform reaction or delirium state with a phenothiazine or haloperidol. The greatest experience has been with chlorpromazine, 25 mg I.M. every 4 to 6 hours, but trifluoperazine, 2 mg. I.M. every 6 hours, has less of a hypotensive effect, and this is often a serious consideration in these critically ill patients. Haloperidol, 2 mg I.M. or I.V. every 6 hours, may be the drug of choice in the elderly, psychotic patient because of its lack of cardiovascular side effects. When a patient is jaundiced or has hepatic dysfunction, haloperidol is the safer drug.

The intensivist is often confronted with a second situation: patients who have been on chronic antipsychotic medication. Omission of drug therapy for several days is usually of no clinical consequence. If the patient is ill for an extended period of time, it will probably be necessary to resume antipsychotic medication. The same concerns about hypotension and jaundice, mentioned above, should be observed. Care should be exercised whenever phenothiazines are used in combination with narcotic analgesics, because of potentiation of sedation, hypotension, and respiratory depression.

SUMMARY

In the intensive care unit, critically ill and/or postoperative patients often require sedation, anxiolysis, analgesia, amnesia, and relief from nausea. These desired goals are often achievable with the judicious use of a narcotic analgesic, a sedative, and an antihistamine; for example, morphine, diazepam, and promethazine or hydroxyzine (Table 1-9). The barbiturates are rapidly being replaced by the benzodiazepines. The phenothiazines should not be used for their sedative action alone.

TABLE 1-9
Sedatives—Tranquilizers

Class	Indications
Benzodiazepines	Sedation; anxiolysis; delirium tremens; hypnosis; status epilepticus
Sedative antihistamines	Nausea; sedation
Barbiturates	General anesthesia; convulsions; occasionally sedation and sleep; cerebral resuscitation
Phenothiazines and butyrophenones	Psychosis—acute or chronic; occasionally nausea

ANTICONVULSANTS

The acute management of seizures whether metabolic or epileptic in origin should be known to all physicians. The diagnostic considerations that must be evaluated whenever one is confronted by a seizure are discussed fully on pages 41–43. The drugs that are most useful in the acute control of convulsions are diazepam, phenobarbital, and phenytoin (Table 1-10). A discussion of the agents effective in the chronic therapy of the epilepsies is beyond the intended scope of this section.

TABLE 1-10
Emergency Control of Status Epilepticus

Drug	Initial Dosage I.V. (mg)	Onset	Maximum Dosage mg/day	Comments
Diazepam (Valium)	5-10	1-2 min	100	Drug of choice in status; short half-life; little maintenance value
Phenytoin (Dilantin)	500*	10-15 min	1000	Alternate drug in status; important maintenance drug
Phenobarbital (Luminal)	150-400	10-15 min	1000	Alternate drug in status; important maintenance drug

* Lower doses should be used in patients maintained on phenytoin.

DIAZEPAM

Diazepam (Valium) is the benzodiazepine that has been used most extensively in the treatment of convulsions.

Indications and Precautions While the clinical usefulness of diazepam and other benzodiazepines for the chronic control of epilepsy is debated, intravenous diazepam is the drug of choice for the treatment of status epilepticus.[23] In the emergency control of convulsions, diazepam is administered slowly intravenously at the rate of up to 5 mg per minute; most seizures will be controlled with 5 to 10 mg of this drug. It can be repeated as necessary up to a maximum dose of 100 mg in 24 hours. Diazepam is rapidly redistributed to other tissues producing a relatively short therapeutic half-life; therefore, it is necessary to start appropriate maintenance medication with other agents such as phenytoin to prevent recurrent convulsions.

The major toxicity of intravenous diazepam is respiratory and cardiovascular depression. Accordingly, the facilities for mechanical ventilation must be at hand when this drug is used.

PHENOBARBITAL

A number of barbiturates, including phenobarbital, pentobarbital, amobarbital, mephobarbital, and metharbital, have been used for the control of acute and chronic convulsions. The relatively long half-life of phenobarbital and its high ratio of anticonvulsant to hypnotic activity make it the barbiturate of choice for treating convulsions.[23]

Routes of Admininstration and Metabolism In the emergency control of convulsions, phenobarbital can be administered intravenously in a dose of 150 to 400 mg at a rate not exceeding 50 mg per minute, with a maximum dose of 1 gm in 24 hours. It must be remembered that even when administered intravenously, it may take 15 min for phenobarbital to equilibrate across the blood-brain barrier and produce its maximum effect. Consequently, it may take this period of time to gauge the effect of a dose of this drug in controlling convulsions. Phenobarbital is also well absorbed after oral administration, and in the chronic management of epileptic states the usual daily dose for adults is 60 to 200 mg orally. More than 50 percent of phenobarbital is conjugated and inactivated by the liver and the remaining portion is excreted by the kidneys.

Anticonvulsant Indications and Precautions While diazepam is the drug of choice for the treatment of status epilepticus, intravenous phenobarbital is also very useful in this situation. Its greatest applicability is in the chronic control of tonic-clonic and focal seizures. When phenytoin inadequately controls tonic-clonic seizures, the addition of small doses of phenobarbital is often effective. In young children phenobarbital is the drug of choice for many seizures because of the frequency of side effects with phenytoin.[23]

As with diazepam, the intravenous administration of phenobarbital may produce respiratory and cardiovascular depression. In the chronic situation the principle side effects are sedation, nystagmus, and ataxia. Osteomalacia and megaloblastic anemia may occur with prolonged treatment. After chronic phenobarbital administration, withdrawal must be gradual to prevent the precipitation of status epilepticus.

PHENYTOIN (DIPHENYLHYDANTOIN)

Over the last 40 years phenytoin (diphenylhydantoin) has established itself as one of the most important drugs for the acute and chronic control of many types of epilepsy. The effects of phenytoin on the central nervous system are quite complex but have been studied extensively and are well summarized in Woodbury and Fingl.[24] The important actions in the I.C.U. relate to the limitation of maximal seizure activity, reducing the spread of the seizure process without causing general depression of the central nervous system. Phenytoin is also useful for the treatment of some cardiac arrhythmias, particularly digitalis-induced tachyarrhythmias. It is of interest that the therapeutic blood levels of phenytoin for arrhythmia control are in the same range as those required for seizures, 10 to 20 μg/ml.

Routes of Administration and Metabolism   In the emergency situation, phenytoin should be administered intravenously. It is available in a special solvent and must be injected slowly without previous dilution at a rate of up to 50 mg per min. Intramuscular administration, because of precipitation and irregular absorption, is unreliable and should rarely be used. Phenytoin has very limited aqueous solubility, and after oral ingestion the absorption is variable but usually adequate for long term, chronic control of seizures.

Phenytoin is extensively metabolized by the hepatic microsomal enzymes with less than 5 percent of it being excreted unchanged in the urine. At low plasma concentrations its elimination is exponential following first order kinetics; however, at higher concentrations of the drug, dose-dependent elimination becomes apparent and the plasma half-life increases with concentration.[25] A number of drugs raise the blood concentration of phenytoin by competing with it for hepatic microsomal metabolism, and these include isoniazid, coumarin anticoagulants, and disulfiram (Antabuse). Other drugs that raise the serum concentration of phenytoin include chloramphenicol (Chloromycetin), chlordiazepoxide (Librium), methylphenidate (Ritalin), and chlorpromazine (Thorazine).[23] Chronic alcoholism decreases the anticonvulsant effect of phenytoin because of increased metabolism of the drug. Due to the wide variability in the rates at which patients absorb and metabolize phenytoin, plasma levels should be determined in all patients who do not respond to the usual therapeutic dosage.[26]

Summary of Therapeutic Indications and Precautions   Phenytoin (Dilantin) has its greatest applicability in the acute and chronic management of seizures.

In adults and older children, phenytoin is the drug of choice for the chronic treatment of most forms of epilepsy except for petit mal seizures. The usual adult dose is from 300 to 400 mg per day. In status epilepticus, intravenous diazepam is the drug of choice, but phenytoin can be used in resistant cases or it can be started acutely for maintenance purposes. It is given intravenously in a loading dose of 10 to 15 mg per kg at a rate not to exceed 50 mg per minute.

Similar to the other drugs used for status epilepticus, an excessively rapid rate of intravenous administration can produce cardiovascular collapse or central nervous system depression. With chronic administration there are numerous side effects that are often more pronounced in children. Frequent problems are nystagmus, ataxia, dysarthria, gingival hyperplasia, and hirsutism. If a morbilliform rash or the Stevens-Johnson syndrome develops, then the drug must be stopped. Other side effects include peripheral neuropathy, a lupus syndrome, megaloblastic anemia, hepatitis, osteomalacia, and gastrointestinal upset.[23]

DRUG INTERACTIONS

In this era of polypharmacology, most hospitalized patients particularly in an I.C.U. receive two or more medications. Increasing experience is accumulating demonstrating how drugs can interact to increase or decrease their intended actions, or even produce totally unexpected reactions.[27] Two of the anticonvulsants, phenobarbital and phenytoin,

TABLE 1-11
Drug Interactions With Anticonvulsants

Interacting Drugs	Adverse Effect	Mechanism
Barbiturates with:		
Alcohol	Decreased sedation with chronic alcohol use	Increased metabolism
	Increased sedation with acute intoxication	Decreased metabolism
Oral anticoagulants	Decreased anticoagulant effect	Microsomal enzyme induction
Tricyclic antidepressants	Decreased antidepressant effect	Microsomal enzyme induction
Corticosteroids	Decreased steroid effect	Microsomal enzyme induction
Quinidine	Decreased quinidine effect	Microsomal enzyme induction
Phenytoin with:		
Alcohol	Decreased anticonvulsant effect with chronic alcohol use	Increased metabolism
	Increased anticonvulsant effect with acute intoxication	Decreased metabolism
Oral anticoagulants	Increased phenytoin toxicity	Inhibition of microsomal enzymes
Chloramphenicol	Increased phenytoin toxicity	Inhibition of microsomal enzymes
Corticosteroids	Decreased steroid effect	Induction of microsomal enzymes
Diazoxide	Decreased anticonvulsant effect	Unknown
Isoniazid	Increased phenytoin toxicity	Inhibition of microsomal enzymes
Quinidine	Decreased quinidine effect	Induction of microsomal enzymes

From Med Lett Drugs Ther 19:5, 1977

have many well-known drug interactions with other medications, although they do not usually affect the blood levels of each other (Table 1-11).

As many of these drugs are frequently used in the I.C.U., the intensivist must be aware of these interactions and manipulate dosages in order to achieve critical therapeutic effects. An example would be an epileptic maintained on phenobarbital who required chronic anticoagulants because of pulmonary emboli. The induction of hepatic microsomal enzyme systems by phenobarbital effectively shortens the half-life of many oral anticoagulants such as warfarin (Coumadin), decreasing the anticoagulant effect of a given dose. Consequently, to attain adequate anticoagulation, higher doses of warfarin may be necessary. If this same epileptic had been receiving chronic phenytoin therapy, initial oral anticoagulant therapy might increase the toxicity of phenytoin by inhibiting other microsomal systems, necessitating decreasing the dose of phenytoin. It is also essential to consider that a patient on phenobarbital or phenytoin who develops an arrhythmia may be relatively resistant to quinidine. Diazoxide (Hyperstat), an important drug in the emergency control of hypertension, can decrease the anticonvulsant effect of phenytoin, possibly precipitating a seizure in an epileptic on chronic phenytoin therapy. Phenobarbital and phenytoin both decrease the effect of corticosteroids. As a result, patients on these drugs who must be treated with steroids may require larger doses of corticosteroids.

A large number of drug interactions have already been described and many more will become apparent with the introduction of new agents. It is impossible to remember all the interactions, but in the I.C.U. where multiple drug therapy is the rule, the possibility of an adverse interaction must always be anticipated. If the desired effect of a drug is not achieved, it may be secondary to altered metabolism, and measuring blood levels of the drug will often assist in correcting the problem.

MUSCLE RELAXANTS

This group of drugs has its greatest applicability in anesthesia. Through various mechanisms, these agents act on the neuromuscular junction inhibiting muscular contraction, and therefore, they should be more specifically classified as neuromuscular blocking agents. While the anesthesiologist most often employs these drugs, any doctor working in an intensive care unit must be familiar with their actions because patients will often return from surgery without full reversal of their muscle relaxants. Also, these agents are occasionally used in other situations.

The neuromuscular blockers can be subdivided into competitive and depolarizing agents (Table 1-12).

TABLE 1-12
Classification of Muscle Relaxants

Drug	Usual Initial Dosage I.V.
Competitive or non-depolar-izing agents	
D-tubocurarine (Tubarine)	3–9 mg
Gallamine (Flaxedil)	1 mg/kg
Pancuronium (Pavulon)	0.05–0.1 mg/kg
Depolarizing agents	
Succinylcholine	0.5–1 mg/kg

MECHANISM OF ACTION

Both groups of drugs produce skeletal muscle paralysis by preventing acetylcholine from depolarizing the postsynaptic membrane at the neuromuscular junction. The nondepolarizing agents combine with receptor sites on the motor end plate, thereby preventing the transmitter activity of acetylcholine. Since these are competitive blocking agents, the administration of an anticholinesterase drug will overcome the competitive inhibition and reverse the block by allowing the accumulation of acetylcholine.

The depolarizing agents resemble acetylcholine in structure and function. They first excite the motor end plate producing muscular fasciculations, but this is soon followed by depolarization and paralysis of the motor end plate. Succinylcholine is hydrolyzed by the pseudocholinesterases, thereby terminating its activity. In contradistinction to the competitive blocking agents, the activity of succinylcholine is not antagonized by anticholinesterases and, in fact, is prolonged by them.

OTHER EFFECTS

All these drugs produce skeletal muscle relaxation, but they also have other side effects which vary somewhat between the various agents. D-tubocurarine has blocking activity at the autonomic ganglia and the adrenal medulla. It also causes the release of histamine. These combined actions account for the hypotension and bronchospasm observed in the clinical use of curare. Gallamine, on the other hand, has an atropine-like effect on the vagus nerve resulting in tachycardia, and either normal or slightly increased blood pressure. Pancuronium has no clinically significant effect on the autonomic ganglia or blood pressure, and along with gallamine, has very little histamine-releasing activity. It is important to remember that no neuromuscular blocker possesses sedative or analgesic properties. Therefore, if they are employed in a setting other than general anesthesia, pain and anxiety must be concomitantly treated. Otherwise, the patient will remain awake and conscious though totally paralyzed. This situation is extremely disturbing because the loss of voluntary muscle control and powerlessness leads to fear and anxiety.

ROUTES OF ADMINISTRATION AND METABOLISM

These muscle relaxants are almost always administered by an intravenous route. D-tubocurarine (3 to 9 mg I.V.) will produce muscular relaxation in most adults. Initially, redistribution throughout the body tissues occurs and is important in terminating the paralytic action of the drug. Consequently, one-half of the loading dose may be repeated within 5 minutes and subsequently as necessary. Over half of the drug is metabolized by the liver and about a third is excreted by the kidney. Gallamine by comparison is excreted almost entirely by the kidney without being metabolized; thus, it is not used in patients with renal failure. The dose of gallamine is about 1 mg per kg of body weight I.V., with an additional dose of half this much in about 45 minutes if necessary. Pancuronium is a relatively new drug which has become increasingly popular because it has few side effects and a relatively long half-life. It is given intravenously in a loading dose of up to 0.1 mg/kg. Supplemental doses of about 0.01 mg/kg can be repeated as necessary. The activity of all these competitive blocking agents can be reversed by anticholinesterases: neostigmine 3 mg I.V. and atropine 1.2 mg I.V. (to minimize undesirable cholinergic side effects).

Succinylcholine is rapidly inactivated by the pseudocholinesterases of the body except in those rare people with a deficiency of this enzyme degradation system.[28] Therefore, its duration of activity is much less than that of the competitive blocking agents. The initial dose in the adult is usually 0.5 to 1.0 mg/kg I.V., but lesser amounts are often effective. If longer relaxation is necessary, an intravenous drip infusion can be used titrating the relaxant effect. The fasciculations induced by succinylcholine can be blocked by a preliminary injection of 3 mg of curare. This, however, may increase the necessary dose of succinylcholine by 50 percent to achieve the required effect.

SUMMARY OF THERAPEUTIC INDICATIONS AND PRECAUTIONS

The major indication for all of these agents is in general anesthesia to facilitate intubation and produce muscular relaxation (Table 1-13). They do have other uses in the intensive care unit, such as occasionally in patients who are convulsing continuously, with status epilepticus or tetanus. The advent of intermittent mandatory ventilation has made the use of these paralyzing agents unusual for the sole purpose of allow-

TABLE 1-13
Muscle Relaxants—Indications and Contraindications

Drugs	Contraindications	Indications
Competitive Agents		
D-tubocurarine	None specific	Similar for all competitive agents: skeletal muscle relaxation during surgery; facilitate mechanical ventilation (occasionally); status epilepticus (rare); tetanus (rare)
Pancuronium	None specific	
Gallamine	Renal failure	
Depolarizing Agents		
Succinylcholine	Plasma cholinesterase deficiency	Endotracheal intubation; muscle relaxation of short duration, e.g., reducing dislocations or electro-convulsive shock therapy

ing a patient to be maintained on a respirator. Occasionally, these agents are necessary so that a young child or an uncooperative adult can be ventilated adequately. Similarly, in some emergency situations, succinylcholine can greatly facilitate endotracheal intubation of a patient. Remember, if these blocking agents are used in patients who are not undergoing general anesthesia, sedation, and/or analgesia should be provided.

The most important side effect of these blocking agents is, of course, respiratory paralysis, but as long as the patient is being adequately ventilated there is no major danger. If it is necessary to paralyze a patient so that he can be maintained on a respirator, he must be carefully supervised to make sure that he does not become detached from the respirator.

ANTIHISTAMINES

Since the first antihistamine was discovered forty years ago, there has been a remarkable proliferation in the numbers of these drugs. The many traditional antihistamines have widespread clinical application, but are of only modest usefulness to the intensive care therapist and therefore will be discussed relatively briefly. The discovery in 1972 by Black et al. of histamine H_2-receptors and subsequently of H_2-receptor antagonists has introduced a new category of antihistamines which may prove to be of much greater benefit to the intensivist.[29]

CLASSIFICATION AND EFFECTS

It is now possible to subdivide the antihistamines into two major groups, the H_1-receptor antagonists and the H_2-receptor antagonists. All antihistamines are competitive blocking agents competing with histamine for binding at specific cell receptors, but the two groups of antihistamines act at different receptor sites producing completely different effects.

The most important activity of the H_2-receptor antagonists is the blocking of gastric acid secretion. This includes not only the inhibition of basal acid secretion, but also blockade of acid secretion stimulated by histamine, gastrin, cholinergic drugs, and food.[30] In large doses, they also block histamine stimulation of the uterus and heart, but these are not clinically important features. Together with H_1-blocking agents, they inhibit the vasodilator effects of large doses of histamine.

The other diverse actions of histamines are mediated through H_1-receptors; the traditional antihistamines can be considered as H_1-receptor antagonists. These agents block the effect of histamine on smooth muscle of blood vessels, bronchi, and the gastrointestinal tract, as well as the effect histamine has on increasing capillary permeability. The H_1-antagonists, such as diphen-hydramine or hydroxyzine, often produce depression of the central nervous system. This sedative activity may be useful clinically or may be an unwanted side effect. A number of antihistamines, including diphenhydramine and promethazine, are good suppressors of motion sickness. This class of antihistamines has no effect whatsoever on gastric acid secretion.

There are hundreds of H_1-receptor blockers with only minor differences between them. Several representative drugs are included in Table 1-14. A more complete categorization by Douglas can be found in Goodman and Gilman's text.[31]

TABLE 1-14
Representative Antihistamines

Drug	Dosage I.M. or P.O.
H_1-receptor antagonists	
Diphenhydramine (Benadryl)	50 mg q 4–6 hr
Promethazine (Phenergan)	25 mg q 4–6 hr
Hydroxyzine (Vistaril)	50 mg q 6–8 hr
Chlorpheniramine (Chlor-trimeton)	4 mg q 4–6 hr
H_2-receptor antagonists	
Cimetidine (Tagamet)	300 mg P.O. or I.V. q 6–12 hr

ROUTES OF ADMINISTRATION AND METABOLISM

H_1 Antagonists The H_1-receptor antagonists are well absorbed orally or after intramuscular injection, but are rarely given intravenously. The intensive care patient is, of course, the exception because perfusion is always in question. The intravenous route, therefore, is still primarily indicated. They are metabolized extensively by the liver and then excreted in the urine.[31]

H_2 Antagonists Cimetidine is well absorbed orally or parenterally. It is mainly excreted in an unchanged form in the urine[30] and, therefore, its half-life is prolonged in renal failure. Accordingly, in patients with severe renal failure, no more than 300 mg every 12 hours should be used.[32]

SUMMARY OF THERAPEUTIC INDICATIONS AND PRECAUTIONS

The H_1-receptor antagonists have wide therapeutic applications in treating many types of allergies including hayfever, urticaria, and allergic dermatitis (Table 1-15). Promethazine is often successfully used in the prevention of motion sickness. In the intensive care unit, however, their usefulness is much more restricted. These antihistamines are of some value in the treatment of minor drug reactions characterized by pruritus and urticaria. Similarly, they may have an adjunctive role in nonhemolytic minor blood transfusion reactions. In life threatening anaphylaxis and angioedema, antihistamines can be administered systemically, but the mainstay of treatment in these situations is epinephrine and endotracheal intubation if necessary. Some of these drugs also have important central effects, as well as blocking the peripheral actions of histamine. Benadryl, Phenergan, and Vistaril have significant sedative and antinau-

TABLE 1-15
Antihistamine Indications

Indication	Antihistamine Class
Allergies Antiemesis Sedation	H_1-blockers
Peptic ulcers Peptic esophagitis Z-E syndrome Stress bleeding?	H_2-blockers

seant properties. They are often administered parenterally in combination with narcotic analgesics in an effort to provide sedation, and to ameliorate the side effects of nausea and vomiting. However, it must be appreciated that the combination of these drugs enhances the sedative and respiratory depressant effects of the narcotic. Apart from sedation there are no serious side effects from H_1-antagonists in the usual therapeutic doses.

Cimetidine, an H_2-receptor antagonist, is being used widely for its inhibitory effects on gastric acid secretion. In double-blind, prospective clinical trials, cimetidine has been shown to accelerate the healing of duodenal ulcers and alleviate ulcer pain symptomatology.[33] Not only is it effective in healing ulcers, but maintenance therapy has been demonstrated to prevent relapse of duodenal ulcers.[34] Cimetidine has also been useful in the treatment of symptomatic gastroesophageal reflux,[35] gastric ulcers,[36] and the medical treatment of the Zollinger-Ellison syndrome.[37]

In the intensive care unit, the development of stress bleeding from the stomach or duodenum is a potentially lethal complication. There are at present few clinical trials demonstrating the efficacy of cimetidine in preventing stress bleeding, although this drug is now being widely used in this role. One study has shown that H_2-receptor antagonism will prevent acute upper gastrointestinal hemorrhage in fulminant hepatic failure.[38]

Cimetidine appears to be an extremely safe drug, with few serious side effects.[39] No incidences of agranulocytosis as seen with the original H_2-antagonist metiamide have yet been reported, but transient neutropenia has been observed. Cimetidine does not have the sedative effects of the H_1-receptor blockers, but C.N.S. symptoms can occur particularly in elderly patients. These include confusion, slurred speech, delirium, and hallucinations. Fever and transient serum creatinine elevations have also been reported. While there is no definite evidence that the cessation of cimetidine therapy produces a rebound acid secretion, there is little question that a significant relapse of ulcers will occur if maintenance therapy of cimetidine or antacids is not continued. Relapses can occur even during long-term maintenance treatment with less than full dosage. To prevent excessive accumulation of the drug, the dose of cimetidine should be reduced in renal failure.

CORTICOSTEROIDS

The adrenal cortex secretes numerous steroid hormones that can be classified into two main groups: the corticosteroids and the adrenal androgens. Those corticosteroids that have a predominant effect on carbohydrate metabolism have been referred to as glucocorticoids, and include cortisol and cortisone. Those whose main effect is on sodium retention, e.g., desoxycorticosterone and aldosterone, have been called mineralocorticoids. The absence of the corticosteroids results in the clinical syndrome of Addison's disease, whereas the overproduction of the glucocorticoids produces Cushing's syndrome. Primary hyperaldosteronism presents clinically as Conn's syndrome.

CORTICOSTEROID EFFECTS

The corticosteroids have many complex physiologic, metabolic, and pharmacologic functions, and these will be outlined in general terms. In the broadest sense, corticosteroids are required for normal living and, without them, survival is possible only in the most strictly controlled laboratory setting. Not only do they have essential activities of their own, but they also have important interactions with other hormonal systems.

Mineralocorticoids such as aldosterone are required for normal fluid and electrolyte balance in the body. They act on the distal tubules of the nephrons to retain sodium, chloride, and water, and facilitate a simultaneous excretion of potassium and hydrogen ions. In an adrenalectomized animal who does not receive mineralocorticoid replacement, hyponatremia, hyperkalemia, and hypovolemia rapidly develop and progress to cardiovascular collapse and death.

The glucocorticoids, such as cortisone, profoundly affect carbohydrate, protein, and lipid metabolism. They inhibit protein anabolism and also accelerate its breakdown, increasing gluconeogenesis. In the light of short-term goals, this results in an increased supply of glucose to satisfy immediate energy requirements—but it is at the expense of muscle mass and tissue synthesis. Carbohydrate utilization by peripheral tissues is decreased and glycogen storage in the liver is increased. Clearly, an excess of glucocorticoids produces a diabetes-like state. The glucocorticoids interact with other hormones, such as epinephrine and norepinephrine to facilitate lipolysis and the mobilization of fat from adipose tissues. Excessive amounts of glucocorticoids also result in the abnormal fat distribution found in Cushing's disease with the resultant moon face, buffalo hump, and thin extremities.

Certain corticosteroids have potent anti-inflammatory properties, and these have extensive clinical applications. They suppress all the classical signs of inflammation including rubor, calor, dolor, and tumor. Although the mechanisms are poorly understood, they clearly stabilize membranes reducing capillary leakage, limiting edema formation. Leukocyte migration, production of collagen by fibroblasts, and scar formation are also inhibited. The corticosteroids have a myriad of other functions as well. Increased levels produce muscle weakness secondary to wasting of skeletal muscle and hypokalemia. Circulating polymorphonuclear leukocytes in the blood increase while lymphocytes, eosinophils, monocytes, and basophils markedly decrease. Similarly, red blood cell synthesis is increased in Cushing's syndrome, often resulting in poly-cythemia. The major cardiovascular effects of the corticosteroids are mediated through salt and water metabolism. Increased or decreased mineralocorticoid activity will result in hyper- or hypotension, respec-tively. The corticosteroids do, however, exert other effects on the cardio-vascular system, particularly in pharmacologic doses. In massive doses, e.g., 30 mg/kg of methylprednisolone, the glucocorticoids appear to in-crease myocardial contractility and cardiac index, as well as decrease peripheral vasoconstriction and capillary permeability.

It is apparent that corticosteroids can be considered as three different classes of drugs, depending on total amount administered: (1) replace-ment of endogenous hormone (up to 300 mg of cortisol equivalent per day), (2) anti-inflammatory action (up to 1000 mg of cortisol equivalent per day), (3) pharmacologic actions (approximately 10,000 mg of cortisol equivalent per dose).

ROUTES OF ADMINISTRATION AND METABOLISM

The corticosteroids have been modified to permit the use of numerous preparations that are active both orally and parenterally. It is also impor-tant to remember that some glucocorticoids, topically applied, can be sufficiently absorbed to produce systemic effects and even adrenal suppression.[40]

The metabolism of corticosteroids is complex. The most important process is conjugation in the liver to water-soluble compounds which are then excreted by the kidneys.

POTENCY

Various corticosteroids have been synthesized to maximize their anti-inflammatory activity and minimize their sodium retaining capacity. Similarly, other steroids have been synthesized that have pronounced sodium retaining activity. The relative potencies of some corticosteroids are summarized in Table 1-16.

THERAPEUTIC USES

Replacement Therapy The most clear cut indication for corticosteroid therapy is replacement in hypoadrenal states, i.e., acute or chronic and primary or secondary. In chronic adrenal insufficiency, most patients can be maintained on oral cortisone acetate, 25 mg in the morning and 12.5 mg in the afternoon. In primary hypoadrenalism, as opposed to a patient with panhypopituitarism, mineralocorticoid activity is also re-

TABLE 1-16
Relative Potencies of Corticosteroids

Corticosteroid	Relative Anti-inflammatory Potency	Relative Sodium Retaining Potency
Hydrocortisone (Cortisol)	1	1
Cortisone	0.8	0.8
Aldosterone	?	3000
Prednisone	4	0.8
Prednisolone	4	0.8
Methylprednisolone	5	0.5
9 α-fluorocortisol	10	125
Dexamethasone	25	0

From Haynes RC, Larner J[40]

quired. This is most easily administered as 9 α-fluorocortisol acetate 0.1 to 0.3 mg daily.

Acute adrenal insufficiency can follow sepsis, trauma, or abrupt cessation of exogenous steroids, and is created commonly by bilateral adrenalectomy. The maximum output of the adrenal glands is about 300 mg of cortisone a day; therefore, replacement in the acute situation should consist of an equivalent amount of corticosteroid. Whenever a patient has been on exogenous steroid therapy one should consider that relative adrenal suppression may have occurred; in the face of any acute illness, the dose of steroid administered parenterally should approximate 300 mg of cortisone per day. It is probably safest to provide acute replacement therapy to all patients treated with steroids within a year (even if they have been tapered) to abort the disasterous occurrence of acute adrenal insufficiency in the postoperative or stress state. Table 1-17 shows one regimen for dealing with the adrenal insufficiency following adrenalectomy; a similar dosage schedule can also be applied to any acute situation. Of course, if any signs of hypoadrenalism become apparent (such as increased temperature, tachycardia, or hypotension) the steroid dosage should be increased once again. A liberal administration of balanced salt solutions may help alleviate the development of cardiovascular instability.

Anti-inflammatory Uses   The list of diseases in which steroids have been used for their anti-inflammatory activities is impressive, particularly when one considers that steroids merely palliate signs and symptoms and rarely are curative. Further, the prolonged use of corticosteroids is attendant with severe side effects. In selecting one of these agents in this clinical situation, a drug is chosen that maximizes the anti-inflammatory activity and minimizes the sodium retention. Further, the

TABLE 1-17

Corticosteroid Replacement Therapy for Adrenalectomy

Day	I.V. Hydrocortisone (mg)	I.M. Cortisone (mg)	P.O. Cortisone (mg)
Preop night		100	
Day 1	100 intraop	100 q 12 hr	
Day 2	50 q 8 hr	50 q 8 hr	
Day 3 and 4	50 q 12 hr	50 q 12 hr	
Day 5* and 6		50 q 12 hr	50
Day 7		25 q 12 hr	50
Day 8			75
Subsequently			37.5–50

* On day 5, 9 α-fluorocortisol 0.1 mg P.O. daily can be started.

drug should be well tolerated orally. Prednisone, prednisolone, and dexamethasone fulfill these criteria. The dose used in each clinical situation varies widely not only with the condition being treated but also with the stage of the disease (Table 1-18). The minimum amount of corticosteroid consistent with an acceptable result should be administered.

Systemic corticosteroids have application in selected instances in the following diseases: collagen vascular diseases (including systemic lupus erythematosus, polyarteritis nodosa, and Wegener's granulomatosis) dermatologic diseases (such as pemphigus vulgaris), inflammatory bowel disease (particularly ulcerative colitis), incapacitating arthritis, some cases of chronic renal disease, chronic active hepatitis, severe allergic states (including bronchial asthma, serum sickness, and anaphylaxis), and as an adjunct to chemotherapy in some malignancies. Corticosteroids have also been used in the acute treatment of cerebral edema and increasing intracranial pressure associated with head trauma, anoxic encephalopathy, and intracranial malignancies. For example, dexamethasone in doses of up to 8 mg every 6 hours can be used acutely in cases of cerebral edema.

There are devastating side effects associated with the prolonged use of corticosteroids (Table 1-19). The most obvious problem is drug-induced adrenal insufficiency. Alternate day administration of steroids may reduce the suppression somewhat. Relative insufficiency may persist for months or years after discontinuation of therapy, and therefore, if a stressful situation occurs during this period, hormonal therapy should be reinstituted. Other complications include a diabetic state, sodium and fluid retention, muscle weakness, osteoporosis, pathologic fractures, impaired wound healing, increased susceptibility to infections, gastrointestinal hemorrhage, cataracts, and a frank Cushingoid state. A further problem is that steroids mask an intercurrent infection

TABLE 1-18
Selected Corticosteroid Uses

Disease	Acute Dosage (per day)	Desired Effect
Periarteritis nodosa	Prednisone, 40–60 mg	Symptomatic improvement
Wegener's granulomatosis	Prednisone, 60 mg	Some symptomatic relief and prolongation of life
Systemic lupus erythematosus, with:		
C.N.S. involvement	Prednisone, 2 mg/kg	Control psychosis and seizures
Severe nephritis	Prednisone, 40–60 mg, occasionally 200 mg	Control but not cure nephritis
Pemphigus vulgaris	Prednisone, 80–300 mg	Induce and maintain remission
Ulcerative colitis or Crohn's disease	Prednisone, 40–60 mg	Symptomatic relief and remission
Chronic active hepatitis	Prednisone, 40–60 mg	Clinical, biochemical, and histologic remission
Acute I.T.P.	Prednisone, 1–2 mg/kg	Increase platelets and capillary integrity
Polymyositis and dermatomyositis	Prednisone, 40–60 mg	Symptomatic improvement
Acute polyneuritis	Prednisone, 40 mg	Reverse muscle weakness
Sarcoidosis	Prednisone, 40 mg	Improved chest x-ray and pulmonary function tests
Chemotherapy		
Acute lymphoblastic leukemia	Prednisone, 2–5 mg/kg	Induce and maintain remission
Lymphomas	Prednisone, 1 mg/kg	Induce and maintain remission
Cerebral edema	Dexamethasone, 4–6 mg q 4–6 hr	Decrease intracranial pressure

or disease process. It is extremely difficult to evaluate a patient with abdominal pain who is receiving steroid therapy because the signs of inflammation are all suppressed. The fact that these patients can even have a perforated viscus with essentially no signs of peritoneal irritation makes it essential that an aggressive diagnostic and surgical approach be adopted if there is any suspicion of a significant intraabdominal problem.

Pharmacologic Uses   The value of corticosteroids in replacement therapy is firmly established; their usefulness as anti-inflammatory agents is

TABLE 1-19
Complications of Corticosteroids

Endocrine	**Immunologic**
Adrenal suppression	Suppression of immune system
Cushing's syndrome	Susceptibility to infections
Diabetic state	Suppression of response to skin
Growth suppression	testing
Fluids and Electrolytes	Suppression of signs of inflammation
Sodium retention	
Fluid retention	**Musculoskeletal**
Hypokalemic alkalosis	Muscle wasting
Congestive heart failure	Muscle weakness
Hypertension	Osteoporosis
	Pathologic fractures
Metabolic	Aseptic necrosis, femoral head
Negative nitrogen balance	
Impaired wound healing	**Miscellaneous**
	G.I. bleeding
	Pancreatitis
	Petechiae and purpura
	Cataracts

accepted, but their therapeutic efficacy in pharmacologic doses is still sharply debated. There are many reasons why the answer to this question is unclear. For several decades a great deal of animal research has been directed toward determining the usefulness of steroids in shock. Unfortunately, shock affects different target organs in the various species studied, and the applicability of this experimental data to humans is unclear. While steroids have often been used in the clinical shock situation, they were frequently given as medical "last rites"—too little and too late. The use of corticosteroids in pharmacologic doses has been advocated in all forms of shock, adult respiratory distress syndrome, postpump perfusion, near drowning, smoke inhalation, myocardial infarction and ischemia, low flow states, and to counteract circulating endotoxins and myocardial depressant factors. Such an impressive list of catastrophic conditions may reflect the desire of the clinician to salvage a desperate situation, rather than any objectively validated efficacy of steroids.

Shock is characterized by inadequate perfusion of critical organs with decreased oxygen delivery and oxygen utilization. This definition intentionally ignores blood pressure, as well as cardiac output, which we now know can be elevated in some forms and/or stages of shock.[41,42] There are many theoretical reasons (with laboratory confirmation) why massive doses of glucocorticoids could be effective in shock. They increase cardiac index and decrease peripheral vascular resistance. They have a protective effect on the microcirculation decreasing capillary permeability. By decreasing arteriolar and venular resistance, they increase visceral and cutaneous blood flow, as well as venous return. They have a diffuse effect on cellular membranes throughout the body, and some believe that they can restore vascular membrane integrity to the capillaries in the lung and other organs. Corticosteroids stabilize lysosomal membranes inhibiting the release of potent lysosomal enzymes, thus eliminating their devastating reactivity. Further, they inhibit the activation of the complement system by endotoxin.[43] Clearly, these and other proposed actions of corticosteroids would be advantageous in shock.

Schumer has reported the first prospective randomized study demonstrating that steroids appear to be useful in the treatment of clinical septic shock.[44] He also analyzed retrospectively his experience with steroids. The corticosteroids used were either 3 mg per kilogram of dexamethasone or 30 mg per kilogram of methylprednisolone, given as a single bolus infusion at the time of diagnosis. If necessary, the dose was repeated once at four hours. In the prospective study, the mortality rate was decreased from 38.4 percent in the controls to 10.4 percent in the steroid group. In the retrospective study the mortality rate in the control group was 42.5 percent versus 14 percent in the steroid treated patients. There was no significant difference in complication rates between the groups. This study must be carefully evaluated before its application is generalized. The most impressive differences appear to be in immunosuppressed patients and those with cancer. Transient septic shock also bears little relationship to the long-term septic patient in whom failure of the immune response, malnutrition, and localized anatomic problems, rather than an acute hemodynamic event, seem to determine survival. The use of pharmacologic doses of glucocorticoids is particularly indicated when there is an acute hemodynamic incident, and if this represents the major threat of the entire illness, such as in septic shock secondary to urologic instrumentation, it would appear that survival is indeed enhanced. Of course, the treatment of septic shock includes the elimination of the source of infection by surgery if necessary, a comprehensive approach to cardiovascular resuscitation, and the institution of appropriate antibiotic therapy. Fluids are administered in whatever volume is necessary to optimize cardiac output and renal function, and other interventions in the respiratory and cardiovascular systems such as endotracheal intubation, PEEP, and the use of inotropic agents, are made as indicated. Long-term therapy includes adequate nutritional support and detailed constant total system care.

Unfortunately, there are no prospective studies demonstrating the usefulness of steroids in severe trauma, hypovolemic shock, or cardiogenic shock. However, if similar microcirculatory and cellular mechanisms are producing "irreversibility" in other forms of shock, then steroids may be useful in these situations as well. There are many anecdotal reports in the literature supporting this; for example, Lozman and Powers demonstrated that administration of methylprednisolone to traumatized patients significantly increases cardiac output and decreases peripheral vascular resistance.[41] However, it must be clearly understood that no objective human clinical evidence supporting such treatment regimes have yet been reported.

Glucocorticoids have also been advocated for the treatment of the adult respiratory distress syndrome and, in particular, shock lung.[45] The many diverse causes of adult respiratory distress syndrome include trauma, aspiration, smoke inhalation, and pancreatitis, among others. In all these clinical situations, a common hypothesis suggests that damage to the pulmonary microcirculation occurs with increased capillary permeability and the accumulation of fluid in the interstitial and alveolar spaces. There is good experimental animal data that methylprednisolone will minimize the pathologic changes normally seen in the canine lung in shock. Whether this has any human relevance is subject to considerable debate since primate models fail to show similar pathologic changes. Human hypovolemic shock does not appear to cause shock lung unless other complications supervene.[46] Sladen,[47] and others,[48] have used methylprednisolone, 30 mg/kg of body weight every 6 hours, for 48 hours after the onset of adult respiratory distress syndrome. Of course, it has to be remembered that steroids, if indeed effective, are only an adjunctive measure. Of greater importance is the management of the precipitating conditions and the use of ventilatory support, especially positive end expiratory pressure (PEEP). Suffice it to say that catastrophic events require heroic efforts: when a therapeutic modality is proved effective, it should be used. The present status of pharmacologic doses of steroids cannot yet be considered "effective" therapy (Table 1-20).

TABLE 1-20
Corticosteroid Uses

Indications	Drug	Dosage
Replacement therapy		
Chronic	Cortisone plus 9α-fluorocortisol	37.5 mg/day; 0.1–0.3 mg/day p.r.n.
Acute stress	Hydrocortisone	300 mg/day
Anti-inflammatory	Prednisone and others	Usually < 100 mg/day
Pharmacologic		
Shock	Methylprednisolone	2000 mg I.V. bolus (30 mg/kg)
Respiratory distress syndrome	Methylprednisolone	2000 mg I.V. q 6 hr × 48 hr (30 mg/kg)

SPECIFIC PATIENT PROBLEMS

NEUROLOGIC DISORDERS

Agitation and Restlessness Almost all patients in an intensive care unit, because of constant monitoring and activity resulting in sleep deprivation, will at some time or another manifest agitation and restlessness (Fig. 1-2). In fact, as the patient improves and becomes more aware of his surroundings, he often becomes very irritable and desires to leave the I.C.U. The frequency of these symptoms and their usual benignity should not lull the intensivist into a false sense of security, because they can occasionally reflect serious underlying pathology.

Incisional pain will often produce irritation and restlessness and this can be managed with an analgesic such as morphine. However, the agitation and uneasiness may be secondary to much more serious problems, including metabolic encephalopathies that accompany liver failure, renal failure, or diabetic ketoacidosis. If a patient on a respirator becomes agitated, one must immediately consider the possibility that he is being inadequately ventilated and that his restlessness is secondary to hypoxia, hypercarbia, or pneumothorax. Impending shock or hypovolemia, sepsis, or heart failure also can produce these symptoms and an early sign of recurrent gastrointestinal hemorrhage may present as

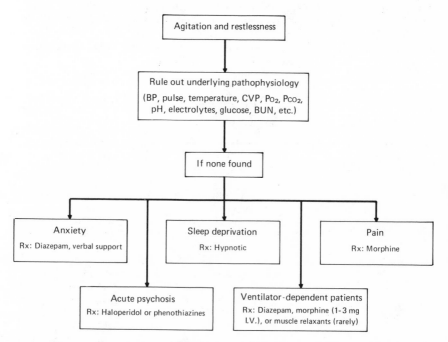

Fig. 1-2. Management principles for agitation and restlessness.

a sense of apprehension on the part of the patient. Other simple but important etiologies that must be ruled out are hypoglycemia and electrolyte abnormalities, including hyponatremia, hypocalcemia, and hypomagnesemia. In county hospitals, with their large populations of alcoholics and drug addicts, nervousness and excitation may be a manifestation of withdrawal from narcotics, barbiturates, or alcohol. There are, of course, many other causes of an agitated patient, including even hyperthyroidism. The important principle is to consider a pathophysiologic cause of agitation and restlessness primarily; if one is found, treat it specifically rather than simply suppressing the symptoms.

In an I.C.U., anxiety and disquietude are most often a normal response of a patient, perhaps in pain and in a strange environment. He is being turned and administered to constantly, precluding uninterrupted sleep. There are people continuously coming and going and the patient does not fully understand the sophisticated monitoring going on around him. In this context, the symptoms can be allayed by assurances and explanations from the staff, combined with the appropriate use of analgesia and sedation. Rarely, a true psychotic episode will occur requiring antipsychotic treatment (see pp. 17–20).

Convulsions   One of the most dramatic clinical situations in medicine is a grand mal seizure. Since this can be a life-threatening condition, all physicians must know how to effect immediate treatment (Table 1-21). Whenever a convulsion occurs, most people immediately think of epilepsy, but, in the critically ill patient in an intensive care unit, a number of other diagnoses must be ruled out.

Seizures represent a paroxysmal disturbance of the electrical activity of the brain. Often this is expressed by alterations in consciousness and convulsions which are a violent, involuntary series of contractions of skeletal muscles. The term *epilepsy* implies a chronic condition with

---

TABLE 1-21
Management Principles for Acute Seizures

No Previous History
Stop seizure with:
  Valium
  Dilantin
  Phenobarbital
  Other drugs including general anaesthesia (rare)
May or may not require chronic anticonvulsants depending on etiology

Known Epileptic
Control as above
Resume chronic anticonvulsants; may have to increase dosages of previous
  medications or add new drugs

---

a tendency to recurrent seizures and is secondary to some form of intra-cranial pathology. From the initial convulsion, it is imperative to distin-guish intracranial from extracranial etiologies, particularly in the I.C.U. setting.

A detailed discussion of epilepsy is beyond the intended scope of this section. However, a classification of convulsive disorders is impor-tant and one useful system groups seizures into generalized and local varieties.[49] Generalized seizures are petit mal (absence attacks) or grand mal (tonic-clonic). In contrast, there can be focal seizures of a simple or a complex variety. It is important to realize that focal seizures may become secondarily generalized in such a rapid manner that the initial focal origin may not be appreciated. Continuous seizure activity without any intervals of consciousness is classified as status epilepticus.

The most common cause of seizures and status epilepticus is the failure of an epileptic patient to receive his anticonvulsants. This may occur in the I.C.U. if little or no patient history was available on admis-sion, or when insufficient information was obtained in the heat of the crisis situation. In the seriously ill or traumatized patient in the I.C.U., several other conditions must be considered especially if there is no previous history of convulsions. Metabolic causes including hypoglyce-mia, hypoxia, uremia, and hepatic encephalopathy must be rigorously excluded by appropriate quantitative tests—blood sugar, Pao_2, and BUN. Water intoxication and electrolyte abnormalities, such as hyponatremia and hypocalcemia, must also be excluded. Withdrawal from alcohol or barbiturates can produce generalized convulsions as well. The possibil-ity of recent or remote head trauma should always be considered as a cause of seizures, particularly in alcoholics who might have been drunk at the time of the trauma and not remember it. The most common cause of seizure disorders beginning after middle age is cerebral vascular disease.[49] Another 10 percent of seizures beginning in adulthood are due to cerebral neoplasms of either a primary or secondary nature. Other etiologies include encephalitis, meningitis, brain abscess, and, occasion-ally, even idiosyncratic reactions to drugs, such as local anesthetics. A patient with tetanus may have generalized convulsions characterized by continuous tonic spasms of muscles, but this is not a seizure and must be distinguished from other convulsive disorders.

When a patient presents with a generalized tonic-clonic seizure, management of the convulsion often precedes diagnosis. Seizures can usually be terminated by the intravenous administration of 5 to 10 mg of diazepam (Valium). Once the seizure has stopped, or indeed, if it has not responded to the diazepam, intravenous phenytoin (Dilantin) can be administered—the first 500 mg of phenytoin should be given slowly at a rate not exceeding 50 mg per min I.V. A second 500 mg should also be given intravenously, to produce a loading dose of one gm. Intravenous phenobarbital in a dose of 150 to 400 mg is another useful drug for the termination of status epilepticus (see pp. 21–22).

During a seizure, the patient should be observed and prevented from injuring himself. A pillow should be placed under his head to protect it and, if possible, a padded tongue depressor should be inserted between his teeth to prevent him from biting his tongue. The patient should not be actively restrained because this can produce soft tissue injury and fractures. He should be turned on his side to avert aspiration. Endotracheal intubation should also be considered since effective airway control can eliminate hypoxic induced convulsions or prevent further damage resulting from the subsequent development of hypoxia.

Once the seizure has been terminated, the etiology must be determined. All the metabolic, physical, and infectious causes listed above must be considered and ruled out. A history of alcoholism or drug abuse is important. Prodromal symptoms or an aura prior to the seizure may help delineate the type of seizure. A description of the seizure itself and whether it started off focally or in a generalized manner, is clearly of diagnostic interest. A careful neurologic exam in the immediate postictal period may be confusing but may also show focal signs which would strongly suggest intracranial pathology. A CAT scan with and without contrast should be strongly considered in all patients who develop acute seizure activity—it should be mandatory if there is any suspicioned trauma. The EEG is a simple bedside noninvasive test that may demonstrate a localized area of cerebral pathology. If infection or hemorrhage are suspected, a lumbar puncture can be performed as long as there are no signs of increased intracranial pressure. Angiography is not usually necessary unless one of the other tests suggests the possibility of a surgically correctable lesion, e.g., a tumor, an arterio-venous malformation, or extracranial cerebrovascular disease.

Clearly, if an extracranial cause for the convulsions can be found, it should be treated. If a metabolic problem is corrected, then long-term anticonvulsant therapy is usually unnecessary. Likewise, if there is a cerebral lesion that is amenable to surgery, it may be possible for the neurosurgeon to eliminate this cause of seizures. Patients for whom no definite cause of the seizures is defined may require anticonvulsant medication—at least throughout the acute hospitalization phase of illness. Thereafter, the neurologic evaluation should be repeated. The picture may then be clarified unless the undiagnosed precipitating cause has already abated (Fig. 1-3).

Hepatic Failure   Hepatocellular failure can complicate almost all forms of liver disease, including alcoholic cirrhosis, viral hepatitis, fatty liver of pregnancy, halothane hepatitis, and chronic cholestasis. Irrespective of etiology, the syndrome is most easily defined on the basis of fairly characteristic features. It is not unusual that an alcoholic patient with spider nevi, gynecomastia, jaundice, and ascites, develops bleeding from esophageal varices. With continued bleeding and transfusions, liver failure is often pronounced and the patient becomes confused, asterixis develops, and eventually frank hepatic coma may ensue (Table 1-22).

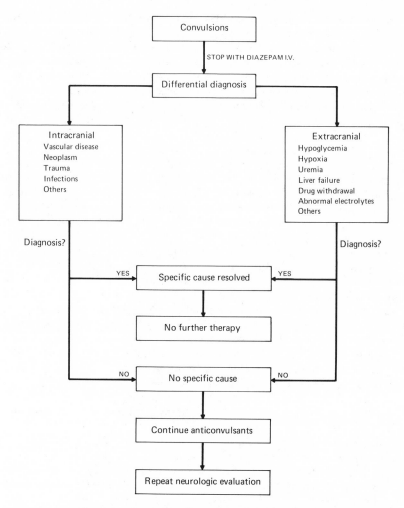

Fig. 1-3.   Summary flow sheet for convulsions.

However, while the clinical syndrome is quite characteristic there are no specific diagnostic tests for it. Although ammonia has been implicated as being an important substance in the production of hepatic coma, there is not a direct correlation between the arterial levels and the severity of the encephalopathy. In fact, at least 10 percent of patients in deep coma have normal ammonia levels. Similarly, although patients in hepatic coma do have an abnormal EEG with slowing of the waves down to the delta range, these are nonspecific findings consistent with any metabolic encephalopathy.

One must remember that even in a patient with known liver disease,

TABLE 1-22
Precipitating Causes of Hepatic Coma

G.I. bleeding
Azotemia, e.g., diuretics or vomiting
Hypokalemic aklalosis
Drugs, e.g., morphine or sedatives
Excessive dietary protein
Portosystemic shunts
Infection
Surgical procedures
Fulminant hepatic necrosis

---

not all coma is hepatic coma. The differential diagnosis includes CO_2 retention, subdural hematoma, hypoglycemia, barbiturate intoxication, and uremia. These alternative possibilities must be ruled out.

The treatment of the hepatic encephalopathy is in large part the reversal of the initiating factor. Azotemia and hypokalemic alkalosis are commonly iatrogenic in origin. If the patient is on potent diuretics for chronic ascites, it is imperative to check potassium and BUN levels.

The liver is important in metabolizing many medications, and therefore, the patient who has liver disease must have the dosage of many drugs modified accordingly. As discussed in preceding sections, morphine and sedatives should be avoided in patients with liver failure because of the tendency to produce hepatic coma. If an analgesic or a sedative is required, reduced dosages of meperidine or oxazepam can be used cautiously.

One of the most common precipitating causes of hepatic coma is G.I. bleeding. Not all bleeding episodes in a cirrhotic are from varices and, of course, specific treatment of the bleeding depends upon making an accurate, rapid diagnosis with endoscopy. While stopping the hemorrhage is vitally important, one must use other modalities as well, to prevent the development of encephalopathy.

The gastrointestinal tract must be emptied of blood, thereby reducing the load of protein available for bacterial degradation. Saline enemas can be administered 2 or 3 times daily to evacuate the colon. Intravenous pitressin is not only beneficial in arresting variceal hemorrhage, but, by stimulating smooth muscle contraction, it creates mass peristalsis and shortens the transit time for blood in the small intestine. Saline cathartics, such as magnesium sulfate or Fleet's Phospho-soda, are also employed to evacuate blood from the G.I. tract. They act as cathartics by osmotically retaining fluid in the bowel lumen, secondarily producing mechanical stimulation of the intestines. These agents are administered once or twice daily and usually result in a bowel movement in about three hours. The single dose for magnesium sulfate is 15 gm, and for

Fleet's Phospho-soda, 30 ml. Magnesium sulfate is contraindicated in renal failure because absorption and accumulation of magnesium can occur.

Neomycin and lactulose are useful in the management of hepatic encephalopathy. Neomycin can be administered orally in a dose of 4 to 6 gm per day; this nonabsorbable antibiotic is very effective in decreasing the bacterial production of ammonia. Lactulose (Cephulac) is a nonnaturally occurring disaccharide and the human intestine does not produce a lactulase that can split it.[50] Consequently, most lactulose reaches the cecum, where it can be degraded by bacteria to lactic acid and small amounts of acetic acid. This reduces the fecal pH favoring the growth of organisms that do not produce ammonia. It also may be effective because the acid pH results in ammonium ion entrapment in the stool and its subsequent excretion. Further, lactulose serves as an effective laxative. In chronic encephalopathy, lactulose may prove to be slightly better than neomycin. Neomycin and lactulose should not be given simultaneously, as the antibacterial effect of neomycin may interfere with the bacterial degradation of lactulose which is essential for its activity.

It has long been recognized that patients in hepatic coma are sensitive to exogenous protein loads. However, these patients are often extremely ill and in negative nitrogen balance. Therefore, nutritional support is extremely important. In recent years special hyperalimentation formulations have been created for these patients, not only to provide calories, but also to serve as a therapeutic modality through provision of specific amino acids. Many patients demonstrate an abnormal plasma amino acid profile: the branched chain amino acids are markedly decreased, whereas the aromatic amino acids are increased. Fischer et al.[51] and others[52] have advocated the use of "liver failure" solutions which are designed to normalize the concentration of the various amino acids in the serum, as well as to provide important calories to the patient. As the encephalopathy improves, the dietary protein can be gradually increased to 40 to 60 gm, or even more, per day.

The use of L-dopa for the treatment of acute and chronic hepatic encephalopathy is controversial. Fischer hypothesized that in hepatic coma, false neurotransmitters are produced in the intestines that bypass the diseased liver, reach the systemic circulation unmodified, and accumulate in the central nervous system.[53] There they compete with dopamine and result in encephalopathy. L-dopa is a normal precursor of dopamine that crosses the blood-brain barrier readily, and perhaps may restore a normal transmitter balance. A number of studies have demonstrated that L-dopa, 500 mg P.O., every 4 to 6 hours, may produce arousal from deep coma within 24 hours.[54,55] However, not even Fischer's work shows any increased survival in acute hepatic coma. The exact role of L-dopa awaits definition by a controlled, prospective clinical trial (Table 1-23).

TABLE 1-23

Management Principles in Acute Hepatic Encephalopathy

Control precipitating cause, e.g., stop bleeding or discontinue drugs
Enemas and cathartics, e.g., magnesium sulfate 15 gm P.O.
Neomycin 1 gm P.O. q 4–6 hr or lactulose 30–45 ml q 6–8 hr
Nutrition:
  "liver failure" solution
  increase dietary protein as tolerated.
Consider L-dopa 500 mg P.O. q 4–6 hr

PERSISTENT POSTOPERATIVE VENTILATORY INSUFFICIENCY

Persistent postoperative ventilatory insufficiency (respiratory paralysis) has many etiologies. The first consideration in all intubated patients who are not breathing "appropriately" must be that there may be a mechanical problem. The clinician must search for and eliminate respirator malfunction; blocking of an endotracheal tube by kinking or a mucous plug; malposition of the endotracheal tube, including "nonintubation," e.g., an extratracheal position; or the opposite extreme, "over intubation" or intubation of the right main-stem bronchus.

Perhaps the most common nonmechanical causes are inadequate reversal of the competitive blocking agents and persistence of the drugs used in producing anesthesia, e.g., fentanyl. Alternatively, the patient may have been hyperventilated during anesthesia producing a marked hypocapnea which results in a loss of the carbon dioxide drive for respiration. One should, however, consider other possibilities. Some people have an atypical or deficient plasma cholinesterase and they inadequately degrade succinylcholine.[28] Therefore, they can have a markedly prolonged activity of the drug. Similarly, drugs such as the aminoglycosides, particularly neomycin and kanamycin, can prolong the activity of the competitive blocking agents.[56] Hypokalemia and rapid rewarming of a patient who has cooled significantly during anesthesia can also result in a potentiation of the effects of competitive blocking agents. D-tubocurarine is partially excreted by the kidneys, and gallamine is totally eliminated by the kidneys; therefore, these drugs must be used cautiously in patients with renal failure (Fig. 1-4).

The treatment of prolonged postoperative ventilatory insufficiency is straightforward—the patient must be adequately mechanically ventilated until he can breathe for himself. Competitive blocking can be reversed with neostigmine and narcotics with naloxone. Direct muscle stimulation will reveal persistent muscular relaxant effects and can be used to guide the dosage of reversing agents. Therapy of the *condition*—

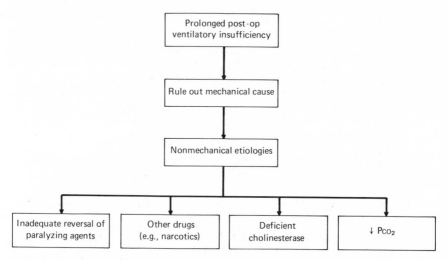

Fig. 1-4. Management principles for prolonged postoperative ventilatory insufficiency.

inadequate spontaneous ventilation—is mandatory; most situations resolve if mechanical ventilation is continued for a few hours.

ALLERGIC REACTIONS

Allergic reactions encompass a large nonhomogenous mixture of immunologically mediated clinical entities. The reactions can be acute or chronic and the precipitating agents are many, including almost all drugs, blood transfusions, radiographic contrast materials, insect stings (not likely in the I.C.U., one hopes) and foreign protein of many types. The broad spectrum of presentations extends from pruritus and urticaria to bronchospasm, laryngeal edema, or even profound anaphylactic shock. While there are many different etiologies of the clinical syndrome, the treatment in the acute situation is fairly standard (Figure 1-5). The management of chronic allergic states is beyond the scope of this text.

Prevention of a complication is always a desirable goal. Many drug reactions can be avoided if a good history is taken from a patient; however, there may not be a history of previous drug sensitization. Similarly, people who have a history of an allergic reaction to radiocontrast materials should not be reexposed to these agents unless it is absolutely essential—and then treated expectantly. Often there is no previous history of allergy and, unfortunately, it is in just such a clinical situation that the severest anaphylactic reactions often occur.

Treatment of any allergic reaction begins by identifying the offending agent, suspending its administration to the patient, and making certain that he will not receive any more of it in the future.

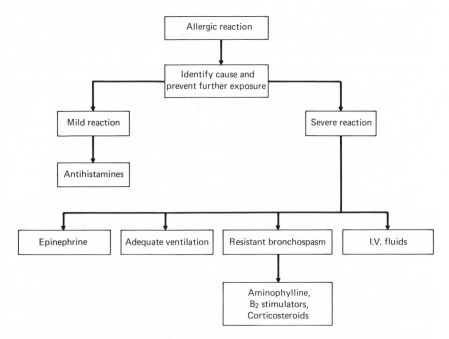

Fig. 1-5. Management principles for allergic reaction.

In mild allergic reactions characterized by pruritus, urticaria, or rhinitis, antihistamines that act by blocking the H_1-receptor sites provide symptomatic relief. For example, diphenhydramine (Benadryl) can be administered in a dose of 25 to 50 mg orally or parenterally. However, in the treatment of a severe systemic anaphylactic reaction, antihistamines play only an accessory role. Epinephrine is the drug of choice for the treatment of all severe allergic reactions. It can be administered in a dose of 0.5 ml of a one part per thousand solution subcutaneously (0.5 mg), and this can be repeated at 10 to 15 minute intervals as necessary. In life threatening reactions, epinephrine can be administered slowly intravenously, but this is not usually necessary.

It is essential to maintain adequate ventilation and airway control in these patients. In severe cases of respiratory insufficiency with bronchospasm and laryngeal edema unresponsive to epinephrine, endotracheal intubation and, rarely, tracheostomy may be required. Emergency tracheostomy *must* be considered a time-consuming procedure—more than 30 minutes usually ensue from time of decision to establishment of adequate ventilation.

If bronchospasm is severe and not responsive to epinephrine, aminophylline can be used. It is administered intravenously, slowly, in a loading dose of 5.6 mg per kilogram followed by 0.9 mg per kilogram per hour.[57] It has been responsible for many I.C.U. deaths and must, therefore, be utilized cautiously in patients suspected of coronary artery disease. Allergic states such as bronchial asthma are characterized by bron-chospasm and respiratory distress. Alternatives to epinephrine for treating this bronchospasm are the newer, selective, β_2-adrenergic stim-ulators (Table 1-24).[58] This group of drugs includes salbutamol, metapro-terenol and terbutaline. Because of their selective effect on β_2-receptors, these drugs are highly effective in producing bronchodilatation and do not add excessive chronotropic stimulation to the already tachycardic heart. Salbutamol and metaproterenol are rapidly effective by aerosol inhalation and have a longer duration of action than does epinephrine or isoproterenol.

In anaphylactic shock, there is functional and absolute intravascular hypovolemia. This should be rapidly corrected using a crystalloid solu-tion (such as Ringer's lactate), monitoring the central venous pressure or pulmonary wedge pressure as indicated.

In acute severe allergic reactions, corticosteroids are not first-line drugs. They may be useful in situations in which the condition may not be readily reversed. In severe bronchospasm, or status asthmaticus, steroids may be administered in doses of up to 500 mg of cortisol equiva-lent every eight hours. However, it must be appreciated that steroids take several hours before they are effective. In life-threatening anaphy-lactic shock, steroids can be administered in very large pharmacologic doses, such as 30 mg per kilogram of methylprednisolone; however, there are no controlled series demonstrating that such therapy is efficacious.

Once the allergic reaction has been treated and the patient has re-covered, he should, of course, be warned to avoid future contact with the precipitating allergen. He should also be advised to wear a Medic-Alert bracelet describing his allergy.

TABLE 1-24
β_2-Stimulators

Drug	Dosage
Terbutaline (Bricanyl or Brethine)	2.5–5 mg P.O. t.i.d. or 0.25 mg S.C. q 4–6 hr
Metaproterenol (Alupent or Meta-prel)	20 mg P.O. q 6 hr or 2–3 inhalations q 3–4 hr (0.65 mg each)
Salbutamol (Ventolin)	2–3 inhalations q 3–4 hr (0.1 mg each)

GENERAL USE MEDICATIONS IN THE PEDIATRIC AGE GROUP

While adults vary somewhat in size and responsiveness to medications, the therapeutic dose for a particular drug tends to fall within a fairly narrow range. This is not at all true in the pediatric age group where age, weight, body surface area, and even maturation of liver enzyme systems have to be taken into consideration. A number of formulae have been developed to help resolve this problem. For example:

$$\text{Approximate dose} = \frac{\text{Surface area (in sq m)}}{1.7} \times \text{adult dose}$$

Clark's Rule:

$$\text{Approximate dose} = \frac{\text{Patient's weight (in lb)}}{150} \times \text{adult dose}$$

The formula relating dose to surface area is the most sensitive, but both of the above are unreliable in premature or newborn infants. The following table of general use medications should serve only as a very rough guideline, and must be tempered by the experience of the clinician and the response of the patient (Table 1-25).

TABLE 1-25
Selected Pediatric Drug Dosages (Parenteral)

Drug	Dosage (mg/kg)	Interval (hr)
Narcotics		
Morphine	0.1–0.2	4
Merperidine (Demerol)	1.0	3–4
Codeine	0.5	4
Methadone (Dolophine)	0.1	4
Narcotic Antagonist		
Naloxone (Narcan)	0.01	p.r.n.
Sedatives and Tranquilizers		
Diazepam (Valium)	0.04–0.2	6–8
Chlordiazepoxide	0.15	6–8
(Librium)	(not indicated for child < 6 yr)	
Phenobarbital	0.5	6
(Luminal)		
Chlorpromazine	0.5	6–8
(Thorazine)	(use with care in child < 6 mo)	
Haloperidol (Haldol)	Not recommended (safety not established in children)	—
Anticonvulsants		
(in status epilepticus)		
Diazepam (Valium)	0.04–0.2	2–4
Phenobarbital	3.5	12–24
(Luminal)		
Phenytoin (Dilantin)	3–8	24
Muscle Relaxants		
D-tubocurarine	0.2–0.4	titrate p.r.n.

(continued)

TABLE 1-25 (continued)
Selected Pediatric Drug Dosages (Parenteral)

Drug	Dosage (mg/kg)	Interval (hr)
Muscle Relaxants *(continued)*		
Pancuronium	0.05–0.1	titrate p.r.n.
(Pavulon)	(in neonates, test with 0.02 first)	
Succinylcholine	1–2	titrate p.r.n.
(Anectine)		
Antihistamines		
Diphenhydramine	1.2	6
(Benadryl)		
Promethazine	0.25–0.5	4–6
(Phenergan)		
Hydroxyzine	0.5–1	6
(Vistaril)		
Chlorpheniramine	0.1	6
(Chlor-Trimeton)		
Cimetidine	5–10	6
(Tagamet)	(very limited pediatric experience)	
Corticosteroids		
Physiologic replacement		
Cortisone acetate	0.7	Daily
Anti-inflammatory		
Prednisone	0.5–4	Daily
Pharmacologic		
Methylprednisolone	30	Usually single dose

CONCLUSION

Although these drugs are probably the most frequently administered, few specific regimes can be unequivocally advocated. The principles described denote the *minimal-drug/minimal-problem* approach. While convincing evidence may well be lacking for certain commonly accepted indications, the consensus of opinion and a frame of reference presented herein is intended to help "today." Refinements and further documentation are anticipated and necessary.

REFERENCES

1. Smith GM, Beecher HK: Measurement of "mental clouding" and other subjective effects of morphine. J Pharmacol Exp Therap 126:50, 1959

2. Goodman LS, Gilman A (eds): The Pharmacological Basis of Therapeutics, 5th ed. New York, Macmillan, 1975

3. Jaffe JH, Martin WR: Narcotic analgesics and antagonists. In Goodman LS, Gilman A (eds): The Pharmacological Basis of Therapeutics, 5th ed. New York, Macmillan, 1975

4. Guillemin R: Endorphins, brain peptides that act like opiates. N Engl J Med 296:226, 1977

5. Hughes J, Smith TW, Kosterlitz HW, et al: Identification of two related pentapeptides from the brain with potent opiate agonist activity. Nature 258:577, 1975

6. Ling N, Burgus R, Guillemin R: Isolation, primary structure, and synthesis of α-endorphin and γ-endorphin, two peptides of hypothalamic-hypophysial origin with morphinomimetic activity. Proc Natl Acad Sci USA 73:3942, 1976

7. Eckenhoff JE, Oech SR: The effects of narcotics and antagonists upon respiration and circulation in man. Clin Pharmacol Ther 1:483, 1960

8. Alderman EL, Barry WH, Graham A, Harrison DC: Hemodynamic effects of morphine and pentazocine differ in cardiac patients. N Engl J Med 287:623, 1972

9. Economou G, Ward-McQuaid JN: A cross-over comparison of the effect of morphine, pethidine, pentazocine, and phenazocine on biliary pressure. Gut 12:218, 1971

10. Way EL, Adler TK: The pharmacologic implications of the fate of morphine and its surrogates. Pharmacol Rev 12:383, 1960

11. Drugs for psychiatric disorders. Med Lett Drugs Ther 18:89, 1976

12. Tyrer P: The benzodiazepine bonanza. Lancet 2:709, 1974

13. Choice of a benzodiazepine for treatment of anxiety or insomnia. Med Lett Drugs Ther 19:49, 1977

14. Hoff JT: Resuscitation in focal brain ischemia. Crit Care Med 6:245, 1978

15. Safar P, Bleyaert A, Nemoto EM, et al: Resuscitation after global brain ischemia-anoxia. Crit Care Med 6:215, 1978

16. Breivik H, Safar P, Sands P, et al: Clinical feasibility trials of barbiturate therapy after cardiac arrest. Crit Care Med 6:228, 1978

17. American Hospital Formulary Service: Current drug therapy—barbiturates. Am J Hosp Pharm 33:333, 1976

18. Matthew H: Barbiturates. Clin Toxicol 8:495, 1975

19. Goodman J, Bischel MD, Wagers PW, Barbour BH: Barbiturate intoxication—morbidity and mortality. West J Med 124:179, 1976

20. Haloperidol in psychiatry. Med Lett Drugs Ther 17:11, 1975

21. Kiely WF: Psychiatric syndromes in critically ill patients. JAMA 235:2759, 1976

22. Nadelson T: The psychiatrist in the surgical intensive care unit. Arch Surg 111:113, 1976

23. Drugs for epilepsy. Med Lett Drugs Ther 18:25–28, 1976

24. Woodbury DM, Fingl E: Drugs effective in the therapy of the epilepsies. In Goodman LS, Gilman A (eds): The Pharmacological Basis of Therapeutics, 5th ed. New York, Macmillan, 1975

25. Hvidberg EF, Dam M: Clinical pharmacokinetics of anticonvulsants. Clin Pharmacokinet 1:161, 1976

26. Gugler R, Manion CV, Azarnoff DL: Phenytoin: Pharmacokinetics and bioavailability. Clin Pharmacol Ther 19:135, 1976

27. Adverse interactions of drugs. Med Lett Drugs Ther 19:5, 1977

28. Kalow W, Gunn DR: The relation between dose of succinylcholine and duration of apnea in man. J Pharmacol Exp Ther 120:203, 1957
29. Black JW, Duncan AM, et al: Definition and antagonism of histamine H_2-receptors. Nature 236:385, 1972
30. Brimblecombe RW, Duncan WAM, Durant GJ, et al: Characterization and development of cimetidine as a histamine H_2-receptor antagonist. Gastroenterology 74:339, 1978
31. Douglas WW: Histamine and antihistamines; 5-hydroxytryptamine and antagonists. In Goodman LS, Gilman A (eds): The Pharmacological Basis of Therapeutics, 5th ed. New York, Macmillan, 1975
32. Ma KW, Brown DC, Malser DS, Silvis SE: Effects of renal failure on blood levels of cimetidine. Gastroenterology 74:473, 1978
33. Binder HJ, Cocco A, Crossley RJ, et al: Cimetidine in the treatment of duodenal ulcer. Gastroenterology 74:380, 1978
34. Hetzel DG, Hansky J, et al: Cimetidine treatment of duodenal ulceration. Gastroenterology 74:389, 1978
35. Behar J, Brand DL, et al: Cimetidine in the treatment of symptomatic gastroesophageal reflux. Gastroenterology 74:441, 1978
36. Freston JW: Cimetidine in the treatment of gastric ulcer. Gastroenterology 74:426, 1978
37. McCarthy DM: Report on the U.S. experience with cimetidine in Zollinger-Ellison syndrome and other hypersecretory states. Gastroenterology 74:453, 1978
38. MacDougall BRD, Williams R: H_2-receptor antagonism in the prevention of acute upper gastrointestinal hemorrhage in fulminant hepatic failure. Gastroenterology 74:464, 1978
39. Cimetidine (Tagamet): update on adverse effects. Med Lett Drugs Ther 20:77, 1978
40. Haynes RC, Larner J: Adrenocorticotrophic hormone; adrenocortical steroids and their synthetic analogs; inhibitors of adrenocortical steroid biosynthesis. In Goodman LS, Gilman A (eds): The Pharmacological Basis of Therapeutics, 5th ed. New York, Macmillan, 1975
41. Lozman J, Dutton RE, English M and Powers S Jr: Cardiopulmonary adjustments following single high dosage administration of methylprednisolone in traumatized man. Ann Surg 181:317, 1975
42. Spath JA Jr, Gorczynski RJ, Lefer AM: Possible mechanisms of the beneficial action of glucocorticoids in circulatory shock. Surg Gynecol Obstet 137:597, 1973
43. O'Flaherty JT, Craddock PR, Jacob HS: Mechanism of anti-complementary activity of corticosteroids in vivo: possible relevance of endotoxic shock (39638). Proc Soc Exp Biol Med 154:206, 1977
44. Schumer W: Steroids in the treatment of clinical septic shock. Ann Surg 184:333, 1976
45. Kusajima K, Wax SD, Webb WR: Effects of methylprednisolone on pulmonary microcirculation. Surg Gynecol Obstet 139:1, 1974
46. Horovitz JH, Carrico CJ, Shires GT: Pulmonary response to major injury. Arch Surg 108:349, 1974
47. Sladen A: Methylprednisolone: pharmacological doses in shock lung syndrome. J Thorac Cardiovasc Surg 71:800, 1976
48. Tomashefski JF, Mahajan V: Managing respiratory distress syndrome in adults. Postgrad Med 59:77, 1976

49. Green L: Convulsive disorders in adults. In Conn HF, Conn RB (eds): Current Diagnosis, 5th ed. Philadelphia, Saunders, 1977
50. Kosman, ME: Lactulose (Cephulac) in portosystemic encephalopathy. JAMA 236:2444, 1976
51. Fischer JE, Funovics JM, Aguirre A, et al: The role of plasma amino acids in hepatic encephalopathy. Surgery 78:276, 1975
52. Maddrey WC, Weber FL, Coulter AW, et al: Effects of keto analogues of essential amino acids in portal-systemic encephalopathy. Gastroenterology 71:190, 1976
53. Fischer JE, Baldessarini RJ: False neurotransmitters and hepatic failure. Lancet 2:75, 1971
54. Fischer JE, Funovics JM, et al: L-dopa in hepatic coma. Ann Surg 183:386, 1976
55. Weiss A, Pitman ER, Javdan P: Arousal response in hepatic encephalopathy with L-dopa. Am J Gastroenterol 62:497, 1974
56. Pittinger C, and Adamson R: Antibiotic blockade of neuromuscular function. Annu Rev Pharmacol 12:169, 1972
57. Mitenko PA, Ogilvie RI: Pharmacokinetics of intravenous theophylline. Clin Pharmacol Ther 14:509, 1973
58. Drugs for asthma. Med Lett Drugs Ther 20:69, 1978

TWO

Infection and Antimicrobials in the Intensive Care Unit

D. Stewart MacIntyre, Jr.

PART I
Infection in the Intensive Care Unit

THE "HOSPITAL FLORA"

There is a clear difference between bacteria acquired by patients in a hospital and bacteria acquired in the community. This difference is seen not only in bacteria which merely colonize, without causing disease, but also in the bacteria which cause disease. Hospital-associated organisms have different species predominance and antibiotic susceptibility patterns from the community-acquired organisms. Furthermore, these hospital strains differ from one hospital to another, and within a given hospital with time.[1-3] One may also see differences in the flora present in a given intensive care unit, with variation from the typical organisms found in the rest of the hospital. Familiarity with the types of organisms in the intensive care unit and the antimicrobial susceptibility patterns of these organisms is of considerable importance in the planning of the antimicrobial management of an individual patient. Ideally, the hospital bacteriology laboratories should issue periodic summaries of the bacterial species isolated from various sources and the antimicrobial susceptibility patterns of these organisms. It is also worthwhile to be aware of the types of organisms causing infection in other patients in the intensive care unit when planning therapy for a given patient.

The principal reservoir of hospital bacteria is in the patients themselves,[4,5] where the bacteria are maintained in their gastrointestinal tracts and on their skin. The respiratory tracts of patients on respirators may act as an additional reservoir. Secondary reservoirs are the hospital personnel (primarily their hands) and any standing water in the hospital, e.g., in respirator tubing, soap dishes, or even flower vases. Acquisition of hospital flora by newly admitted patients frequently occurs within 3 days.[6,7] A number of studies have shown that the administration of antimicrobials accelerates this acquisition.[5-8]

The patterns of antimicrobial susceptibility within a hospital are strongly affected by the patterns of antimicrobial usage within the hospital. When specific antimicrobials have been controlled, microbial resistance to these agents has tended to become less prevalent. Rising inhospital bacterial resistance to a newly introduced antimicrobial occurs as usage of the antimicrobial becomes widespread within the hospital.[9]

The problem of bacterial resistance becomes particularly acute in intensive care units due to the concentration of "high-risk" patients in one area. Intensive care unit patients generally have impaired host defenses, including extra portals of entry for bacteria such as surgical or traumatic wounds, invasive monitoring lines, and catheters; antimicrobial usage is also widespread. Thus, there are several reasons for using antimicrobials sparingly.

In some circumstances one may consider adopting an antimicrobial "policy" within an intensive care unit, using certain antimicrobials preferentially and holding others for individual cases of infection presumptively or proven to be due to organisms resistant to the preferential antimicrobials. More stringent restrictions may at times be advisable if the flora in the intensive care unit has become extremely resistant.[10]

METHODS OF "SPARING" ANTIMICROBIALS

1. Use the least number of agents in a patient's regimen as possible. However, synergistic combinations may occasionally be necessary to treat certain serious infections.
2. Attempt to make an etiologic diagnosis of infection and use the narrowest spectrum antimicrobial regimen which is available for the infecting agent.
3. Use full doses of antimicrobials, and do not taper dosage before discontinuing. Insufficient dosage levels encourage development of resistance by bacteria.
4. Avoid prophylactic use of antimicrobials in situations in which prophylaxis has been shown not to be efficacious. An attempt should be made to use defined protocols of prophylaxis.
5. Discontinue antimicrobials when their clear indication (prophylactic or therapeutic) has terminated. Do not attempt to prolong therapy to increase effect; the longer an antimicrobial is administered, the more likely resistant organisms will be selected and the greater the suppression of normal organisms which act as a host defense mechanism.

EPIDEMIOLOGIC DATA NEEDED FOR PLANNING
INDIVIDUAL PATIENT THERAPY

1. Is this a new admission without recent hospitalization (may be presumed to be carrying community flora)?
2. Are there recent cultures available of a normal flora-bearing site which often is the source of bacteria causing this infection (e.g., a tracheal culture before onset of a new pneumonia)?
3. What organisms are colonizing other patients in the intensive care unit and what are their antimicrobial susceptibility patterns?
4. Is this a new infection in a patient currently receiving an antimicrobial regimen (increased possibility of resistance to the agents being administered)?

GENERAL TYPES OF INFECTION

A large proportion of the infections observed in an intensive care unit are not primary infections due to organisms from outside the body (exogenous infection) but are due to the extension of infectious agents from sites of the body where they colonize but do not cause disease (endogenous infection). Endogenous infection can be classified by the source body site. These sources are the normal flora-bearing areas of the body: the skin, the intestinal tract, the mouth and pharynx, and the distal female genital tract. Urinary tract infections represent a special case of endogenous infection due to intestinal tract organisms. The normal flora-bearing areas can be and frequently are colonized by new organisms originating in the environment of the patient; these organisms can then go on to cause endogenous infection. These cases thus represent endogenous infection by originally exogenous organisms.[4] Thus, knowledge of the colonizing organisms in normal flora-bearing areas can be of value in planning therapy of infections due to organisms arising from these areas. Likewise, therapy of exogenous infections can be aided by any information available as to the organisms present in outside sources of infecting agents.

ENDOGENOUS INFECTION

Skin Flora   The normal flora of the skin consists of *Staphylococcus epidermidis, Bacillus* spp., and diphteroids (mainly anaerobic).[11] *Staphylococcus aureus* is not universally present but is a frequent colonizer.[12] These organisms are generally susceptible to penicillinase-resistant semisynthetic penicillins or cephalosporins (but see pp. 60–61). Colonization with aerobic gram-negative bacilli (*E. coli, Klebsiella, Proteus,* etc.) occurs occasionally, mainly from fecal or urine contact. It should be noted that many yeasts are found on the skin, but *Candida albicans* is not part of the normal skin flora.[11,13]

Organisms of the true normal skin flora seldom cause disease. When they do, frequently a foreign body is involved. In some cases severe or life-threatening infection has occurred.[14] Thus, *S. epidermidis* is a characteristic cause of infection of shunts used to relieve hydrocephalus.[14,15] Infection of access sites used for hemodialysis is occasionally due to *S. epidermidis* or to *Bacillus* sp.[16,17] Surgical wound infections yielding pure cultures of *S. epidermidis* occur, and this probably represents true invasive infection in some of these cases.[18]

The most frequent sites of colonization by *S. aureus* are the anterior nares, the perineum, and the axillae in that order. In most surveys, around 10 to 40 percent of normal people have been shown to carry *S. aureus.*[12] In newborns, the umbilical stump is a frequent site of colonization.[11] The mere presence of *S. aureus* in a normal skin site culture does not necessarily represent a risk of endogenous infection due to *S. aureus* or a risk of transmitting *S. aureus* to other people, since strains vary greatly in invasiveness. Presence of a lesion resulting from staphylococcal invasion, such as a furuncle, paronychia, etc., is a clue that suggests skin colonization with an invasive strain.

Endogenous infections from skin flora in an intensive care unit are mainly surgical or traumatic wound infections and infections related to the use of invasive monitoring lines and catheters. Attention must be paid to all possible breaks in the skin which could carry skin flora into the tissues or the circulation, including such easy to miss portals of entry as intramuscular injection sites or minor traumatic wounds.

Surgical Wound Infection   Surgical wound infections are predominantly endogenous. They are frequently related to organisms contaminating the wound at the time of operation. Postoperative contamination is also of some importance, particularly in the first two days, before the wound edges have sealed.[19,20] Organisms present in the structures which are actually incised at operation would be expected to predominate as the causes of postoperative infection. Thus, in procedures which involve incision of skin but no other contaminated tissues, *S. aureus* is the predominant pathogen. If a foreign body is left in place, the possibility of infection due to *S. epidermidis, Bacillus* sp., or diptheroids is increased. If the procedure also involves incision of bowel, bowel flora become more likely as causative agents in wound infection (see pp. 64–69). If the patient has an active infection at a site remote from the incision at the time of operation, the organism (or organisms) causing the remote infection becomes more likely as a cause of wound infection.

The above considerations have some predictive value in planning antimicrobial therapy should a wound infection occur. However, the best immediately available means of directing antimicrobial therapy is the microscopic examination of Gram-stained material from the infected site. This gives semiquantitative data as to the type and number of organisms, which can be correlated with the above considerations and with the later culture results.

Catheter-Related Infection   This can be due to skin flora (endogenous) or to organisms contaminating the parenteral fluid or the fluid line (exogenous). The subject is discussed in more detail on pages 78–79.

Oxacillin-Resistant Staphylococcus aureus   Strains of *S. aureus* resistant to methicillin, oxacillin, the other penicillinase-resistant semisynthetic panicillins, and also generally to cephalosporins, long widespread in Europe,[21] are now becoming more common in the United States. The European experience was that these strains tended to be hospital-associated, with few isolates appearing directly from the community outside the hospital; they tended to appear and remain concentrated in specific hospitals, not affecting others in the same community. The limited experience in the United States has been similar, with good documentation of patient-to-patient spread in the hospital.[22,23] Thus, infections due to these organisms are generally exogenous, although many probably result from prior colonization at a normal flora-bearing site by the oxacillin-resistant strain of *S. aureus,* followed by development of disease at another site, as is the usual case with staphylococcal infections. Disease due to these organisms has been similar to disease due to oxacillin-susceptible *S. aureus,* with serious and life-threatening infections being possible.

Laboratory detection of resistance to the penicillinase-resistant semisynthetic penicillins and the cephalosporins is difficult, and laboratory reports can be misleading.[21,24] These strains appear to be resistant to all penicillins and cephalosporins. Although disc susceptibility testing may indicate susceptibility to one or more of these agents, tube-dilution susceptibility testing usually reveals resistance, and clinical response to administration of the agent often has been poor. This false susceptibility result is most common with the cephalosporins. Thus, if a strain is shown by disc susceptibility testing to be resistant to oxacillin (or methicillin) and susceptible to cephalosporins, the cephalosporins should not be used unless tube dilution studies confirm the susceptibility. The false susceptibility result is seen less with the oxacillin disc than the others, so this disc is best for screening for this type of resistance (hence the terminology "oxacillin-resistant *S. aureus*"; these strains are often called "methicillin-resistant *S. aureus*" in the literature). Some other technical factors in the microbiology laboratory, such as incubating at 35 C instead of 37 C, will minimize the false susceptibility readings.[24]

For treatment of severe or life-threatening infections due to oxacillin-resistant *S. aureus,* the only reliable agent available is vancomycin. For less severe infections, bacteriostatic agents such as erythromycin, clindamycin, tetracyclines, or chloramphenicol may be used according to the susceptibility pattern of the individual strain. In general, treatment of staphylococcal infection with aminoglycosides has been disappointing in spite of the disc susceptibilities.

If a patient is colonized or infected with oxacillin-resistant *S. aureus,* care must be taken to prevent spread to other patients. This is particularly difficult in an intensive care unit. Transmission by hands of personnel and by objects passed patient-to-patient is of main importance. Some hospitals have used strict isolation procedures for containment of oxacillin-resistant *S. aureus,*[23] while others have used the equivalent of wound and skin precautions with approximately equivalent success.[22,25]

***Oxacillin-Resistant* Staphylococcus epidermidis** Resistance to the penicillinase-resistant semisynthetic penicillins and to the cephalosporins among strains of *S. epidermidis* has been widespread longer than similar resistance of *S. aureus.* Various surveys show approximately 10 percent of isolates of *S. epidermidis* to have this resistance pattern.[26] The problem of false susceptibility reports from disc susceptibility testing appears to occur with *S. epidermidis* as it does with *S. aureus.*[27]

Oral and Pharyngeal Flora This consists almost exclusively of anaerobic bacteria, with a notable lack of *Bacteroides fragilis.* In ill patients nonspecifically, and in hospitalized patients, gram-negative aerobes such as *E. coli* or *Klebsiella* colonize the oropharyngeal area.[3,7,8,28] Two other important aerobes, *Streptococcus pneumoniae* and *Hemophilus influenzae,* sometimes colonize the pharynx. These frequently appear as major pathogens in infections of areas directly related to the pharynx, such as the middle ear, as well as common causes of pneumonia.

Penicillin is the drug of choice for infections due to the normal, mainly anaerobic, mouth and pharyngeal flora. Clindamycin is also adequate. Cephalosporins are somewhat less useful for this purpose.[29]

Infections from the pharyngeal flora occur by direct extension from the upper airways, e.g., dental abscesses, cervical lymphadenitis, retropharyngeal abscess.[29] In the intubated patient, purulent parotitis may be seen. A special case of oropharyngeal organism infection is human bite.[30]

Pneumonia Infection in the lung occurs either by hematogenous access of organisms or by direct access via the airway. The latter is by far the most common route.[31] Most pneumonias are caused by aspiration of oropharyngeal contents, with the bacteriology of the eventual infection in the lung being a function of the size of the inoculum of organisms—and, hence, the size of the aspiration, the virulence of the organisms in it, and the host's intrapulmonary defenses. A relatively small aspiration, or direct inhalation, of *Streptococcus pneumoniae* or of a virulent strain of *Klebsiella pneumoniae* will result in a pneumonia. To produce a mixed anaerobic pneumonia due to relatively avirulent components of the mouth flora, a large aspiration is necessary.[32]

In an intensive care unit, the risk of a hospital-acquired pneumonia is aggravated by several factors: (1) the mechanical cleaning functions of the lung and bronchi, such as ciliary function and cough, are often compromised, making aspiration of mouth contents more likely; (2) the oropharyngeal flora is changed with emergence of gram-negative aerobes, as mentioned above; (3) the frequent necessity of intubation or tracheostomy further compromises the mechanical cleaning mechanisms; and (4) finally, a new risk appears, that of direct passage of an aerosol of microorganisms from respiratory therapy equipment into the lungs. This last risk has recently been recognized, and when measures are taken against it, the risk can be minimized.[33,34] Sudden onset of widespread (multilobar) pneumonia, frequently with cavitation, in a patient on ventilatory support, should raise the question of aerosolization of organisms contaminating the respiratory therapy equipment.

The precise etiologic diagnosis of pneumonia is difficult,[35] particularly in a patient with previously abnormal lungs.[36] There are two steps to this diagnosis: the establishment that there is inflammation in the lung, and the establishment of the cause of the inflammation. To establish the presence of inflammation, a new infiltrate should be seen radiographically and purulent sputum should be present. The latter may be lacking in a granulocytopenic patient.[37] Fever is usually seen except in very ill patients who are hypothermic or unable to mount a febrile response. Without inflammation in the lung, the need for antibiotic therapy directed at bacteria found in sputum is questionable. With inflammation present, an attempt should be made to establish the identity of the infecting agent. Blood cultures should be taken and if pleural fluid is present, it should be examined microscopically after Gram staining, and it should be cultured. In all cases, an attempt should be made to obtain a specimen of sputum as nearly representative as possible of the sputum emerging from the area of inflammation. The microscopic examination of the Gram-stained specimen of this sputum and its culture are of crucial importance in obtaining an etiologic diagnosis. In the non-intubated patient, a cough sputum specimen may be adequate, but cough specimens are frequently nondiagnostic. A diagnostic sputum specimen is one in which, when Gram stained and examined microscopically, there are areas of abundant polymorphonuclear neutrophils without squamous epithelial cells.[31] The presence of only one type of bacteria in such areas of the sputum smear enhances the diagnostic likelihood, although in a mixed anaerobic pneumonia many morphologic types of organisms will be seen. If a cough specimen is not adequate in a nonintubated, seriously ill patient, consideration should be given to transtracheal aspiration of sputum,[31] even if intubation is planned. In the intubated patient, sputum should be aspirated from as deep as possible; however, the diagnostic value of sputum in the intubated patient is never as good as in the nonintubated patient, since the oropharynx and trachea are essentially in continuity, and the tracheal flora will generally reflect the oropharyngeal flora. Again, in sputum from an intubated patient, the presence of a single morphologic type of organism on microscopic examination of a Gram-stained smear increases the diagnostic implications of the specimen.

Therapy of pneumonia in the intensive care unit should be directed at the infecting organism or organisms as precisely as possible using all the information at hand, including the clinical picture, sputum microscopic examination, and any epidemiologic information available, such as previous colonizing organisms in the pharynx and organisms present elsewhere in the unit. Sputum culture results may later modify the therapeutic regimen; the chronologic progression of the pulmonary infiltrate may modify the diagnosis, even eliminating the diagnosis of pneumonia in spite of sputum culture results. Bactericidal antibiotics (penicillins or cephalosporins) are preferred unless bacterial resistance is shown or presumed, or unless these drugs are excluded by a history of severe patient allergy. Chloramphenicol shows good activity in lung and may be useful for certain organisms resistant to the bactericidal antibiotics; but *Pseudomonas aeruginosa* is generally resistant, and other gram-negative aerobes in an intensive care unit may be resistant. Carbenicillin or ticarcillin are also useful in lung infection, but probably should not be used alone due to the rapid development of bacterial resistance. The aminoglycosides often show poor results when given alone, even though they appear in bronchial secretions; the poor results may be related to inactivation of these drugs by components of pus.[38] Amino-glycosides are most often used in conjunction with carbenicillin or ticar-cillin, although they may need to be used alone if they are the only agents available for the infecting organism. For mixed anaerobic pneu-monia, penicillin is generally adequate, even if *Bacteroides fragilis* is present. Alternatives are clindamycin or chloramphenicol.[39]

Bowel Flora   The stomach in normal people is sterile.[40] The normal small bowel has a relatively sparse bacterial population, with both aerobes and anaerobes present in approximately equal numbers.[41] The large bowel is the principal reservoir of organisms, with increased coloniza-tion of the upper tract occurring in the presence of local dysfunction[42] or lower general host resistance. Anaerobes predominate in the large bowel contents of normal individuals, with multiple species including *Clostridium* spp. and *Bacteroides fragilis.* Anaerobic gram-negative ba-cilli present in smaller numbers include *Escherichia coli, Klebsiella,* and *Proteus* spp. Enterococcus represents an important member of the bowel flora. *Candida albicans* also occurs as normal bowel flora.[43] *Staphylococcus* sp. occurs in stool of 20 to 40 percent of people.[12] Organ-isms infecting the biliary tract appear to parallel the organisms found in the lower bowel, although anaerobes are less common.[44]

Infections due to bowel flora are usually secondary to trauma or direct extension from the bowel (e.g., appendicitis, perirectal abscess, diverticulitis). The importance of surgical management of these infec-tions must be stressed.[45,46] Gram-stained smears and cultures of infected material should be obtained at the time of operation to direct postopera-tive antimicrobial therapy. The Gram stain is of particular importance since results are immediate[44] and are more quantitative than culture results.

It has always been difficult to devise an antimicrobial regimen active against all the organisms that comprise the normal bowel flora. Animal studies suggest that the anaerobic component of the bowel flora is mainly responsible for abscess formation, whereas the aerobic gram-negative bacilli are responsible for bacteremias and early death.[39] There are few controlled clinical studies comparing regimens for presumptive therapy of infection due to bowel flora. One would reasonably use an agent active against the gram-negative aerobes (usually gentamicin) as well as an-aerobes (penicillin, clindamycin, or chloramphenicol). Often a triple regimen of penicillin, clindamycin, and an aminoglycoside is used to provide activity against enterococci (penicillin plus aminoglycoside) and *B. fragilis* (frequently resistant to penicillin).

Fever after Abdominal Surgery   This represents a common and frequently perplexing problem in an intensive care unit.[47] The source of fever may remain obscure, forcing a decision as to treatment for presumed infection.

Initial diagnostic procedures should include a physical examination, chest X-ray, white blood cell count, urinalysis, and cultures of blood and urine. Sputum cultures are not generally useful unless a pulmonary infiltrate is present. Special attention in the examination must be given to the wound, the abdomen in general, the possibility of venous thrombosis in the lower extremities, and to any invasive monitoring lines or parenteral fluid lines. These procedures, following the old mnemonic of "wind, water, walkers, and wound," will reveal the source of most temperature elevations. The possibility of drug fever must also always be kept in mind, with consideration of the possibility of discontinuing specific agents. Any indwelling foreign body, whether surgically placed or present for monitoring purposes, should be under suspicion as a focus of infection.

For the fever not clarified by initial studies, the possibility of an intra-abdominal site of infection (i.e., abscess or phlegmon) and empirical antimicrobial therapy must be considered. Empirical antimicrobial therapy should be individualized as much as possible, considering: (1) the normal flora of the structures involved in the surgical procedure; (2) the possible alterations of this flora by colonization by new organisms in the intensive care unit environment; and (3) the effect of previous administration of antimicrobials. In general, therapy directed against bowel flora, as outlined in the previous section, will be warranted. However, antimicrobial therapy cannot be used as a diagnostic test.

If empirical antimicrobial therapy is begun, it must be coupled with diagnostic efforts aimed at finding the presumed site of infection. The flat and upright abdominal roentgenograms remain an important simple study. The gallium-67 radionuclide scan has become widely used as a means of detecting infected foci.[48] However, secretion of gallium-67 into the colonic contents results in difficulties of interpretation of the scans and may necessitate bowel cleansing.[49] Also, false negatives occur.[50] Ultrasound scanning of the abdomen is a promising noninvasive technique which is now widely available,[51,52] and which can be used to guide needle aspirations[53] (Figs. 2-1 and 2-2).

Crepitant Infections A number of organisms can cause infections resulting in tissue emphysema.[39,54] *Clostridium* sp. is the classic cause of such infections; however, many other aerobes and facultative organisms, such as enteric gram-negative bacilli, can also produce gas in tissue. Essentially any bacterium growing anaerobically can produce gas which is sufficiently insoluble to become clinically or radiographically evident in tissue. Most of these infections are related to bowel flora or to exogenous contamination of trauma sites with soil or fecal organisms. Illicit drug injection is associated with some cases. Frequently, diabetes mellitus is often a contributing factor.

In the differential diagnosis of tissue emphysema, noninfective causes must be considered.[54] In an intensive care unit, tissue emphysema due to positive pressure ventilatory assistance is common. Other causes are introduction of air into tissue during surgical manipulation and perforation of a viscus, particularly the esophagus. If gas in tissue is bacteriologically produced, one expects signs of inflammation, locally

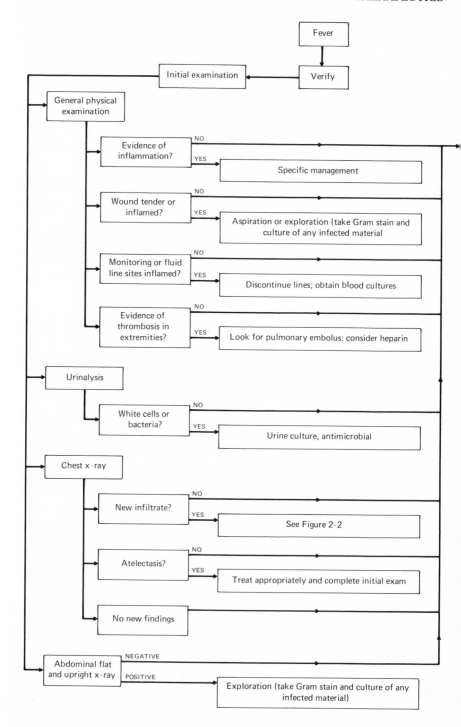

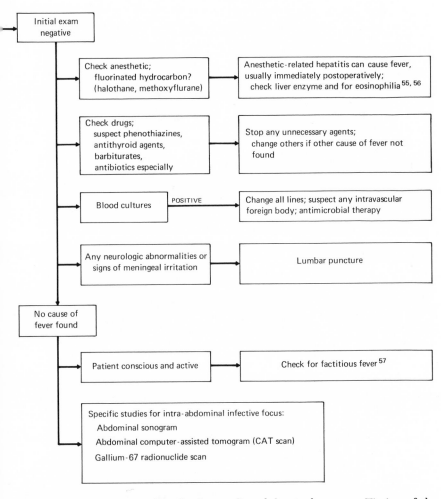

Fig. 2-1. Diagnostic outline for fever after abdominal surgery. Timing of the onset of fever is of help in diagnosis.[47] New fever appearing two or more weeks postoperatively may result from transfusion-related infections.[58,59] In some cases, fever resolves without diagnosis or intervention.

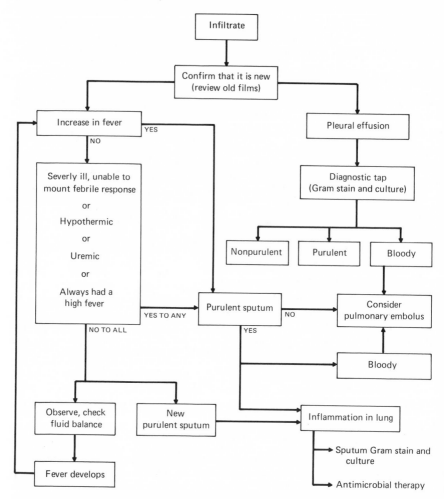

Fig. 2-2. Diagnostic outline for new pulmonary infiltrate. A new pulmonary infiltrate that lasts for only 24 to 48 hours is not pneumonia; consider fluid overload, pulmonary embolus, or noninfected aspiration. In obscure cases, an acute increase in right-to-left shunt (as reflected by decreased arterial oxygenation) may suggest a new infiltrate.

(erythema, tenderness, edema, occasionally formation of bullae) or systemically (fever, mental status changes, "toxicity"). Classically, these infections are divided into two groups: anaerobic myonecrosis (gas gangrene), in which muscle necrosis occurs, and anaerobic cellulitis, in which infection, is confined to skin and subcutaneous tissue.[39,60]

In crepitant infections, as in others, an attempt at a rapid etiologic diagnosis should be made. Aspiration of material from the infected area must be performed promptly, using a syringe with excluded air. Immediate Gram stain of the material is of paramount importance. For culture, the material should be placed in an anaerobic transport tube, or sent to the laboratory in the original syringe with air expelled and a cap placed, as is done with specimens for blood gas determinations.

Surgery remains the mainstay of treatment, with prompt and total debridement of the infected area leaving only healthy tissue. This applies to both anaerobic cellulitis and anaerobic myonecrosis.[59,60] In the case of anaerobic myonecrosis, the use of a hyperbaric chamber can be considered after surgery.[61,62] Clostridial antitoxin is not considered effective alone.[60]

Antimicrobial therapy should be directed by the result of a Gram stain of aspirated material or of a direct touch imprint of infected material on a slide. In almost all cases, high-dose intravenous penicillin is indicated. This is the drug of choice for gram-positive rods (suspect *Clostridium* sp.) or gram-positive cocci (suspect *Peptostreptococcus* sp.). If gram-negative rods are seen (suspect *Bacteroides* sp. or enteric facultative organisms), chloramphenicol or the combination of clindamycin and an aminoglycoside may be added. The dangerously penicillin-allergic patient should probably receive a cephalosporin or chloramphenicol. With cephalosporins, there is a risk of allergic cross-reactivity with penicillin, and cephalosporins are frequently not as active against anaerobic organisms as penicillin.

Necrotizing fasciitis (Fournier's disease) is a rapidly progressive infection which selectively involves fascia.[39] It is typically seen in diabetics and is frequently associated with perirectal abscess, female genital tract infection, trauma, or surgery. Organisms involved are generally streptococci, usually anaerobic (*Peptostreptococcus* sp.). *Staphylococcus aureus* is sometimes cultured. Fever, local pain, spreading erythema, and clinically necrotic fascial layers, often with separation of overlying skin and subcutaneous tissue, are seen. Although the local lesion is similar to that of anaerobic myonecrosis (gas gangrene), tissue emphysema is not seen.

Treatment of necrotizing fasciitis is surgical. Wide debridement is necessary, with resection up to healthy tissue at the limit of the infection. Repeated debridement is often necessary. Antimicrobial drug management should include penicillin in high dosage intravenously (Table 2-1).

Infection Due to *Candida albicans* and Allied Yeasts   A number of yeasts which form part of the normal flora can act as pathogens in an intensive care unit setting. The most common and the most virulent of these is *Candida albicans*. Others that are seen are *C. tropicalis, C. parapsilosis,* other *Candida* spp., and *Torulopsis glabrata.*[63] Most of these fungi exist in two phases: a yeast phase consisting of unicellular ovoid organisms which reproduce by budding, and a mycelial phase consisting of "pseudohyphae," which are branching chains of elongated cells. *C. albicans*

TABLE 2-1

Rapidly Spreading Anerobic Infections

Entity	Physical Signs	Gram Stain	Cause	Initial Antimicrobial
Anaerobic cellulitis	Local inflammation	Gram-positive rods	*Clostridium*	Penicillin
	Tissue gas Fever usual	Gram-positive cocci	*Peptostreptococcus*	Penicillin
	Minimal toxicity	Gram-negative rods	*Bacteroides* enteric bacilli	Penicillin plus clindamycin plus aminoglycoside*
Anaerobic myonecrosis	Local inflammation, local edema and skin necrosis, tissue gas, severe toxicity, delirium	Same as anaerobic cellulitis		
Necrotizing fasciitis	Local inflammation, separation of fascial planes, no tissue gas	Gram-positive cocci	*Peptostreptococcus*†	Penicillin

Caveats: All these infections must be treated by prompt and extensive surgical debridement back to healthy tissue; antimicrobial drug therapy alone has no effect. Antimicrobial drug therapy must be based initially on Gram stain results and modified later according to culture results. Close control of the diabetes mellitus which frequently underlies these infections aids in therapy.

* Chloramphenicol may replace clindamycin plus aminoglycoside.

† Other bowel flora or *Staphylococcus* sometimes present requiring additional antimicrobials.

and some other species can also produce true septate hyphae with terminal chlamydospores.[64] The ability to form hyphae or pseudohyphae in tissue, seen in *C. albicans* and *C. tropicalis,* may be a virulence factor in yeasts.[63]

Candida spp. and allied yeasts are strict aerobes. They grow rapidly on standard bacteriologic media, so that a laboratory can usually report the presence of "yeast" in a specimen within 48 to 72 hours. Identification of the specific species takes longer. The production, under certain conditions, of "germ tubes" (i.e., tubular structures projecting from the yeast cells which grow to hyphae) is one means of rapidly differentiating *C. albicans* or *C. stellatoidea* from the others.[64]

Candida albicans is a common yeast component of the enteric normal flora of man, occurring in 20 to 40 percent of individuals without evidence of disease.[43,64] It is also found in the mouth and vagina. *C. albicans* does not appear to colonize intact dry skin, but many other yeasts do.[11] A number of factors appear to encourage growth of yeasts, including increased glucose (as in uncontrolled diabetes mellitus), steroid therapy (perhaps again by increasing glucose), and antimicrobial therapy, particularly with the broader spectrum agents. With an increase of the yeast population, colonization of new areas (skin, urine) occurs as well as overgrowth in normally colonized areas, all of which can eventually lead to tissue invasion.[65] Thus, most yeast infections are endogenous and are preceded by overgrowth in normally colonized areas. The progress of gastrointestinal overgrowth leading to spread to new mucous membrane or cutaneous areas,[13] and then to invasion, can frequently be observed in intensive care unit patients. *C. albicans* appears in the mouth as white patches surrounded by erythema (thrush) and as perianal and perineal red elevated areas with sharply demarcated margins and satellite lesions (cutaneous candidiasis). Further skin extension to other intertriginous areas, such as the axillae, under the breasts, or sometimes the back of a chronically supine patient, occurs. In cutaneous candidiasis, the whitish appearance seen in mucous membrane candidiasis, which gives the organism its name, will also frequently be seen in moist intertriginous areas. Candidal vaginitis has a physical appearance similar to thrush. Extension into the urinary tract will manifest itself as urine cultures which yield yeast and yeast cells seen on urinalysis.

Invasion can occur at any site with a heavy superficial growth of yeast. Local trauma, ulceration, or impaired systemic host defenses probably contribute.[63,65,66] Most common sites of invasion are the esophagus and the urinary tract. Candidal pyelonephritis occurs with occasional formation of mycelial masses (fungus balls) in the renal pelvis. *C. albicans* pneumonia[67] occurs, probably through aspiration of yeast from the oropharynx.

Invasion of the circulation from a site of local invasive yeast infection leads to fungemia and possibly metastatic yeast infections. This occurs most commonly as pyelonephritis, but also as meningitis, mycotic aneurysm, or endocarditis.[65,66,68]

Yeast infections are occasionally exogenous, related to a contaminated parenteral solution, particularly parenteral hyperalimentation fluid.[69,70]

The frequent occurrence of yeasts as normal flora and the frequent noninvasive overgrowth seen in hospitalized patients lead to severe difficulties in interpretation of yeasts isolated in culture.[65,66,71] In general, growth of yeast in a culture taken from a site where the yeast occurs as normal flora is not meaningful. Visible lesions at a site where the yeast occurs as normal flora (e.g., *C. albicans* in the mouth or vagina or a positive culture in urine or sputum) have about the same meaning—

that of overgrowth, but not necessarily invasion. A commonly used rule of thumb is that the presence of budding yeast and hyphal elements, visualized on Gram stain, potassium hydroxide preparation, or other direct smear or tissue section, correlates with invasion. This has been demonstrated in oral thrush and in intestinal lesions.[66,71] It may be also true with sputum and catheterized urine specimens.

Culture of yeast from a normally sterile area, with the exception of urine, must be taken to mean invasion. However, presence of yeast in a blood culture presents a diagnostic problem, particularly if a parenteral line is in place. A transient fungemia may not require specific antimicrobial treatment if the offending line is promptly discontinued.[72] Small inocula of C. albicans can be overcome by phagocytosis and by fungistatic mechanisms in blood.[65,66] Persistent positive blood cultures for yeast, particularly when accompanied by deterioration in the patient's condition or evidence of invasive yeast infection in a local area, must be treated.

Treatment of noninvasive yeast overgrowth is directed at reduction of the total yeast population at visible sites of growth and also in the intestinal reservoir.[66] An important consideration is the attempt to eliminate as many growth-promoting factors as possible by (1) control of diabetes; (2) reduction or discontinuation of antibiotics, corticosteroids, and cancer chemotherapeutic agents; and (3) discontinuation or change of invasive lines or catheters. Nystatin (Mycostatin) should be applied topically to affected areas four times a day and should also be given orally, 400,000 to 600,000 units four times a day to minimize the gastrointestinal reservoir. An advantage of nystatin is its narrow antifungal spectrum and the lack of resistance developed by yeast species. If a nasogastric tube, orogastric tube, or a gastrostomy is in place, the nystatin oral solution can be instilled in the tube; but some of the dosage may be given directly into the mouth in order to come into contact with the oral mucosa and the esophagus. For yeast in the urine, the elimination of an indwelling catheter will usually suffice. When the catheter cannot be removed, bladder irrigation with a triple-lumen catheter, using nystatin or amphotericin B, has been used as local treatment (although this is not an approved use of these drugs in the United States). In cases of yeast overgrowth in urine, oral nystatin should be given as well.

For treatment of invasive or disseminated yeast infections, systemic amphotericin B therapy is recommended. An oral agent, flucytosine (Ancobon), is also available as an adjunct to amphotericin B in some cases. For a discussion of the use of amphotericin B, see pages 124–28.

Another yeast, Cryptococcus neoformans, is a cause of pulmonary and of disseminated disease, particularly meningitis. These infections are exogenous and generally community-acquired; while they are beyond the scope of this discussion, they are discussed elsewhere.[73,74]

Urinary Tract Infection   These are usually endogenous infections caused by aerobic organisms from the colonic reservoir.[75] Anaerobes are rarely implicated in urinary tract infection.[76] Probably the infecting organism first colonizes the perineal and introital areas, and then gains access to the bladder urine.[77,78] The resulting infection is nearly always due to a single strain of bacteria (pure culture) except in severely abnormal urinary tracts with frequent direct external contamination. The likelihood of a given species and antimicrobial resistance pattern roughly parallels the relative abundance of that species and antimicrobial resistance pattern among the aerobic bacteria in the colonic reservoir. Thus, the great majority of uncomplicated, community-acquired urinary tract infection is caused by *E. coli* susceptible to a broad range of antimicrobials. Any urologic abnormality causing obstruction or stasis of urine is associated with an increased incidence of infection and an increasing degree of antimicrobial resistance in the infecting organisms.[79,80] One factor contributing to this trend is the frequent use of antimicrobials in patients with such abnormalities. Such patients may bring resistant organisms into the intensive care unit with them. Also, it is probably true that a new urinary tract infection acquired in an intensive care unit is more likely to be due to antimicrobial-resistant organisms because of prior colonization of the colon by these organisms originating in the environment of the unit, particularly from other patients.

Another complicating factor in urinary tract infection is the frequent necessity for an indwelling bladder catheter.[81] Although the use of closed system drainage has decreased the incidence of infections in catheterized patients, one still can expect about a 5 to 10 percent increase in the incidence of infection for each day of catheterization. Some infections of the urinary tract associated with catheters are terminated by merely removing the catheter. Thus, the indications for catheter placement should be reviewed carefully on an individual basis with consideration of alternate methods of achieving the same end, such as the use of a condom catheter or diapers for incontinence, voluntary voiding for monitoring of urine output, or intermittent in-and-out catheterization for urine stasis.[82,83]

Urinary tract infection is one of the classical predisposing factors for acute bacteremia leading to the syndrome of septic shock (pp. 79–81). Bacteremia in urinary tract infection is usually associated with a physical abnormality of the urinary tract, frequently with obstruction of urine. A urethral catheter is often associated with the condition. Also, bacteremia occurs with instrumentation of an infected urinary tract (see p. 84).

The method of treating a urinary tract infection in an intensive care unit depends on the severity of the infection and on the antimicrobial susceptibilities of the infecting organism. The most severe infections, those which can be presumed to have escaped the urinary tract, need to be treated with an antimicrobial regimen which produces serum levels of an antimicrobial adequate to inhibit the infecting organism. Infections with marked fever, suggestive of bacteremia or abscess formation, fall into this category. In these infections, the "urinary tract antiseptics"—nitrofurantoin, nalidixic acid, or methenamine—are inadequate.

If possible, a bactericidal antibiotic should be used, preferably a penicillin, cephalosporin, or, if required by bacterial resistance, an aminoglycoside.

URINARY ANTISEPTICS*

Agent	Advantages	Disadvantages
Nitrofurantoin (Furadantin, Macrodantin)	Bacterial resistance development unlikely	Inactive against many bacteria found in intensive care units; neuropathy with high dose or any renal failure
Methenamine (Mandelamine, Hiprex)	Extremely broad spectrum (active principle is formaldehyde)	Urine pH must be kept below 5.5 for effect; poor results in eradicating established infection
Naladixic acid (NegGram)	Active against many strains resistant to other agents	Rapid in vivo development of resistance

* These are antimicrobial agents which are given systemically, but which achieve adequate concentrations to be effective in the urine only. Disc susceptibility testing screens for susceptibility to concentrations achieved in urine only.

Infections confined to the urinary tract can be treated with antimicrobial regimens which give urine levels adequate to inhibit the infecting organism.[84,85] This applies whether infection involves the lower tract only or both lower and upper tract as long as the infection is confined to the urinary tract. The choice of antimicrobial to use while urine culture is pending should be dictated by the potential organisms in the colonic reservoir. In uncomplicated, community-acquired infection, a sulfonamide (e.g., sulfisoxazole [Gantrisin], sulfamethoxyzole [Gantanol], or ampicillin is usually adequate. Other agents, including aminoglycosides or the combination of trimethoprim and sulfamethoxyzole (Bactrim or Septra) should be reserved for patients with infections that include potentially resistant organisms.

A third group of urinary tract infections includes those which are related to an indwelling catheter in the bladder or an abnormality of the lower urinary tract and which are asymptomatic. These infections can frequently be treated by removal of the catheter or correction of the underlying anatomical or functional abnormality. If this is impossible, suppression of infection by irrigation of the bladder with an antimicrobial solution using a triple-lumen catheter is a possible alternative.[86] Approximately 1 liter per day of fluid is used, irrigating at a continuous rate. This method is compatible with strict input-and-output measurement but makes urinary electrolyte and other chemical determinations uninterpretable. Many of this third group of infections may not require specific treatment. If such an infection is persistent after a treatment course with a relatively nontoxic antimicrobial, or if the organism is resistant, it may be better to leave the infection untreated.

BLADDER IRRIGATION AGENTS

Agent	Uses	Disadvantages
Neomycin-poly-myxin (Neosporin GU Irrigant)[75,86]	Treatment of uncomplicated bladder infections due to susceptible organisms; prophylaxis of infection when frequent catheter opening is necessary (e.g., post transurethral surgery)	The agent is selective; some bacterial strains are resistant or partially resistant and may be selected out
Povidone-iodine (Betadine, Pharmadine, others)	Prophylaxis of infection if frequent catheterization is necessary	Possible systemic iodine absorption; not approved for this use by Food and Drug Administration —safety and efficacy studies are lacking
Acetic acid 0.25% in normal saline[75]	Prophylaxis of infection when frequent catheter opening is necessary; intermittent suppression of infection in long-term catheter patients	Mainly of use for *Pseudomonas;* less effective against other gram-negatives
Amphotericin B, 5.0 mg/liter in sterile water[75]	Treatment of candidiasis of the bladder	Care must be taken to avoid missing diagnosis of candidal pyelonephritis; not approved for this use by Food and Drug Administration

Female Genital Tract Flora The vagina and introitus contain a complex and varying microbial flora, consisting predominantly of anaerobes.[87-89] This flora varies with age, menstrual cycle, sexual practices, antimicrobial drug administration, and other factors. The most important of the normal vaginal flora is *Lactobacillus* sp. (Doderlein's bacillus), which is rarely associated with invasive infection and may act to suppress growth of other, potentially more pathogenic bacteria. Other anaerobes which occur in the lower female genital tract are those which occur in the colonic flora, including *Clostridium* spp., *Bacteroides fragilis,* and anaerobic streptococci. Colonizing aerobic flora are primarily skin organisms and group B beta-hemolytic streptococci. This latter organism seldom causes important infection in an adult, but is an important cause of generalized sepsis or meningitis in neonates.[90] Anaerobic enteric bacilli and yeasts also occasionally colonize the vagina. Bacteria colonization normally stops at the cervix; the uterine cavity is therefore normally sterile.

Organisms from the female genital tract flora which cause invasive infection thus are similar to those from the intestinal flora, i.e., mostly anaerobes, including *Clostridium* spp. and penicillin-resistant *Bacteroides fragilis.* Anaerobic enteric bacilli such as *Escherichia coli* also must be considered.

Acute infections associated with genital tract trauma, manipulation, or parturition (obstetric infections) range from minor endometritis to fulminant uterine clostridial myonecrosis.[29,39] Because these infections can be rapidly progressive, immediate institution of therapy is important. Prompt surgical removal of necrotic tissue is mandatory. Although it should be done in any case, the Gram stain of vaginal secretions is usually of limited usefulness except in the unusual case of a pure culture infection due to a gram-positive coccus (e.g., *Staphylococcus aureus*). Cultures are of great importance and should be taken of vaginal secretions, if possible, using anaerobic technique (see p. 68); blood cultures should also be taken.

Initial antimicrobial drug therapy should be similar to that used for initial treatment of infection due to bowel flora, with special attention to *Clostridium* sp. Thus, a three-drug regimen of penicillin in high dosage (for most anaerobes, including *Clostridium* sp.), an aminoglycoside (for aerobic enteric bacilli), and clindamycin (for *Bacteroides fragilis*) is often used.

Chronic gynecologic infection (pelvic inflammatory disease) can have acute complications necessitating the intensive care unit setting. Although pyosalpinx, tubo-ovarian abscesses, and parametritis are often primarily caused by gonorrhea, the infections encountered in the intensive care unit usually involve secondary invasion by anaerobic organisms and aerobic enteric bacilli.[39,87] Cervical Gram stains and cultures are of limited use, except to exclude *Neisseria gonorrheae.* Culdocentesis, with anaerobic culture of aspirated material, may be useful.[39]

Initial antimicrobial therapy should be directed against anaerobes and aerobic enteric bacilli; thus, a combination of clindamycin and an aminoglycoside is frequently used in serious cases. Ampicillin may suffice in mild cases. Surgical drainage of pus is the key part of therapy.

EXOGENOUS INFECTION

Tuberculosis Tuberculosis is the only disease of importance in the intensive care unit that is spread by a true airborne route. Droplet nuclei carrying tubercle bacilli, produced from the respiratory tracts of patients, can follow air currents for long distances, including passage through air conditioning and heating ducts. The possibility of undiagnosed tuberculosis in an intensive care unit represents a distinct danger, not only to the patient involved, but also to other patients and to the staff.[91,92] Tuberculosis can present in many different ways, including adult respiratory distress syndrome.[93] Patients with pulmonary infiltrates who are admitted to an intensive care unit should have acid-fast smears done on sputum on an emergency basis. Also, any intensive care unit should have a respiratory isolation room with air pressure lower than the surrounding areas and with all exhaust air delivered outdoors.

There is no emergency in the specific antimicrobial treatment of tuberculosis except, perhaps, in tuberculous meningitis. With this one exception, the therapy of all forms of tuberculosis can be delayed for two to three days while appropriate cultures are taken and skin tests done. If large numbers of tubercle bacilli are present, particularly in pulmonary tuberculosis with cavities, three tuberculostatic drugs should be administered simultaneously if this is possible.[94] However, only isoniazid and aminoglycosides are available for parenteral administration if the patient is unable to take oral medications.

ANTITUBERCULOUS DRUGS AVAILABLE FOR PARENTERAL USE

Agent	Daily dose	Dose in renal failure	Major toxicity
Isoniazid*	300–600 mg	Limit 300 mg	Hepatotoxic, neuropathy
Aminoglycosides			
Streptomycin	1.0 gm	0.5 gm every three days	Nephrotoxic, ototoxic
Capreomycin	1.0 gm	Do not use	Nephrotoxic, ototoxic
Viomycin	1.0–2.0 gm	Do not use	Nephrotoxic, ototoxic
Kanamycin†	1.0 gm		
Gentamicin†	240 mg		

* Add pyridoxine 50 mg/day in poorly nourished patients.
† For dosage, see p. 112; for toxicity, p. 111.

Two aminoglycosides should not be used together. Cases of tuberculosis with lower numbers of organisms, e.g., pulmonary tuberculosis with negative sputum smears or most cases of extrapulmonary tuberculosis, generally require only two drugs; however, no case of active tuberculosis should ever be treated with one tuberculostatic drug alone, due to the risk of resistance development. Generally, isoniazid is included in any regimen. If an aminoglycoside is already in use, it will suffice for an adjunctive drug in tuberculosis management and no change is necessary. Aminoglycoside doses for tuberculosis can be given in a single daily injection.

The use of steroids in tuberculosis is controversial.[95] They have been used with some success for the following indications:

1. Systemic "toxicity" (fever, weight loss)
2. Poor oxygenation

3. Minimization of fibrosis and obstruction in endobronchial tuberculosis
4. Minimization of obstructive complications in tuberculous meningitis.

Water Organisms Gram-negative bacilli, such as *Pseudomonas aeruginosa* and allied species, can exist and grow in any standing water within the intensive care unit,[96] with transfer to patients by hands of personnel, invasive monitoring equipment, or respiratory therapy equipment.[97] A continued attempt must be made to avoid standing water in the unit. Any medication, irrigating solution, or nebulizer fluid must be changed every 24 hours. Flowers or plants, which may have potentially pathogenic bacteria in high concentration in soil or water, should be avoided in the unit.[98]

Infection Mediated by Intravenous or Intra-arterial Lines "Catheter sepsis" represents an important danger to the intensive care unit patient.[99] Organisms involved include *Staphylococcus aureus, S. epidermidis,* aerobic gram-negative bacilli associated with water sources (see above), *Candida* sp., and allied yeasts.

Catheter associated infection presents in two ways: as local phlebitis or as an acute systemic change in condition with new or increased fever. The cases which present as local suppuration are more likely endogenous, related to either normally or abnormally colonizing skin flora. Systemic reaction may be due to contamination of the intravenous fluid in manufacture or in local in-hospital handling, although skin organisms may also be involved.

Therapy for suppurative thrombophlebitis is primarily surgical; the entire suppurative vein must be removed.[100] Antimicrobial therapy should be based on the Gram stain of pus aspirated from the vein. Gram-positive cocci suggest the use of a penicillinase-resistant semisynthetic penicillin or a cephalosporin. Gram-negative rods suggest the use of an aminoglycoside, pending culture. Anaerobic infection in this context is rare.

The intensive care unit should have a prepared standard procedure for cases of acute change in condition with fever in a patient with intravenous or intra-arterial lines.[101]

SUGGESTED STANDARD PROCEDURE FOR SUSPECTED "CATHETER SEPSIS"

1. Blood cultures are drawn through all intravenous or intra-arterial lines and one or two peripheral sites.
2. All lines are discontinued or changed.
3. Sites are inspected, with attempt to milk pus from any inflamed areas. Any pus encountered is sent to the laboratory for immediate Gram stain and culture.
4. Tubing, catheters, and fluids are sent to the microbiology laboratory to hold for culture if blood cultures are positive.[101]

5. Catheter tips may be semiquantitatively cultured by cutting off the distal 3 cm with sterile scissors and rolling it over a blood agar plate.[102] If this is done with a suspect line, the blood culture drawn through that line may be omitted, but at least two separate blood cultures from sites separate from the line should be obtained.

6. An antimicrobial regimen is begun which is active against presumed skin flora (oxacillin, nafcillin, or a cephalosporin) and against gram-negative aerobic bacilli (usually gentamicin). This should be modified according to Gram stain findings from any pus encountered.

ACUTE BACTEREMIA AND THE SEPTIC SHOCK SYNDROME

Varying degrees of vasomotor instability are associated with bacteremia. This instability varies from the mild hypotension frequently seen with acute onset of bacteremia to a profound state of vasomotor collapse. These effects are mediated by several different mechanisms, many of which remain totally unclear. The septic shock syndrome cannot be considered to be a single pathogenic entity, but rather a series of events frequently seen in cases of bacteremia.[103-106] The bacteremia involved is most commonly due to gram-negative organisms (approximately 70 percent), but can also be due to *Staphylococcus aureus* or to other gram-positive organisms. The effects consist of both peripheral vasomotor instability and frequently a direct myocardial depression. Other complications such as diffuse intravascular coagulation, adult respiratory distress syndrome, or renal failure may supervene, necessitating additional specific treatment. The peripheral vasomotor effects may include an early vasodilatation, but this ultimately is followed by tissue hypoxia and eventually leakage of intravascular fluid into tissues. Central perfusion generally is maintained longer than peripheral utilization of delivered oxygen. Cardiac output is often initially high—the "hyperdynamic state"—but the heart itself is subject to poor tissue oxygenation and ultimately fails; this reduction obviously correlates with poor prognosis.[106] As one would expect with varying mechanisms operating, varying effects on circulatory parameters such as arterial pressure, peripheral resistance and central venous pressure are seen. The pulmonary artery pressures, resistance, and pulmonary artery occlusion pressure, may also reflect varying stages: hypovolemia, pulmonary edema, and tissue hypoxia. Thus, it is impossible to outline a typical course of septic shock.

For management of septic shock, appropriate monitoring is essential. Monitoring of arterial blood pressure alone will not suffice to differentiate the various events occurring or to show response to therapy. If true hemodynamic instability is encountered, then complete monitoring is mandatory to interpret the pathophysiologic events: central venous pressure, pulmonary artery, and pulmonary capillary wedge pressures and cardiac output should also be followed. In addition, stroke work, resistance, stroke volume, and intrapulmonary shunt need to be calculated. Close following of urinary output aids in assessing tissue perfusion. Arterial and pulmonary artery blood gases need careful attention for information relative to oxygen delivery and extraction by the tissues as well as pH and Pco_2 to determine acid-base status—particularly with reference to the development of anaerobic metabolism. Also, direct observations of the extremities for evidence of impaired peripheral perfusion is necessary. Care should be taken to use no more invasive monitoring than is necessary and to discontinue the monitoring as soon as possible to limit the risk of acquisition of new infection.

There are three principal modalities of therapy for the septic shock syndrome, namely (1) direct treatment of impaired cardiovascular parameters such as volume replacement and the use of vasoactive drugs, (2) appropriate intravenous antimicrobial drug therapy, and (3) adequate surgical therapy of underlying disease. The use of glucocorticoids is also frequently advocated.

Direct management of abnormal physiologic parameters usually begins with a trial of fluid loading. Central venous pressure might be used to gauge the response but it has inherent documented limitations in sepsis; wedge pressure must be used if a desired response is not immediately obtained. As noted above, care must be taken to avoid fluid overload because of the direct myocardial depressive effects frequently seen in the septic shock syndrome. Wedge pressures in the range of 12 to 15 torr indicate adequate volume replacement without risk of causing pulmonary edema. Normal saline or Ringer's Lactate are generally used for volume expansion since they replace both intravascular volume and functional extracellular space losses. Colloid has no advantage since increased capillary permeability is the rule. Digitalization is generally indicated unless the patient has already received adequate doses of digitalis glycoside. Dopamine in low to moderate doses (up to approximately 10 to 15 μg/kg/min, at which dose α-adrenergic effects begin to appear), may be used to support cardiac output. If peripheral vasoconstriction is evident, a beta adrenergic agent such as isoproterenol should be given (1 to 2 μg/min total dose in adults). A pulse rate rising to over 120/min or the presence of ectopic beats will limit the dosage of isoproterenol. The use of the α-adrenergic blocking agent phenoxybenzamine has also been suggested to combat vasoconstriction. Hypotension and vasodilatation at a late stage may be irreversible. At this point an α-adrenergic agent, such as norepinephrine, metaraminol, or dopamine, in higher doses may be used, but survival is unlikely. The main strategy of the direct treatment of impaired cardiovascular parameters is the tailoring of the treatment according to the observed responses of the patient. No general recipe of therapy is available.

Antimicrobial drug therapy must be prompt and must be by the intravenous route. Blood cultures as well as cultures from any presumptive sources of bacteremia, such as urine or intravenous lines, should be taken prior to the start of the antimicrobial therapy. Initial antimicrobial therapy usually must be "shotgun," often with use of multiple drugs, but it should be directed at the possible infecting agents and the presumptive sources of bacteremia. Thus, for instance, if the urine is the presumed source, therapy should be directed at organisms recently cultured from urine. In addition, antimicrobial therapy should be modified according to the microbial flora known to be present in the intensive care unit, if the presumed acute bacteremia occurs in a patient who has been in the unit for 24 hours or more. Bacteriocidal antimicrobials should be used if possible, always in full dosage. In cases in which the source organisms are not known, combinations of drugs are usually necessary, usually involving a penicillin or cephalosporin combined with an aminoglycoside. Cephalothin and gentamicin is a frequently used combination; cephalothin is directed at the possibility of *S. aureus* as a causative agent. If gentamicin-resistant gram-negative aerobes are present in the intensive care unit, amikacin may be used to replace gentamicin in selected patients with probable unit-acquired bacteremia. If *Pseudomonas aeruginosa* is suspected, usually in a granulocytopenic or leukemic patient, carbenicillin may be added. If *Bacteroides fragilis* is suspected, as in a bacteremia potentially deriving from the colon reservoir, clindamycin or chloramphenicol may be added.

The possibility that high-dose corticosteroids may alleviate some manifestations of the septic shock syndrome remains controversial in spite of many studies.[106,107] If a corticosteriod drug is used, it should be administered promptly, in large doses, and for a short course, 2 to 3 days at the longest. Various agents have been recommended, including dexamethasone (Decadron), 1 mg/kg initially followed by 2 to 3 mg/kg/day,[103] 1.0 gm hydrocortisone or equivalent initially followed by 1.0 gm every 4 to 6 hrs,[108] or methylprednisolone (Medrol) 30 mg/kg as a single dose.[109]

PROPHYLACTIC USE OF ANTIMICROBIALS

General Principles The subject of prophylactic use of antimicrobials has long been a controversial one and continues to be so. The obvious hope of stopping an infection before it starts has led to continued heavy use of many antimicrobials with varying success in preventing infections. However, with the realization that antimicrobial use is associated with a number of adverse effects, it has become necessary to justify specific prophylactic uses. This necessity is especially acute in the intensive care unit, since development of antimicrobial drug resistance by bacteria within the unit has severe consequences.[110] Ideally, antimicrobials would be used prophylactically only in specific cases for which there is true scientific evidence of efficacy and in which the reduction in total

number of infections brought about by the particular prophylactic protocol is large enough to justify the additional exposure of intensive care
unit patients and their bacteria to the antimicrobials. Obviously, this
ideal can be met only rarely. Recently, however, large reviews of the
available literature have made it easier to sort out the merit of studies
which have been reported and to designate which surgical procedures
have been associated with efficacious prophylaxis.[111,112]

With or without specific evidence of efficacy, it is first necessary
to consider general principles of prophylaxis.[113] In order to aid in prevention of an infection, an antimicrobial agent must be present in *adequate*
levels in tissue at the *site* of the contamination at the *time* of the contamination. Antimicrobials given for a prolonged time before the contamination is expected can only have the effect of changing the host's own
resident flora in a direction of increased resistance to antimicrobials.
Antimicrobials given for a prolonged time after the contamination must
either be for the purpose of therapy of an established infection or of a
presumed infection. Otherwise, their only effect, again, would be the
changing of the host's resident flora in the direction of increased resistance. In addition, an antimicrobial regimen should be used which has
the narrowest spectrum possible directed at the contaminating organisms. It should be pointed out that a number of antimicrobial usages
which are generally considered to be prophylactic are in reality treatment of a presumed infection or preventive treatment of a subclinical
but established infection. An example of therapy of presumptive infection is the use of antimicrobials after abdominal trauma with a potentially ruptured viscus. An example of preventive therapy of a subclinical
but established infection is the use of isoniazid for persons showing
evidence of tuberculosis infection by a positive tuberculin test, but with
no evidence of clinical disease.

Surgical Prophylaxis   In the case of a surgical procedure, the time of
contamination of the host by potentially infectious organisms is well
known, i.e., during the period of the operation itself and perhaps shortly
thereafter, but not longer than 24 hours. The nature of the contaminating
organisms also can be deduced with some degree of certainty from the
surfaces which will be transected during the procedure. If a skin incision
is made, these contaminating organisms include members of the skin
flora. If a contaminated internal structure, e.g., the gastrointestinal tract,
is transected, contaminating organisms will include those resident in
that structure. Thus, application of the general principles outlined above
leads to a protocol of prophylaxis involving a dose of an antimicrobial
agent shortly before the planned surgery, continuation of dosage during
surgery, and completion of the regimen no longer than 24 to 48 hours
postoperatively. This short protocol of prophylaxis will result in a minimal effect on the normal flora of the host and yet satisfy the principles
stated initially.[113] Prospective controlled studies have shown that this
form of prophylaxis is efficacious in abdominal and vaginal hysterec-

tomy, cesarean section, biliary surgery, total hip replacement, and microneurosurgery.[111] In addition, surgical procedures resulting in transection of the gastrointestinal tract also probably represent procedures in which antimicrobial prophylaxis is efficacious.[114]

In general, antimicrobial prophylaxis is not efficacious in clean surgery, i.e., surgery in an uninfected patient without transection of a normal flora-bearing structure other than skin. Examples of this would be breast surgery, most orthopedic surgery, hernia repairs, and most neurosurgery. Although there have been studies indicating efficaciousness of antimicrobial prophylaxis in some of these procedures, it will be noted that in such studies one usually is dealing with a rather high rate of infection in the placebo or control group. Procedures which carry an infection rate of 2 to 4 percent would not normally require a prophylactic regimen, since the reduction in number of infections would not be clinically worthwhile compared to the problems of prophylaxis.

There is a group of surgical procedures for which prophylactic antimicrobials are usually recommended, although the infection risk is low, because an infection, if it occurs, has disastrous results. Any small reduction in infection rate from antimicrobial prophylaxis thus results in a substantial saving of morbidity. The best example of this is total hip arthroplasty with insertion of a prosthesis.[115] Many neurosurgical procedures probably fall into this category as well. In these cases, unfortunately, scientific basis for the prophylaxis is less solid. However, adherence to a short-term protocol of prophylaxis following the principles outlined above minimizes the adverse effects of the prophylaxis.

An additional group of procedures for which antimicrobial prophylaxis has been advocated is that in which a therapeutic foreign body is implanted. There is a strong body of opinion that some form of antimicrobial prophylaxis should be applied for a longer period of time than usual in these cases, because of the possibility of transient bacteremias or other contaminations occurring postoperatively, resulting in infection at the site of the foreign body. Proof of efficacy of longer term prophylaxis in this group of procedures is still lacking. Vascular prostheses and heart valves are the obvious examples of such procedures.

Pneumonia Prophylaxis Antimicrobial agents have been used much in the past for high-risk patients in an intensive care setting for the prevention of pneumonia. However, this is not recommended due to the lack of efficaciousness in controlled studies.[116] This failure is reasonable in the light of the principles outlined above. One must consider a broad range of organisms for prophylaxis, not only those forming the normal mouth and pharyngeal flora, but also abnormal colonizers frequently seen in the mouth and pharynx and especially about endotracheal tubes or tracheostomy sites in patients in an intensive care unit. Consequently, a broad spectrum protocol would be required. In addition, a prolonged application of antimicrobial prophylaxis would be necessary, probably for the entire time of the patient's residence in the intensive care unit.

Thus, in order to attempt prophylaxis of pneumonia, nearly all patients in an intensive care unit would be receiving broad spectrum antimicrobial prophylaxis nearly all of the time. One could expect rapid development of antimicrobial resistance in the flora in the intensive care unit to the antimicrobials being used, with colonization by resistant organisms of the mouth and pharynx, and tracheostomy site, if present, of every patient. The risk of pneumonia would continue, with a different flora being responsible for that risk.

A possible exception to the lack of efficaciousness of pneumonia prophylaxis is the use of aerosolized polymyxin in selected patients requiring controlled ventilation when infection with *Pseudomonas aeruginosa* is endemic within the intensive care unit.[117] However, the longer *continuous* prophylaxis has been followed, the more difficulties with resistant organisms have been encountered.

Bacteremia Prophylaxis   In many cases, manipulation of an infected site or structure will result in access of bacteria from that site to the circulation. Frequently, the underlying infection in these cases is minor and does not require specific treatment. However, if a manipulation is to occur, it is reasonable to use an antimicrobial regimen active against the infecting organisms at the site to prevent potentially damaging bacteremia. This, more precisely, is preventive therapy rather than prophylaxis. The most common example is the use of antimicrobials during urologic manipulations in the presence of infected urine.[118] Other examples would be use of antimicrobials during incision and drainage of an abscess or furuncle, even though antimicrobial therapy is not being considered for definitive therapy. For therapy to be effective in preventing bacteremia, one should know the infecting organisms by culture in advance of the manipulation and use an antimicrobial regimen effective against them.

Endocarditis Prophylaxis   In patients with valvular or septal heart abnormalities which predispose to infective endocarditis and in patients with foreign bodies in the circulation, any bacteremia represents a threat even though the organism involved may ordinarily not be pathogenic. Thus, in these patients, the considerations previously outlined for bacteremia prophylaxis also apply to manipulations of noninfected, normal flora-bearing areas.[116,119,120] This is especially true for manipulations in the oral cavity. The necessity for endocarditis prophylaxis for predisposed patients who are to have manipulations of the urogenital or gastrointestinal tract is less well established, but frequently recommended. Prophylaxis for endocarditis during manipulations in the oral cavity is directed against the normal oral flora. In generally healthy people, this flora is almost universally susceptible to penicillin. One recommended regimen[121] is 2.4 million units of procaine penicillin given intramuscularly or crystalline penicillin G given intravenously 30 to 60 minutes before the procedure, with repetition of the dose 12 hours after the procedure. Some authorities recommend addition of an aminoglycoside, e.g., 1.0 gm streptomycin, given at the time of each penicillin dose. For genitourinary tract procedures, the regimen should be directed against enterococci; gram-negative organisms show little tendency to colonize heart valves. In this case, one recommended regimen is 2.4 million units of procaine penicillin plus 1.0 gm streptomycin, given intramuscularly 30 to 60 minutes before the procedure (or the same dose of crystalline penicillin G plus streptomycin given intravenously), and the same dose repeated every 12 hours for 2 days. A similar regimen can be used for manipulation of the gastrointestinal tract. Whether endocarditis prophylaxis is necessary for proctoscopy or sigmoidoscopy remains controversial. For patients allergic to penicillin, vancomycin 10 mg/kg body weight every 8 hours for 2 days can be given as a substitute for the penicillin in the above regimens. The cephalosporins are not recommended for this type of prophylaxis because of relative ineffectiveness against enterococci.

In an intensive care unit, abnormal colonization may have occurred at any of the normal flora-bearing areas. Thus, modifications of the above regimens may be necessary according to available culture data.

Not all heart abnormalities can be considered as predisposing to infective endocarditis. In general, any abnormality that results in a high pressure gradient across an orifice predisposes to this infection. Thus, lesions of the aortic or mitral valve are especially predisposing, as is a ventricular septal defect. Right-sided valvular lesions probably also have an increased risk. Atrial septal defects appear to not confer increased risk of endocarditis. The syndrome of mitral valve prolapse probably does carry some risk of endocarditis, so that prophylaxis is recommended if this lesion is present.

Prophylaxis for Patients with Intravenous and Intra-arterial Catheters
Although the presence of a foreign body in the circulation is cited as a possible reason for antimicrobial prophylaxis, in many cases of therapeutic foreign bodies placed in the intensive care unit for purposes of fluid administration or monitoring, e.g., umbilical catheters,[122] intravenous catheters,[99] or temporary intravenous pacemakers,[123] there is evidence that prophylaxis is not efficacious. Thus, it is not recommended and could result in a substantial increase in usage of antibiotics in an intensive care unit. In the case of external ventriculostomies, prophylaxis has been advocated only on the basis of retrospective data.[124]

REFERENCES—PART 1

1. McGowan JE, Finland M: Infection and antibiotic usage at Boston City Hospital: Changes in prevalence during the decade 1964–1973. J Infect Dis 129:421, 1974

2. Moody ML, Burke JP: Infections and antibiotic use in a large private hospital, January 1971. Arch Intern Med 130:261, 1972
3. Rose HD, Babcock JB: Colonization of intensive care unit patients with Gram-negative bacilli. Am J Epidemiol 101:495, 1975
4. Eickhoff TC: Nosocomial infections. In Hoeprich PD (ed): Infectious Diseases, 2nd ed. Hagerstown, Md: Harper & Row, 1977, pp. 27–33
5. Selden R, Lee S, et al: Nosocomial *Klebsiella* infections: intestinal colonization as a reservoir. Ann Intern Med 74:657, 1971
6. Tillotson JR, Finland M: Bacterial colonization and clinical superinfection of the respiratory tract complicating antibiotic treatment of pneumonia. J Infect Dis 119:597, 1969
7. Pollack M, Charache P, et al: Factors influencing colonization and antibiotic-resistance patterns of Gram-negative bacteria in hospital patients. Lancet 2:668, 1972
8. Johnson WG Jr, Pierce AK, et al: Nosocomial respiratory infections with Gram-negative bacilli. The significance of colonization of the respiratory tract. Ann Intern Med 77:701, 1972
9. Finland M: Changing patterns of susceptibility of common bacterial pathogens to antimicrobial agents. Ann Intern Med 76:1009, 1972
10. Price DJE, Sleigh JD: Control of infection due to *Klebsiella aerogenes* in a neurosurgical unit by withdrawal of all antibiotics. Lancet 2:1213, 1970
11. Noble WC, Somerville DA: Microbiology of Human Skin. Philadelphia: Saunders, 1974
12. Nahmias AJ, Eickhoff TC: Staphylococcal infection in hospitals. Recent developments in epidemiologic and laboratory investigation. N Engl J Med 265:74, 120, 177, 1961
13. Baxter DL: Candidiasis. In Moschella SL, Pillsbury DM, Hurley HJ (eds.): Dermatology. Philadelphia: Saunders, 1975
14. Andriole VT, Lyons RW: Coagulase-negative *Staphylococcus.* Ann NY Acad Sci 174:533, 1970
15. Schoenbaum SC, Gardner P, Shillito J: Infections of cerebrospinal fluid shunts: epidemiology, clinical manifestations, and therapy. J Infect Dis 131:543, 1975
16. Ihde DC, Armstrong D: Clinical spectrum of infection due to *Bacillus* species. Am J Med 55:839, 1973
17. Dobkin JF, Miller MH, Steigbigel NH: Septicemia in patients on chronic hemodialysis. Ann Intern Med 88:28, 1978
18. Wilson TS, Stuart RD: *Staphylococcus albus* in wound infection and in septicemia. Can Med Assoc J 93:8, 1965
19. Dixon RE: The role of airborne bacteria in theater-acquired surgical wound infection. Cleve Clin Q 40:115, 1973
20. Altemeier WA, Burke JF, Pruitt BA et al (eds.): Manual on Control of Infection in Surgical Patients. Philadelphia: Lippincott, 1976
21. Finland M: Perspective. Hospital-acquired infections: the problems of methicillin-resistant *Staphylococcus aureus* and infections with *Klebsiella pneumoniae.* Am J Med Sci 264:207, 1972
22. O'Toole RD, Drew WL, Dahlgren BJ et al: An outbreak of methicillin-resistant *Staphylococcus aureus* infection. Observations in hospital and nursing home. JAMA 213:257, 1970
23. Klimek JJ, Marsik FJ, Bartlett RC et al: Clinical epidemiologic, and bacteriologic observations of an outbreak of methicillin-resistant *Staphylococcus aureus* at a large community hospital. Am J Med 61:340, 1976

24. Plorde JJ, Sherris JC: Staphylococcal resistance to antibiotics: origin, measurement, and epidemiology. Ann NY Acad Sci 236:413, 1974

25. MacIntyre DS, Bolyard EA, Cleary T: Experience with oxacillin-resistant *Staphylococcus aureus* in a large county hospital (abstract). Presented at 1978 Annual Meeting, American Society of Microbiology, Las Vegas, May 14–19, 1978

26. Sabath LD, Barrett FF, Wilcox C et al: Methicillin resistance of *Staphylococcus aureus* and *Staphylococcus epidermidis*. In Hobby GL (ed): Antimicrobial Agents and Chemotherapy—1968. Bethesda, Md: American Society for Microbiology, 1969

27. Laverdiere M, Peterson PK, Verhoef J et al: *In vitro* activity of cephalosporins against methicillin-resistant, coagulase-negative staphylococci. J Infect Dis 137:245, 1978

28. Johanson WG, Pierce AK, Sanford JP: Changing pharyngeal bacterial flora of hospitalized patients. Emergence of Gram-negative bacilli. N Engl J Med 281:1137, 1969

29. Finegold SM, Rosenblatt JE: Practical aspects of anaerobic sepsis. Medicine (Baltimore) 52:311, 1973

30. Shields C, Patzakis JM, Meyers MH et al: Hand infections secondary to human bites. J Trauma 15:235, 1975

31. Hoeprich PD: Bacterial pneumonias. In Hoeprich PD (ed): Infectious Diseases, 2nd ed. Hagerstown, Md: Harper & Row, 1977

32. Bartlett JG, Gorbach SL, Finegold SM: The bacteriology of aspiration pneumonia. Am J Med 56:202, 1974

33. Pierce AK, Sanford JP, Thomas GD et al: Evaluation of decontamination of inhalation-therapy equipment. N Engl J Med 282:528, 1970

34. Pierce AK, Sanford JP: Bacterial contamination of aerosols. Arch Intern Med 131:156, 1973

35. Shulman JA, Phillips LA, Petersdorf RG: Errors and hazards in the diagnosis and treatment of bacterial pneumonias. Ann Intern Med 62:41, 1965

36. Ziskind MM, Schwarz MI, George RB et al: Incomplete consolidation in pneumococcal lobar pneumonia complicating pulmonary emphysema. Ann Intern Med 72:835, 1970

37. Sickles EA, Young VM, Greene WH et al: Pneumonia in acute leukemia. Ann Intern Med 79:528, 1973

38. Bryant RE, Hammond D: Interaction of purulent material with antibiotics used to treat Pseudomonas infections. Antimicrob Agents Chemother 6:702, 1974

39. Finegold SM, Bartlett J, Chow AW et al: Management of anaerobic infections (UCLA Conference). Ann Intern Med 83:375, 1975

40. Gorbach SL: Intestinal microflora. Gastroenterology 60:1110, 1971

41. Kalser MH, Cohen R, Arteaga I et al: Normal viral and bacterial flora of the human small and large intestine. N Engl J Med 274:500, 558, 1966

42. Nichols RL, Miller B, Smith JW: Septic complications following gastric surgery: relationship to the endogenous gastric microflora. Surg Clin North Am 55:1367, 1975

43. Cohen R, Roth FJ, Delgado E et al: Fungal flora of the normal human small and large intestine. N Engl J Med 280:638, 1969

44. Keighley MRB, Drysdale RB, Quoraishi AH et al: Antibiotic treatment of biliary sepsis. Surg Clin North Am 55:1379, 1975

45. Altemeier WA, Culbertson WR, Fullen WD et al: Intra-abdominal abcesses. Am J Surg 125:70, 1973

46. Lorber B, Swenson RM: The bacteriology of intra-abdominal infections. Surg Clin North Am 55:1349, 1975

47. Silen W, Weinberg AN: Fever. In Skillman JJ (ed): Intensive Care. Boston: Little, Brown, 1975

48. Littenberg RL, Taketa RM, Alazraki NP et al: Gallium-67 for localization of septic lesions. Ann Intern Med 79:403, 1973

49. Silberstein EB: Gallium detection of inflammation (letter). Ann Intern Med 80:774, 1974

50. Podoloff DA: Gallium-67 and infections (letter). Ann Intern Med 82:848, 1975

51. Bartrum RJ: Practical considerations in abdominal ultrasonic scanning. N Engl J Med 291:1068, 1974

52. Smith EH, Bartrum RJ: Ultrasonic evaluation of pararenal masses. JAMA 231:51, 1975

53. Smith EH, Bartrum RJ, Chang YC et al: Percutaneous aspiration biopsy of the pancreas under ultrasonic guidance. N Engl J Med 292:825, 1975

54. Nichols RL, Smith JW: Gas in the wound: what does it mean? Surg Clin North Am 55:1289, 1975

55. Klion FM, Schaffner F, Papper H: Hepatitis after exposure to halothane. Ann Intern Med 71:467, 1969

56. Brenner AI, Kaplan MM: Recurrent hepatitis due to methoxyflurane anesthesia. N Engl J Med 284:961, 1971

57. Murray HW, Tuazon CA, Guerrero IC et al: Urinary temperature: a clue to early diagnosis of factitious fever. N Engl J Med 296:23, 1977

58. Gerding DN, Menge PAR, Hall WH: Detection of factitious fever. Use of the electronic thermometer. Minn Med 60:163, 1977

59. Feinstone SM, Kapikian AZ, Purcell RH et al: Transfusion-associated hepatitis not due to viral hepatitis type A or B. N Engl J Med 292:767, 1975

60. Dineen P: Gas gangrene. In Hoeprich PD (ed): Infectious Diseases, 2nd ed. Hagerstown, Md: Harper & Row, 1977

61. Hitchcock CL, Demello FJ, Haglin JJ: Gangrene infection. New approaches to an old disease. Surg Clin North Am 55:1403, 1975

62. Holland JA, Hill GB, Wolfe WG et al: Experimental and clinical experience with hyperbaric oxygen in the treatment of clostridial myonecrosis. Surgery 77:75, 1975

63. Goldstein E, Hoeprich PD: Candidosis. In Hoeprich PD (ed): Infectious Diseases, 2nd ed. Hagerstown, Md: Harper & Row, 1977

64. Silva-Hutner M, Cooper BH: Medically important yeasts. In Lennette EH, Spaulding EH, Truant JP (eds): Manual of Clinical Microbiology, 2nd ed. Washington, DC: American Society for Microbiology, 1974

65. Edwards JE, Lehrer RI, Steihm ER et al: Severe candidal infections. Clinical perspective, immune defense mechanisms, and current concepts of therapy (UCLA Conference). Ann Intern Med 89:91, 1978

66. Taschdjian CL, Kozinn PJ, Tomi EF: Opportunistic yeast infections with special reference to candidiasis. Ann N Y Acad Sci 174:606, 1970

67. Louria DB, Stiff DP, Bennett B: Disseminated moniliasis in the adult. Medicine (Baltimore) 41:307, 1962

68. Andriole VT, Kravetz HM, Roberts WC et al: Candida endocarditis. Clinical and pathologic studies. Am J Med 32:251, 1962

69. Goldmann DA, Martin WT, Worthington JW: Growth of bacteria and fungi in total parenteral nutrition solutions. Am J Surg 126:314, 1973

70. Goldmann DA, Maki DG: Infection control in total parenteral nutrition. JAMA 223:1360, 1973

71. Kozinn PJ, Taschdjian CL: *Candida albicans:* saphrophyte or pathogen? A diagnostic guideline. JAMA 198:170, 1966
72. Ellis CA, Spivack ML: The significance of candidemia. Ann Intern Med 67:511, 1967
73. Hoeprich PD: Cryptococcosis. In Hoeprich PD (ed): Infectious Diseases, 2nd ed. Hagerstown, Md: Harper & Row, 1977, pp 902–910
74. Lewis JL, Rabinovich SH: The wide spectrum of cryptococcal infections. Am J Med 53:315, 1972
75. Kunin CM: Detection, Prevention, and Management of Urinary Tract Infections, 2d ed. Philadelphia: Lea and Febiger, 1974
76. Segura JW, Kalalis PP, Martin WJ et al: Anaerobic bacteria in the urinary tract. Mayo Clin Proc 47:30, 1972
77. Stamey TA, Timothy M, Millar M et al: Recurrent urinary tract infections in adult women: the role of introital enterobacteria. Calif Med 115, 1:1, 1971
78. Bailey RR, Gower PE, Roberts AP et al: Urinary tract infection in nonpregnant women. Lancet 2:275, 1973
79. Gould JC: The comparative bacteriology of acute and chronic urinary tract infection. In O'Grady F, Brumfitt W (eds): Urinary Tract Infections. London: Oxford University Press, 1968
80. Rocha H: Epidemiology of urinary tract infection in adults. In Kaye D (ed): Urinary Tract Infection and its Management. St. Louis: C V Mosby Co, 1972
81. Stamm WE: Guidelines for prevention of catheter-associated urinary tract infections. Ann Intern Med 82:386, 1975
82. Lapides J, Diokno AC, Silber SJ et al: Clean, intermittent self-catheterization in the treatment of urinary tract disease. J Urol 107:458, 1972
83. Hinman F Jr: Intermittant catheterization and vesical defenses. J Urol 117:57, 1977
84. Stamey TA, Govan DE, Palmer JM: The localization and treatment of urinary tract infections: the role of bactericidal urine levels as opposed to serum levels. Medicine (Baltimore) 44:1, 1965
85. Stamey TA, Fair WR, Timothy MM et al: Serum versus urinary antimicrobial concentrations and urinary tract infections. N Engl J Med 291:1159, 1974
86. Thornton GF, Lytton B, Antriole VT: Bacteriuria during indwelling catheter drainage. Effect of constant bladder rinse. JAMA 195:179, 1966
87. Lawrence RM: Infections of the female genital tract. In Hoeprich PD (ed): Infectious Diseases, 2nd ed. Hagerstown, Md: Harper & Row, 1977, pp 443–454
88. Neary MP, Allen J, Okubadejo OA: Preoperative vaginal bacteria and postoperative infections in gynocologic patients. Lancet 2:1291, 1973
89. Bartlett JG, Onderdonk AB, Drude E et al: Quantitative bacteriology of the vaginal flora. J Infect Dis 136:271, 1977
90. Yow M: Group B streptococci: a serious threat to the neonate (editorial). JAMA 230:1177, 1974
91. Ehrenkranz NJ, Kicklighter JL: Tuberculosis outbreak in a general hospital: evidence for airborne spread of infection. Ann Intern Med 77:377, 1972
92. MacIntyre DS, Goldstein MS, Collier C: Outbreak of tuberculosis infection associated with an intensive care patient with undiagnosed tuberculosis (abstract). Am Rev Respir Dis 115 (suppl):403, 1977
93. Homan W, Harman E, Braun NM et al: Military tuberculosis presenting as acute respiratory failure: treatment by membrane oxygenator and ventricle pump. Chest 67:366, 1975
94. Stead WW: Tuberculosis. In Wintrobe MW, Thorn GW, Adams RD et al (eds):

Harrison's Principles of Internal Medicine, 7th ed. New York: McGraw-Hill, 1974

95. American Thoracic Society Committee on Therapy: Adrenal corticosteroids and tuberculosis. Am Rev Respir Dis 97:484, 1968

96. Favero MS, Carson, LA, Bond WW et al: *Pseudomonas aeruginosa:* growth in distilled water from hospitals. Science 173:836, 1971

97. Pierce AK, Sanford JP: Bacterial contamination of aerosols. Arch Intern Med 131:156, 1973

98. Taplin D, Mertz PM: Flower vases in hospitals as reservoirs of pathogens. Lancet 2:1279, 1973

99. Maki DG, Goldmann DA, Rhame FS: Infection control in intravenous therapy. Ann Intern Med 79:867, 1973

100. Munster AM: Septic thrombophlebitis. A surgical disorder. JAMA 230:1010, 1974

101. National Coordinating Committee on Large Volume Parenterals: Recommended procedures for in-use testing of large volume parenterals suspected of contamination or of producing a reaction in a patient. Am J Hosp Pharm 35:678, 1978

102. Maki DG, Weise CE, Sarafin HW: A semiquantitative culture method for identifying intravenous catheter related infection. N Engl J Med 296:1305, 1977

103. Hoeprich PD, Boggs DR: Manifestations of infectious disease. In Hoeprich PD (ed): Infectious Diseases, 2nd ed. Hagerstown, Md: Harper & Row, 1977

104. Mason JW, Kleebert U, Dolan P et al: Plasma kallikrein and Hageman factor in Gram-negative bacteremia. Ann Intern Med 73:545, 1970

105. McCabe WR: Endotoxin and bacteremia due to Gram-negative organisms (editorial). N Engl J Med 283:1342, 1970

106. Schumer W: Steroids in the treatment of clinical septic shock. Ann Surg 184:333, 1976

107. Weil MH, Nishijima H: Cardiac output in bacterial shock (editorial). Am J Med 64:920, 1978

108. Christy JH: Treatment of Gram-negative shock. Am J Med 50:77, 1971

109. Lillehei RC, Dietzman RH: Circulatory collapse and shock. In Schwartz SI (ed): Principles of Surgery, 2nd ed. New York: McGraw-Hill, 1974

110. Stoddard JC: Gram-negative infections in the ICU. Crit Care Med 2:17, 1974

111. Chodak GW, Plaut ME: Use of systemic antibiotics for prophylaxis in surgery. Arch Surg 112:326, 1977

112. Veterans' Administration Ad Hoc Interdisciplinary Advisory Committee on Antimicrobial Drug Usage. Guidelines for peer review. I Prophylaxis in surgery. JAMA 237:1003, 1977

113. Burke JF: Preoperative antibiotics. Surg Clin North Am 43:665, 1963

114. Polk HC Jr, Lopez-Mayor JF: Postoperative wound infection: a prospective study of determinant factors and prevention. Surgery 66:97, 1969

115. Rangno RE: The rationale of antibiotic prophylaxis in total hip replacement arthroplasty. Clin Orthop 96:206, 1973

116. Veterans' Administration Ad Hoc Interdisciplinary Advisory Committee on Antimicrobial Drug Usage. Guidelines for peer review. 2. Nonsurgical prophylaxis. JAMA 237:1134, 1977

117. Greenfield S, Teres D, Bushnell LS et al: Prevention of Gram-negative bacillary pneumonia using aerosol polymyxin as prophylaxis. J Clin Invest 52:2935, 1973

118. McGuire EJ: Antibacterial prophylaxis in prostatectomy patients. J Urol 111:794, 1974
119. Kaplan EL, Anthony BF, Bisno A et al: AHA committee report. Prevention of bacterial endocarditis. Circulation 56:139A, 1977
120. Petersdorf RG: Antimicrobial prophylaxis of bacterial endocarditis. Prudent caution or overkill? Am J Med 65:220, 1978
121. Hoeprich PD: Chemoprophylaxis of infectious diseases. In Hoeprich PD (ed): Infectious Diseases, 2nd ed. Hagerstown, Md: Harper & Row, 1977
122. Anagnostakis D, Kamba A, Petrochilou V et al: Risk of infection associated with umbilical vein catheterization. A prospective study of 75 newborn infants. J Peds 86:759, 1975
123. Patton KD, Kenamore B, Stein E: Antibiotic prophylaxis for temporary transvenous pacemakers. N Engl J Med 281:1106, 1969
124. Wyler AR, Kelly WA: Use of antibiotics with external ventriculostomies. J Neurosurg 37:185, 1972

PART II

Antimicrobials in the Intensive Care Unit

In the intensive care unit, a wide and often confusing range of antimicrobial agents applicable to a specific illness in a specific patient is available. The choice of an antimicrobial regimen is further complicated by the need to consider the available routes of administration, the often impaired function of body systems with concomitant alteration of pharmacology and potential toxicity, and the simultaneous administration of other drugs. In addition to these individual patient factors, an equally important consideration is the effect of the antimicrobial regimen on the overall microbial ecology of the intensive care unit, a factor unique to the antimicrobials.

In the following discussion, antimicrobial agents are considered in groups. For each group there is a discussion of advantages, disadvantages, and dosages. Our objective is not to provide "the answer" for each specific instance, but rather to establish the appropriate criteria that form the necessary data base for the unique problems that the clinician faces.

Advantages include organisms or infections for which the drug is best used—*drug of choice;* organisms or infections for which the drug may be used if another, better drug is for some reason contraindicated—*drug of alternate choice;* situations in which the drug may be used with another to gain improved microbial suppression or killing—*use in synergistic combinations;* and other specific advantages. It should be pointed out that the synergistic combinations are specific for organism or infection and *not* attempts to broaden coverage in clinical situations where the infecting agent is not specifically known or in polymicrobial infections (see Part 1).

Disadvantages include adverse reactions, problems of administration (restricted availability of routes of administration, major incompatibilities, high incidence of phlebitis, etc), cation contents which may adversely affect patients with fluid and electrolyte retention or instability, and also major groups of organisms which are not treatable with the agent.

Dosage includes adult dosage, pediatric dosage, and use in renal failure.

In some cases, discussion of choice of specific agents in the group is included. Frequently, however, specific agents within a group are so similar that choice should be made on the basis of cost.

Some groups of agents are not discussed due to minimal usefulness in an intensive care unit. One such group is the tetracyclines. They are bacteriostatic agents (not bactericidal). Many organisms in intensive care units are already resistant to them and they frequently have substantial adverse effects, particularly when given intravenously. In a rare case, doxycycline (Vibramycin, Doxy-II, and others) may be useful for a known infection with a known susceptible organism. It may be used in renal failure.[1] Whether its fat solubility confers a clinical advantage of penetrability is controversial.

Erythromycin, trioleandomycin (TAO), and the urinary antiseptics (nalidixic acid, nitrofurantoin, and methenamine) also are of limited usefulness in an intensive care unit for reasons similar to those for the tetracyclines. A new use of erythromycin in treatment of presumed Legionnaire's disease[2,3] may require its use on occasion by intravenous route in an intensive care unit. Oral administration (or administration through a nasogastric tube), is preferable to intravenous administration if it is possible, since intravenous administration is difficult and requires large fluid volumes; details in the manufacturers' package inserts should be consulted.

Trimethoprim-sulfamethoxyzole (co-trimoxyzole, Bactrim, Septra) and metronidazole (Flagyl) are not available for intravenous use in the United States. Although these drugs may in the future be important in the intensive care unit,[4] they are not discussed here.

PENICILLIN

Major advantage	Low toxicity, high doses possible
Major disadvantage	Allergy
Primary indications	Gram-positive cocci except staphylococci, many anaerobes
Caveats	Care must be taken with the possibility of allergic reactions; very high dosage can lead to neurotoxicity

The oldest antibiotic continues to be a cornerstone for the therapy of infection, including that encountered in the intensive care unit. Many formulations are available for different routes of administration and durations of action, but in an intensive care unit setting, only intravenous crystalline sodium or potassium penicillin is likely to be of use.

ADVANTAGES

Drug of Choice Penicillin is the drug of choice for infections due to the following organisms:

GRAM-POSITIVE AEROBES

Streptococcus pneumoniae (pneumococcus)—a few cases of resistance have been reported, especially in South Africa[5]
Streptococcus pyogenes (Group A, β-hemolytic)
Other nonenterococcal streptococci ("Viridans," etc.)
Penicillin-susceptible *Staphylococcus* sp.
Listeria monocytogenes

GRAM-NEGATIVE AEROBES

Neisseria meningitidis (meningococcus)
Neisseria gonorrheae (gonococcus)—development of relative resistance is requiring higher doses for genital infections; however, strains causing bacteremia have tended to remain susceptible

ANAEROBES

Essentially all obligate anaerobic bacteria except *Bacteroides fragilis*[6]

Drug of Alternate Choice This situation does not occur; penicillin is the drug of first choice for all infections due to susceptible organisms.

Use in Synergistic Combinations Enterococci (*Streptococcus faecalis* and *S. faecium,* i.e., most, but not all, group D streptococci)—penicillin is used with gentamicin for these difficult to treat organisms when they are the cause of serious infections.[7,8] For less severe infections, ampicillin can be used. Enterococci often have misleading in vitro disc susceptibility tests which generally can be disregarded.

High Therapeutic-to-Toxic Ratio The serum levels of penicillin necessary to show toxic effects on the host are extremely high compared to the bactericidal levels for susceptible bacteria. This most important advantage allows use of penicillin in extremely high doses that permit acceptable amounts of drug to diffuse into tissues and tissue space, such as the central nervous system, joints, etc.

Bactericidal Effect Penicillin acts on the cell wall of growing cells, resulting in rapid cell death, not just suppression of growth. Thus, penicillin is of particular use in situations in which host defense mechanisms cannot be expected to eradicate susceptible organisms, e.g., infective endocarditis, infections in granulocytopenic hosts.

DISADVANTAGES

Inactivation by Bacterial Penicillinase   Enzymes produced by several species of bacteria, especially *Staphylococcus* sp., inactivate penicillin, rendering it ineffective against such organisms. In the case of *Staphylococcus* sp., penicillinase production is so prevalent that these organisms must be considered resistant to penicillin until proven otherwise, even in community-acquired infections.

Allergic Reactions   Allergy to penicillin is the most frequent contraindication to its use. Prevalence of penicillin allergy ranges from 5 to 10 percent in various surveys.[9] All penicillin derivatives are cross-allergenic. The most dangerous types of allergy take the form of anaphylactoid reactions or of exfoliative erythroderms. A careful history is the best way of ascertaining the risk of a dangerous allergic reaction to penicillin. A history of reaction occurring promptly (within minutes to hours) after penicillin administration, or a history of generalized urticaria (hives), is a particularly strong contraindication to the use of penicillin because of the risk of an anaphylactoid reaction. However, any history of allergy to penicillin or to one of its derivatives should prompt selection of a suitable alternate agent if available (see also cephalosporins, pp. 104–8). Skin testing for penicillin allergy has been evaluated extensively in field trials[10,11] but no satisfactory skin test agents are currently available for clinical use.

Cation Content   Penicillin for intravenous use is available either as the sodium or potassium salt. Both have approximately 1 mEq of ion per gram of penicillin. The sodium salt, when given in large doses, can present a meaningful sodium load in cases of congestive heart failure or of hepatic cirrhosis. The potassium salt can raise serum potassium levels in renal failure or other hyperkalemic states. Also, bolus injection of potassium penicillin through a central venous line may lead to arrhythmias due to transient intracardiac and intracoronary hyperkalemia.[12] Administration over 5 to 30 minutes permits dilution and equilibration.

Coombs-Positive Hemolytic Anemia   This occurs rarely with penicillin.[13] Although mechanistically an allergic reaction, it is dose related and does not predictably recur with retreatment with penicillin. The occurrence of this reaction does not necessarily preclude use of penicillin at a future time.

Neurotoxicity   At very high levels, penicillin acts to excite neural tissue.[14,15] The neurotoxicity generally occurs only at doses higher than 50 million units per 24 hours, or in renal failure patients in whom lower doses may not be adequately cleared. Symptoms begin with depressed mental status and myoclonic jerks, particularly in the face, neck, and upper extremities, and progress with continued high-dosage penicillin to grand-mal seizures and coma. Symptoms reverse with discontinuation of the penicillin. All penicillin derivatives are potentially neurotoxic and the effects are additive. Care must be taken to limit total dosage when two penicillin derivatives are being administered simultaneously.

DOSAGE

Unfortunately, for historical reasons penicillin dosage is measured in activity units rather than by weight; the conversion factor may be expressed as approximately 1.6 million units to 1 gm.

Low Dosage Range 400,000 to 600,000 units (250 to 375 mg) every 12 hours. This is sufficient for pneumococcal pneumonia and mild streptococcal cellulitis. Dosage below 3 million units per day is less likely to promote acquisition of antibiotic resistant flora by the patient than are higher doses.[16]

Middle Dosage Range 1 million units (0.625 gm) every 4 to 6 hours (4 to 6 million units per day). This is used for lung abscess and for wound infections.

High Dosage Range Dosage can be raised to as high as 40 million units per day for serious infections, particularly those in anatomically protected areas such as in the central nervous system, pleural or peritoneal cavities, or on heart valves. In high concentration, penicillin also has a broader spectrum of activity, resembling that of ampicillin.

Usage in Renal Failure In patients with impaired renal function (creatinine clearance of less than 30 ml/min, serum creatinine greater than 4 mg/100 ml, or oliguria), dosage should be cut in half. Penicillin is hemodialyzable, so normal dosage can be used during a hemodialysis run. Penicillin is not predictably removed during peritoneal dialysis; penicillin can be added to the dialysate to maintain desired serum levels.[17]

PENICILLINASE-RESISTANT SEMISYNTHETIC PENICILLINS

Major advantage	Action against penicillinase-producing staphylococci
Major disadvantage	Relatively low activity against organisms susceptible to penicillin (compared to activity of penicillin itself); allergic reactions
Primary indication	Staphylococcal infections

Caveats	Watch for staphylococcal strains which are resistant to this group of antibiotics as well ("methicillin-resistant" or "oxacillin-resistant"); the penicillinase-resistant semisynthetic penicillins are cross-allergenic with penicillin

There are several penicillinase-resistant semisynthetic penicillins currently available: methicillin (Staphcillin, Celbenin), oxacillin (Prostaphlin, Bactocil), nafcillin (Unipen, Nafcil), cloxacillin (Tegopen, Cloxapen), and dicloxacillin. All have the same antibacterial spectrum. They differ somewhat in pharmacologic parameters, mainly oral absorption, protein binding, and serum half-life. The usefulness of methicillin is limited by renal toxicity (interstitial nephritis) and hemolytic anemia. Cloxacillin and dicloxacillin are available only for oral use. Oxacillin and nafcillin are very similar and are among the most useful drugs in the intensive care unit. Cost considerations may enter into the choice between them (1976 costs were approximately equivalent).[18]

ADVANTAGES

Drug of Choice Oxacillin or nafcillin is the drug of choice for infections due to the following penicillin-resistant organisms:

Staphylococcus aureus
Staphylococcus epidermidis

Note that all *S. aureus* and *S. epidermidis* must be considered penicillin-resistant until susceptibility testing is available, whether the infection originated in the hospital or in the community. Also, strains of staphylococci resistant to the penicillinase-resistant semisynthetic penicillins are being identified with increasing frequency in hospitals in the United States (see disadvantages).

Drug of Alternate Choice This situation does not occur. Oxacillin or nafcillin is the drug of choice in those situations in which it is indicated.

Use in Synergistic Combinations Gentamicin is sometimes used with oxacillin or nafcillin for treatment of staphylococcal endocarditis (oxacillin or nafcillin is the primary drug) because of evidence from an animal study which suggests greater efficacy of the combination.[19] However, in the special case of staphylococcal endocarditis in intravenous drug addicts, the combination may not offer any advantage clinically over oxacillin or nafcillin.[20]

High Therapeutic-to-Toxic Ratio Same as penicillin.

Bactericidal Effect Same as penicillin.

DISADVANTAGES

Allergic Reactions Same as penicillin. All penicillin derivatives must be considered to be cross-allergenic with penicillin (p. 95). However, skin test reagents used to test for penicillin allergy cannot be used to test for penicillin-derivative allergy; reagents made from the specific derivative must be used.

Lower Activity than Penicillin The penicillinase-resistant semisynthetic penicillins are not as active on a weight basis as is penicillin itself against organisms susceptible to penicillin. Therefore, if laboratory testing shows penicillin susceptibility of the organism responsible for an infection, penicillin should be used.

Oxacillin-Resistant (Methicillin-Resistant) Staphylococci Some strains of *S. aureus* show resistance not only to penicillin, but also to the penicillinase-resistant semisynthetic penicillins. This resistance may occur through a different mechanism, not the elaboration of an antibiotic-inactivating enzyme. Such strains have been rare in the United States and relatively common in Europe; recently, however, they have been reported in hospital-associated outbreaks in many widely separated locations in the United States.[21,22] Such strains can cause severe infection. They are considered uniformly resistant to all penicillin derivatives and also to all cephalosporin derivatives, even if disc susceptibility testing shows susceptibility to certain of these agents.[23] The drug of choice for serious infections due to these strains is vancomycin (pp. 121–24).
     Strains of *S. epidermidis* resistant to oxacillin and nafcillin are relatively common. In this case, the cross-resistance among all penicillin and cephalosporin derivatives is not as marked as in oxacillin-resistant *S. aureus;* however, disc susceptibility testing can be unreliable[24] and should be confirmed by other means of determining minimal bactericidal concentrations of antibiotic.

Hemolytic Anemia This has been reported with oxacillin.[25]

Granulocytopenia This has been reported with oxacillin.[25]

Interstitial Nephritis Although this is primarily a problem with methicillin,[26] it has been reported with oxacillin[27] and with nafcillin[28] as well. It is an idiosyncratic, non-dose-related reaction, presenting as fever, hematuria, and proteinuria, frequently with rash and eosinophilia. In newborns, it may be more common with oxacillin.

Neurotoxicity This is seen with either oxacillin or nafcillin in very high doses or in renal failure, similar to penicillin.

Lack of Activity Against Gram-Negative Organisms and Enterococci Penicillinase-resistant semisynthetic penicillins have no useful activity against *Neisseria gonorrheae, N. meningitidis, Escherichia coli,* some *Proteus mirabilis,* and enterococci, although penicillin or ampicillin is frequently useful in infections due to these organisms. The characteristic resistance of enterococci to oxacillin and to clindamycin on disc susceptibility testing can act as an early hint that a suspected streptococcus is an enterococcus before all biochemical testing is complete in the laboratory.[29]

Irritation of Veins Oxacillin and nafcillin are severely irritating to veins, frequently leading to phlebitis when given through peripheral veins. In the intensive care unit, most antimicrobials are appropriately administered by central venous infusion, using appropriate dilutions.

Cation Content

Methicillin—2.8 mEq sodium per gram
Oxacillin—2.9 mEq sodium per gram
Nafcillin—3.0 mEq sodium per gram

DOSAGE

Severe Infections Dosage is 6 to 18 gm per day divided into 3- to 6-hour intervals, intravenously.

Pediatric Dosage Dosage is 100 mg/kg/day; may go higher.

Usage in Renal Failure In patients with impaired renal function (creatinine clearance of less than 30 ml/min, serum creatinine greater than 4 mg/100 ml, or oliguria), dosage may be reduced, usually by half. These drugs are not well dialyzed, so a reduced dosage should be used in patients during, as well as between, runs of hemodialysis or peritoneal dialysis.[30]

BROAD-SPECTRUM SEMISYNTHETIC PENICILLINS

Major advantages	Activity against many gram-negative aerobic organisms; low toxicity and potential of very high dosage as with penicillin
Major disadvantage	Development of bacterial resistance
Primary indication	Infection due to, or presumptively due to, susceptible gram-negative aerobes
Caveats	Strains of *Hemophilus influenzae* resistant to ampicillin are sufficiently widespread to make

its use in severe infections due to this organism dangerous unless microbial susceptibility is documented. Carbenicillin requires high dosage for *Pseudomonas* sp.; cation loading may be a problem. These agents are all inactivated by penicillinase and cannot be used for penicillin-resistant staphylococci

These antibiotics were developed in an attempt to widen the spectrum of penicillin to include various gram-negative organisms, although these agents are not as active as penicillin against most gram-positive bacteria. Agents of this group which find use in the intensive care unit are ampicillin (Amcill, Penbritin, Principen, Polycillin, Omnipen), carbenicillin (Geopen), and ticarcillin (Ticar). A new agent in this series, piperacillin, is undergoing clinical testing. In addition to these, several oral agents are available. These should be used in hospitalized patients only in certain selected cases, because of the possibility of resistant organisms developing, especially in the case of oral carbenicillin.

ADVANTAGES

Drug of Choice   The broad-spectrum semisynthetic penicillins are presumed to be the drugs of choice when treating infection due to susceptible organisms, unless (1) resistance is shown by laboratory testing, (2) resistance is suggested by the clinical situation of the patient (e.g., new infection in a patient already receiving the agent), or (3) resistance is suggested by the epidemiologic situation (e.g., new infection while a resistant organism is prevalent in the patient's immediate environment, the intensive care unit).

GRAM-POSITIVE AEROBES

Enterococci, in urinary tract infection or other non-life-threatening infection (in serious infections, a combination of penicillin and gentamicin should be used)

GRAM-NEGATIVE AEROBES

Shigella sp.
Salmonella sp. (including *S. typhi*)
Escherichia coli
Proteus mirabilis
Hemophilus influenzae—Note that resistance is progressively developing in these bacteria and that in many localities this has eliminated ampicillin as a drug of first choice for presumptive serious infection due to *H. influenzae*. Of special importance is the fact that ampicillin

is no longer drug of first choice for *H. influenzae* meningitis.[31,32] Resistance of *Salmonella* sp. and *Shigella* sp. is also becoming meaningful in some localities, especially outside of the United States.

Proteus sp., indole positive *(P. vulgaris, P. rettgeri, P. morganii)*—carbenicillin and ticarcillin

Pseudomonas aeruginosa—carbenicillin and ticarcillin

Other gram-negative aerobes according to susceptibility testing

ANAEROBES

None.

Note that because of cost considerations and development and selection of resistance, ampicillin should be used against the organisms susceptible to it, and carbenicillin and ticarcillin reserved as first choice agents for *Pseudomonas aeruginosa*, indole positive *Proteus* sp., and other gram-negative aerobes resistant to ampicillin and susceptible to carbenicillin or ticarcillin.

Drug of Alternate Choice   The broad-spectrum semisynthetic penicillins are used as an alternate, second choice drug for the following indications, i.e., when a better agent is available but it cannot be used.

Gram-positive aerobes—all those susceptible to penicillin, penicillin being the drug of first choice

Gram-negative aerobes—all those susceptible to penicillin, penicillin being the drug of first choice

Anaerobes—all those susceptible to penicillin, penicillin being the drug of first choice; note that carbenicillin and ticarcillin may have increased activity against *Bacteroides fragilis* compared to penicillin, although clindamycin or chloramphenicol remain the drugs of first choice for infections due to these organisms[33,34]

Use in Synergistic Combinations   In many cases, synergism can be demonstrated between aminoglycosides and carbenicillin or ticarcillin against strains of gram-negative aerobes susceptible to both classes of agents. In life-threatening infections or in infections of closed spaces with poor antimicrobial penetration, an agent from each of the two classes should be used. (See also resistance development, p. 111.) In addition, synergism is sometimes seen against strains showing resistance to one of the two classes of antibiotics; thus, in special cases of difficult-to-eradicate infection, evidence of such synergism should be sought by special laboratory testing.[32,35,36]

High Therapeutic-to-Toxic Ratio   Same as penicillin.

Bactericidal Effect   Same as penicillin.

Effect on Bacteremia in the Leukopenic Patient   In patients with absolute granulocyte counts below 1000 per ml (the absolute granulocyte count is the total white blood cell count multiplied by the sum of the percents of mature granulocytes and of band forms), there is some evidence that in usual dosage carbenicillin (and, presumably, ticarcillin) and an aminoglycoside are associated with a higher cure rate of bacteremia due to organisms susceptible to both classes of agents.[37]

DISADVANTAGES

Allergic Reactions   Same as penicillin. All penicillin derivatives must be considered to be cross-allergenic (see penicillins p. 95). However, it must be remembered that skin test reagents used to test for penicillin allergy cannot be used to test for penicillin-derivative allergy; reagents must be made from the specific derivative to be used, and these may not be clinically reliable.

Lower Activity than Penicillin   The broad-spectrum semisynthetic penicillins are frequently not as active on a weight basis as is penicillin itself against penicillin-susceptible organisms, and thus must not be considered the drugs of choice. It is natural, however, for the clinician to desire a "totally effective" drug that just doesn't exist.

Inactivation by Bacterial Penicillinase   Ampicillin, carbenicillin, and ticarcillin are inactivated by penicillinase as is penicillin, and are not used against *Staphylococcus* sp. without documented susceptibility.

Rapid Bacterial Resistance Development   In the treatment of *P. aeruginosa* infection with carbenicillin or ticarcillin, the rapid appearance of resistance is a special problem.[38,39] If the agents are used in full dosage, this effect may be minimized. Except for the urinary tract infection, it is often preferable to use, in addition, an aminoglycoside active against the infecting agent as an adjunctive drug.

Resistant Gram-Negatives   Susceptibility of gram-negative aerobic bacilli is by no means universal and should be confirmed by disc susceptibility testing whenever possible. In particular, *Klebsiella* sp. are resistant to all currently available penicillin derivatives. Piperacillin (T-1220), currently under investigation, may have useful activity against *Klebsiella.*[40]

Platelet Dysfunction with Carbenicillin and Ticarcillin   A nearly universal platelet dysfunction has been shown with high doses of carbenicillin and ticarcillin.[41,42] This becomes manifest in the form of increased bleeding time and decreased clot retraction with normal platelet counts. This effect must be considered if a clinical bleeding diathesis occurs in a patient receiving carbenicillin or ticarcillin.

Agranulocytosis This has been reported with ampicillin.[43]

Interstitial Nephritis This has been reported with ampicillin.

Pseudomembranous Colitis This has been reported with ampicillin,[45] and presumably could occur with carbenicillin or ticarcillin (see clindamycin, pp. 119–20).

Neurotoxicity This may occur with high doses or in renal failure, as with penicillin. Because of the very high doses necessary to treat *P. aeruginosa* infections, this toxic manifestation is more likely to be seen. Therefore, careful neurologic monitoring of the individual patient is prudent.

Irritation of Veins Carbenicillin and ticarcillin are irritating to veins; the high doses usually given must, therefore, be administered through a central vein.

Cation Content

Ampicillin—sodium salt (for intravenous use), 2.8 to 3.4 mEq per gram
Carbenicillin—4.7 mEq per gram
Ticarcillin—5.2 to 6.5 mEq per gram

Note that when compared with carbenicillin, the lower dosage of ticarcillin used for *P. aeruginosa* infections, results in a net saving of sodium load; this has been cited as an advantage of ticarcillin over carbenicillin.[42]

Hypokalemia This has occurred with carbenicillin and with ticarcillin.[42] Hyponatremia and water intoxication have also occurred; therefore, total electrolyte surveillance seems appropriate.

Teratogenicity Ticarcillin should not be used in pregnant women since it has been shown to be teratogenic in mice.[42]

DOSAGE

Ampicillin For serious infections (e.g., gram-negative bacteremia, biliary tract infection), 8 to 16 gm every 24 hours, divided into doses every 3 to 4 hours (pediatric dose: 100 to 400 mg/kg/24 hr).

Carbenicillin For serious infections, including *Pseudomonas aeruginosa*, 20 to 30 gm every 24 hours, divided into doses every 3 to 4 hours (pediatric dose: 400 to 600 mg/kg/24 hr).

Ticarcillin   For serious infections, including *Pseudomonas aeruginosa,*
14 to 21 gm every 24 hours, divided into doses every 3 to 4 hours (pediatric
dose: 200 to 300 mg/kg/24 hr; for neonates, a special dosage schedule
is used: under 2000 gm, 225 mg/kg/24 hr; over 2000 gm, 300 to 450 mg/
kg/24 hr; and for all over 7 days of age, 600 mg/kg/24 hr).

Urinary Tract Infection   Approximately one-quarter of the above adult
dosages are used.

Usage in Renal Failure   Dosages of these agents are reduced by one-half
in moderate renal failure (creatinine clearance less than 30 ml/min,
serum creatinine greater than 4 mg/100 ml), and to one-fourth in patients requiring dialysis.[46] The dose of carbenicillin in anuric patients
is 2 gm every 12 hours. These drugs are dialyzable.

CEPHALOSPORINS

Major advantage	Low toxicity, very high doses possible
Major disadvantage	Allergy
Primary indication	Infections due to susceptible *Klebsiella*
Secondary indication	Infections due to gram-positive cocci, primarily staphylococci
Caveats	Cross-reaction with penicillins may occur in allergic patients. The indications for these drugs are limited; there has been a tendency to overuse these drugs

A plethora of drugs from this group is available with minimal differences between them;[47] this group, furthermore, has been subjected to
the most conspicuous overuse of any group of antibiotics. The cephalosporins are in many ways very similar to the penicillins. Cephalothin
(Keflin), cefazolin (Kefzol, Ancef), cephaloridine (Loridine), cephapirin
(Cefadyl), and cephradine (Velosef) are available for parenteral use.
A number of others are available for oral use. Due to its renal toxicity,
cephaloridine is not advocated for use in an intensive care unit.

Recently, two new cephalosporin-like drugs have become available
which have somewhat different antibacterial spectra from the above
older agents, all of which can be considered to be antimicrobially
identical.[48,49] One of these is cefamandole (Mandol), a true cephalosporin
and the other, cefoxitin (Mefoxin) a cephamycin which is for all practical purposes a cephalosporin. These agents have greater in vitro activity
against certain gram-negative aerobes, specifically *Hemophilus influenzae, Enterobacter* sp., indole-positive *Proteus* sp., and possibly also some

gram-negative anaerobes. Thus, separate discs are used to test susceptibility to these agents.[48] In selected cases, these agents may provide useful
activity in infections due to organisms resistant to other cephalosporins
and susceptible to one of them. However, they offer no clear advantage
over other cephalosporins for infections due to organisms susceptible
to all cephalosporins. Also, one must exercise caution using these agents
in cases of meningitis (p. 106).[50]

ADVANTAGES

Drug of Choice Cephalosporins are the drugs of choice for a limited
group of bacterial pathogens.

GRAM-NEGATIVE AEROBES

Klebsiella sp.—when shown to be susceptible or presumed to be so from
    clinical or epidemiologic data
Certain strains of other gram-negative aerobes, such as *E. coli, Entero-*
    bacter sp., or *Proteus* sp., which have been shown to be susceptible.

Note that for the above gram-negative aerobes, ampicillin is the drug
of first choice; cephalosporins may be used in selected cases with a history of penicillin allergy (see below) if susceptibility of the organism
to cephalosporins has been shown or can be presumed.

Drug of Alternate Choice All anaerobes susceptible to penicillin; penicillin is the drug of first choice in such cases. Cephalosporins may be substantially less active than penicillin on a weight basis against many
strains of anaerobes.[51]

Use in Synergistic Combinations

GRAM-POSITIVE AEROBES

Staphylococcus aureus endocarditis—gentamicin is sometimes used
    with a cephalosporin for treatment of this condition, as it is with
    oxacillin or nafcillin

GRAM-NEGATIVE AEROBES

Klebsiella pneumoniae pneumonia—gentamicin is used with a cepha-
    losporin for this condition in an attempt to achieve rapid killing
    of organisms in a very dangerous infection, although no studies have
    shown an advantage

Penicillinase Resistance The cephalosporins are resistant to bacterial
penicillinase, thus making them drugs of alternate choice for staphylo-

coccal infections. Cefazolin, however, is partially inactivated by penicillinase.[52]

High Therapeutic-to-Toxic Ratio Same as penicillin.

Bactericidal Effect Same as penicillin.

Substitution for Penicillin in the Allergic Patient One frequent use of cephalosporins is as a substitute for penicillin or penicillin derivatives in the patient allergic to penicillin.[53] There is clearly some allergic cross-reactivity between cephalosporins and penicillins, but it does not appear to be as complete as the cross-reactivity among the penicillin derivatives themselves (or among the cephalosporins themselves). With history of anaphylaxis or of generalized urticaria, prudence would dictate avoidance of cephalosporins as well as of penicillins (p. 95).[51]

DISADVANTAGES

Allergic Reactions As in the case of penicillin, allergic reactions represent the largest single group of adverse effects. Prevalence is about as high as penicillin allergy.[53] The same precautions should be maintained with cephalosporins as with penicillins in order to avoid life-threatening reactions. No skin-test reagents are currently available for detection of cephalosporin allergy. All cephalosporins are cross-allergenic.

Ineffectiveness in Meningitis The clinical record of cephalosporins in the treatment of meningitis caused by susceptible organisms is poor, even when some penetration of the blood-brain barrier can be demonstrated. The reason for this is not clearly understood. In addition, there are cases reported of patients developing meningitis due to various organisms susceptible to cephalosporins while receiving intravenous cephalosporin therapy (3 to 12 gm/24 hr).[54] Cephamandole has been ineffective in treatment of meningitis due to susceptible *Hemophilus influenzae*.[50]

Ineffectiveness Against Neisseria Although in vitro susceptibility occurs, cephalosporins are not dependable for treatment of meningococcal meningitis or of gonorrhea.

Oxacillin-Resistant (Methicillin-Resistant) Staphylococci Strains of *S. aureus* which are resistant to the penicillinase-resistant semisynthetic penicillins (methicillin, oxacillin, nafcillin) are not dependably susceptible to cephalosporins, even if indicated to be so by disc susceptibility testing.[23,55] For all general purposes, cephalosporins are useless against these organisms.

False-Positive Direct Coomb's Test A positive direct Coomb's test becomes nearly uniformly present with cephalothin administration at high doses or in patients with renal failure.[56] This complicates blood-banking, since it interferes with the crossmatch. This is a nonimmunologic phenomenon and is not accompanied by hemolytic anemia. The false-positive Coomb's test probably occurs with all cephalosporins.

Acute Tubular Necrosis with Cephaloridine This unique problem of renal toxicity occurs at dosages greater than 4 gm/24 hr or in patients with renal failure; it may also be potentiated by renal-active or renal-toxic drugs frequently used in an intensive care unit (e.g., furosemide, aminoglycoside antibiotics). This problem, combined with the lack of particular advantages of cephaloridine over the other available antibiotics, seems to limit its usefulness.[57] Rare cases of acute renal failure, probably similar to interstitial nephritis seen with penicillin derivatives, have been reported with other cephalosporins.[58,59]

Hemolytic Anemia This has been reported with cephalothin.[60]

Granulocytopenia This has been reported with all parenteral cephalosporins.[61]

Pseudomembranous Colitis This has been reported with cephalosporins.

Thrombocytopenia This has been reported with cephalothin.[62]

Irritation of Veins Cephalothin is very irritating to veins; the other parenteral cephalosporins are less so.

Cation Content

Cephalothin—2.8 mEq sodium per gram
Cefazolin—2.1 mEq sodium per gram
Cephapirin—2.4 mEq sodium per gram
Cephradine—6 mEq sodium per gram
Cefamandole—3.3 mEq sodium per gram
Cefoxitin—2.3 mEq sodium per gram

DOSAGE

Cephalothin In severe infections, 6 to 12 gm per day divided into 3- to 4-hour intervals (pediatric dosage: 80 to 160 mg/kg/24 hr).

Cefazolin In severe infections, 4 to 6 gm per day divided into 3- to 6-hour intervals (pediatric dosage: 100 mg/kg/24 hr). Cefazolin has a somewhat longer serum half-life (0.8 to 2.2 hours in normal individuals) than the other cephalosporins.

Cephapirin Similar to cephalothin.

Cephradine Similar to cefazolin.

Cefamandole Similar to cephalothin.

Cefoxitin Similar to cephalothin. (Cefoxitin has not been officially released for use in infants and children.)

Usage in Renal Failure In patients with very poor renal function (creatinine clearance of less than 30 ml/min, serum creatinine greater than 4 mg/100 ml, or oliguria), dosage should be cut by one-fourth to one-half. In anuric patients, the serum half-life of cephalothin is 3 to 18 hours, and that of cefazolin 18 to 36 hours.[63] These drugs are dialyzable, so the normal dosage is used in patients while peritoneal or hemodialysis is being carried out.

AMINOGLYCOSIDES

Major advantage	Effective against many gram-negative aerobes not susceptible to other classes of agents
Major disadvantage	Toxicity (nephrotoxicity and ototoxicity) limits dosage and the ability to facilitate diffusion into closed spaces or antimicrobial action in the presence of purulent exudate
Primary indication	Serious infection due to susceptible gram-negative aerobes (e.g., *E. coli, Klebsiella* sp., *Serratia* sp., *Pseudomonas* sp.) which are not susceptible to penicillins or cephalosporins
Caveats	In diminished renal function, careful dosage adjustment and monitoring of drug levels is necessary

Though of great utility, this series of antibiotics represents the best example of the race between development of new drugs and the emergence of resistant microbial strains. Each time a new drug of this group is introduced, with an increased antimicrobial spectrum, bacterial resistance to it becomes more widespread, especially in hospitals and most particularly in intensive care units.[64-66] Streptomycin, neomycin, kanamycin (Kantrex), gentamicin (Garamycin), tobramycin (Nebcin), and amikacin (Amikin) are the available aminoglycosides; however only the last four are still of general use in intensive care units.[67]

ADVANTAGES

Drug of Choice An aminoglycoside is the drug of choice for infections due to the following organisms:

GRAM-POSITIVE AEROBES

None.

GRAM-NEGATIVE AEROBES

Escherichia coli—resistant to penicillins and cephalosporins
Klebsiella sp.—resistant to cephalosporins
Enterbacter sp.—resistant to penicillins and cephalosporins
Serratia sp.—resistant to penicillins and cephalosporins
Proteus sp.—resistant to penicillins and cephalosporins
Pseudomonas aeruginosa
Other less common gram-negative aerobes, e.g., *Acinetobacter* sp., resistant to penicillins and cephalosporins

Note that the susceptibilities of these organisms to aminoglycosides are by no means universal, especially in hospital-acquired infections, and the organisms should be shown to be susceptible to the particular aminoglycoside by disc susceptibility testing. *P. aeruginosa* and indole-positive *Proteus* sp. (*P. vulgaris, P. rettgeri,* and *P. morganii*) are generally susceptible only to gentamicin, tobramycin, and amikacin.

ANAEROBES

None.

Drug of Alternate Choice   This situation does not occur. Although strains of *Staphylococcus* sp. are generally susceptible to aminoglycosides in vitro,[68] aminoglycosides are of very limited clinical usefulness against these organisms.

Use in Synergistic Combinations

ENTEROCOCCI

(*Streptococcus faecalis* and *S. faecium,* i.e., most Group D streptococci)

Aminoglycosides are used with penicillin for serious infections caused by these organisms. Disc susceptibility testing of these organisms is difficult to interpret; often the penicillin-gentamicin combination is useful even though the organism may show resistance to gentamicin in the disc testing. Approximately one-third of the strains of enterococci are resistant to the streptomycin-penicillin combination even when tested by quantitative methods; this resistance seems to correlate with lack of clinical efficaciousness. Thus, the penicillin-gentamicin regimen is generally recommended.[69] Occasionally, aminoglycosides are used in combination with vancomycin[70] for serious infections due to enterococci in patients in whom penicillin is contraindicated.

STAPHYLOCOCCUS AUREUS ENDOCARDITIS

Gentamicin is sometimes used with a penicillinase-resistant semisynthetic penicillin or a cephalosporin for treatment of this condition.[71]

KLEBSIELLA PENUMONIAE PNEUMONIA

Gentamicin is used with a cephalosporin for this condition; although no controlled studies have shown clinical advantage of the combination, it is nevertheless generally used since pneumonia due to this organism is such a dangerous disease.

OTHER SERIOUS INFECTIONS DUE TO GRAM-NEGATIVE AEROBES

Aminoglycosides are sometimes used in combination with carbenicillin or ticarcillin for synergism in these infections.

PSEUDOMONAS SP. INFECTIONS

Gentamicin, tobramycin, or amikacin may be used as an adjunct to carbenicillin or ticarcillin for treatment of *Pseudomonas* infections in order to retard the development of resistance to the carbenicillin or ticarcillin.

High Urinary Concentrations   The aminoglycosides are excreted by the kidneys, resulting in high urinary concentrations relative to serum concentrations. Therefore, these drugs are especially effective in urinary tract infection provided that renal function is adequate (creatinine clearance greater than 30 ml/min) and that there is no urinary tract obstruction. However, penicillin or a cephalosporin should be used in cases where urinary pathogens are susceptible to these drugs.[72]

Bactericidal Activity   Aminoglycosides are bactericidal to susceptible organisms and thus may be superior to bacteriostatic agents such as chloramphenicol in bacteremias or in infections in compromised hosts.

Tuberculostatic Activity   The aminoglycosides are all tuberculostatic and can act as parenteral adjunctive agents in the treatment of tuberculosis. There is no need to use streptomycin for tuberculosis if another aminoglycoside is in use, and the toxicities are additive.

DISADVANTAGES

Important Pathogens Are Not Affected   The aminoglycosides are not broad-spectrum. They are not active against anaerobic organisms and against some important gram-positive aerobes such as *Streptococcus pneumo-*

niae. Although in vitro activity is demonstrated against some other gram-positive aerobes, such as staphylococci and some streptococci, this is of limited clinical usefulness. The question as to whether an aminoglycoside should be used as part of a regimen for presumptive acute bacteremia if *Staphylococcus* sp. is one of the possible causative agents is controversial. Other agents should be selected if the possibility of staphylococcal etiology is high.

Development of Bacterial Resistance The spread of bacterial resistance to these agents in the "hospital flora" has tended to follow their introduction and heavy use. Much of this resistance is mediated by specific enzymes elaborated by the microorganisms, analogous to penicillinase, which render the antibiotic inactive by chemical alteration at specific sites on the molecule. The ability to manufacture these enzymes is usually mediated by episomes (R-factors) which can be passed between species, genera, and even families of bacteria. These episomes predated use of antibiotics, but with increasing antibiotic use, bacterial strains carrying them have been selected.[73] Attempts have been made to develop new aminoglycosides which are resistant to these enzymes; however, each available aminoglycoside is rendered inactive by at least one known enzyme.[74] Thus, the newer aminoglycosides should be reserved for cases of serious infection by organisms known, i.e., by disc susceptibility testing, or presumed, i.e., by clinical or epidemiologic data, to be resistant to other agents. Presumption of resistance in clinical circumstances may be indicated by the development of a new infection in a patient already receiving an aminoglycoside. Epidemiologic presumption of resistance can be defined as the development of a new infection at the time when organisms resistant to a patient's antibiotics are resident in the same patient area, and thus patient-to-patient transmission of the resistant organism is presumed.

Renal Toxicity and Ototoxicity These well-known effects of aminoglycosides are dose related and occur at dosages not far above therapeutic dosage. This narrow therapeutic index restricts the usefulness of aminoglycosides compared to penicillins and cephalosporins, which show toxicity only at extremely high dosage levels. It is still unclear if these toxic effects are strictly related to serum or tissue levels of antibiotic, or whether they are more related to *peak levels* or to *trough levels* (the highest level after a dose or the lowest level before a dose, respectively).[75] Both renal and ototoxicity are probably cumulative over long periods of time, so that they probably are more likely to become manifest in a patient who has previously received aminoglycosides.[76] There is a possibility of increased nephrotoxicity with the concurrent administration of aminoglycosides and cephalosporins.[77-79]

Neuromuscular Blockade The curare-like effect of aminoglycosides is rarely seen except with intraperitoneal instillation of the drugs in high doses, now seldom done since this problem has been recognized. It remains a risk especially when other neuromuscular blocking drugs are being used.[76]

Inactivation by Pus and at Acid pH   Aminoglycosides are reversibly bound and rendered inactive by components of pus.[80] In addition, activity falls with falling pH. This may explain the difficulty of treating closed-space infections, such as septic arthritis with aminoglycosides even though drug can be demonstrated within the closed space.

Poor Penetration into the Central Nervous System   Aminoglycosides cross the blood-brain barrier extremely poorly, even if the meninges are inflamed. Thus, to be of any effect in meningitis, these drugs must be given by intrathecal or intraventricular route.[81]

Increased Clearance of Drug in Burn Patients   It has become empirically evident in centers caring for burn patients that high doses of aminoglycosides are frequently necessary to maintain serum drug levels in the therapeutic range in patients with large body-surface-area burns. Necessary dosages have been as high as three to four times the usual dosages in adult patients. The mechanism of this increased drug clearance is not clear; skin loss of drug may occur, and increased glomerular filtration, affecting drug clearance, has been demonstrated in burn patients.[82]

DOSAGE

Kanamycin   Dosage is 1.0 to 1.5 gm per day (15 mg/kg/day) divided into doses every 8 to 12 hours; pediatric dosage: 15 mg/kg/day.

Gentamicin   Dosage is 240 to 300 mg per day (3 to 5 mg/kg/day) divided into doses every 8 hours; serum levels obtained 1 hour after a one-half hour intravenous infusion should not exceed 10 μg/ml; predose levels should not exceed 2 μg/ml for prolonged periods of time;[76,82] pediatric dosage: 6 to 7 mg/kg/day.

Tobramycin   Similar to gentamicin.

Amikacin   Similar to kanamycin. Serum postdose levels obtained as outlined above should not exceed 30 μg/ml, and predose levels should not exceed 4 to 8 μg/ml.[75]

Dosage in Urinary Tract Infection   Due to the excretion of aminoglycosides in high concentration in the urine, lower doses are sufficient for treatment of urinary tract infection. Urinary tract infection dosage for gentamicin and tobramycin is 60 to 80 mg per day (1 mg/kg/day) divided into doses every 8 hours; for kanamycin and amikacin, it is 500 mg per day (7.5 mg/kg/day) divided into doses every 12 hours. These lower doses should be used for infection which is confined to the urinary tract, without presumptive bacteremia or abscess. The dosage regimen described below for use in renal failure should also be used for urinary tract infection in renal failure.

Intraperitoneal Dosage   There is no advantage of intraperitoneal dosage for local peritoneal infection. However, adding an aminoglycoside to dialysate during peritoneal dialysis will aid in maintaining a stable serum level. The dialysate is prepared containing aminoglycoside at the desired serum level, and additional intravenous doses need not be given.[83]

Usage in Renal Failure   Because of the toxicity of aminoglycosides, dosage must be carefully adjusted in renal failure. A loading dose (5.0 mg/kg for kanamycin or amikacin, or 1 to 1.5 mg/kg for gentamicin or tobramycin) is given when therapy is initiated. A serum sample for creatinine determination should be drawn at that time unless a recent (within 24 hours) value is available. For maintenance dosage, one practical method is to use the same dose as the loading dose, giving it at increased intervals based on the serum creatinine or, more exactly, on creatinine clearance. For gentamicin and tobramycin, a between-dose interval in hours equal to eight times the serum creatinine will approximate an appropriate serum drug level; e.g., for a serum creatinine of 3.0 mg/100 ml, give the loading dose every 8 times 3 hours, that is, every 24 hours. For amikacin and kanamycin, the factor of 9 times creatinine should be used.[84] Serum drug levels should be monitored in any case of impaired renal function, with further dosage modification directed at maintaining the levels mentioned above.[85]

Intrathecal or Intraventricular Dosage[81]   Gentamicin: 4 to 8 mg/day (children 1 to 3 mg/day); tobramycin: same as gentamicin; amikacin: 20 mg/day (no reports of use in children). Note that care must be taken so that only the low dose is administered; doses similar to these given intravenously have been associated with neuropathy when given intrathecally.

SELECTION OF SPECIFIC AGENTS WITHIN THE GROUP

Kanamycin   The intrinsic ineffectiveness of this drug against *Pseudomonas aeruginosa* and the high prevalence of resistance of hospital strains of bacteria limit its usefulness at the present time. It has been suggested that kanamycin be used in infection due to kanamycin-susceptible gram-negative aerobes preferentially over the other aminoglycosides, in an effort to diminish the widespread use of the other, anti-*Pseudomonas* agents. Whether this will retard the further increase in prevalence of organisms resistant to the other aminoglycosides is unclear. The general principle is sound; however, decisions as to antimicrobial usage in an intensive care unit should be based on the conditions and antimicrobial susceptibility patterns in that unit.

Gentamicin This agent is effective against *Pseudomonas aeruginosa*, and resistance of this and other gram-negative aerobes is not yet common in most areas. However, in certain large hospitals, enzyme-mediated resistance to gentamicin is widespread and unfortunately tends to concentrate in intensive care units. In infections due to *Serratia marcescens*, susceptible to both gentamicin and tobramycin, gentamicin is preferred since it is on the average 2 to 4 times more active on a weight basis than tobramycin.[86]

Tobramycin This agent is inactivated by most of the same enzymes as gentamicin, so that it is essentially the same in antimicrobial spectrum. Some strains of *Pseudomonas aeruginosa* and rare strains of other gram-negative aerobes which are resistant to gentamicin may be susceptible to tobramycin. Among strains of *Pseudomonas aeruginosa* susceptible to both antibiotics, tobramycin may have an advantage over gentamicin, being 2 to 4 times more active on a weight basis.[87]

Amikacin[88] This recently released antibiotic is inactivated by only one of the enzymes which inactivate other aminoglycosides and thus has activity against many gram-negative aerobes resistant to other aminoglycosides. These strains are usually hospital associated. However, for strains susceptible to other aminoglycosides, amikacin has no advantage, and in the case of *Pseudomonas aeruginosa,* it appears to have somewhat less activity. In an intensive care unit, it may be wise to limit the use of this agent to serious infections caused by organisms that are resistant to gentamicin and tobramycin, proven by disc susceptibility testing, or strongly suspected on a clinical or epidemiologic basis. When usage is limited, amikacin can retain its advantage in treatment of infections due to organisms now resistant to other antibiotics. As noted above, such antimicrobial usage policies should be formulated for an individual intensive care unit based on conditions in that unit.

CHLORAMPHENICOL

Major advantage	Broad spectrum of activity and wide distribution in body spaces
Major disadvantages	Development of bacterial resistance; serious idiosyncratic hemotoxicity
Primary indications	Central nervous system infections due to *Haemophilus influenzae* and other gram-negative aerobes

Secondary indications	Severe systemic infections due to anaerobes and gram-negative aerobes, as well as mixed infections, not treatable with bactericidal antimicrobials
Caveats	Hematologic parameters must be watched; chloramphenicol must be given in reduced dosage in prematures and newborns to avoid the "gray syndrome"

Chloramphenicol (Chloromycetin) has maintained an important place in the care of severely ill patients. Its rare but severe hemotoxicity has resulted in a sharp curtailment in its use in the community setting, and for less severe infections, in a hospital setting. Paradoxically, this curtailment has made the antibiotics more valuable in the intensive care unit, since hospital associated organisms have frequently maintained susceptibility to it.

ADVANTAGES

Drug of Choice Chloramphenicol cannot be considered drug of first choice for any situations commonly occurring in an intensive care unit; it is a drug of choice for enteric fever due to *Salmonella* sp., particularly *S. typhi.*

Drug of Alternate Choice

GRAM-POSITIVE AEROBES

Streptococcus pneumoniae meningitis—penicillin is the drug of choice; chloramphenicol is used in cases of penicillin allergy
Others—chloramphenicol is active against a wide range of gram-positive aerobes, but bactericidal agents (penicillins, cephalosporins, vancomycin) are almost always perferable

GRAM-NEGATIVE AEROBES

Escherichia coli
Klebsiella sp.
Enterobacter sp.
Serratia marcescens
Proteus sp.
Occasionally other gram-negative aerobes such as *Acinetobacter* sp.

Note that in infections due to these gram-negative aerobes, penicillin derivatives, cephalosporins, or aminoglycosides are usually drugs of choice. Chloramphenicol is used in meningitis due to these organisms if they are resistant to the bactericidal antibiotics, penicillin, or broad-spectrum semisynthetic penicillins, or in some cases of infection by multiple organisms at other sites, in an attempt to treat several organisms with a single drug.

ANAEROBES

Chloramphenicol is a drug of alternate choice for many anaerobic bacteria. Penicillin is drug of choice for most, with the exception of *Bacteroides fragilis.* For *B. fragilis,* clindamycin is considered drug of choice, although chloramphenicol is nearly of equal value; the choice must be made on the basis of risk of toxicity.[89-91]

Use in Synergistic Combinations   None.

Wide Distribution in Body Fluids   Chloramphenicol, as a lipid-soluble drug, is distributed so well in body compartments that one can expect tissue levels to reflect serum levels in most parts of the body, including the central nervous system.[92]

No Modification of Dosage in Renal Failure   Chloramphenicol is metabolized to inactive conjugates in the liver; this metabolism is independent of renal function, so that the half-life of active drug is the same in the anephric patient as in the patient with normal renal function.[93] Only in the case of concurrent severe renal and hepatic failure should chloramphenicol dosage be modified; in these cases it probably should be cut in half.[94]

DISADVANTAGES

Bacteriostatic Effect   The effect of chloramphenicol on bacteria is to inhibit protein synthesis reversibly; thus organisms cannot grow, but will survive.[92] One must depend on host defense mechanisms for eradication of the organisms. This limits the usefulness of chloramphenicol in the granulocytopenic patient and in infections at sites protected from host defense mechanisms, such as endocarditis.

Resistance Development   Bacterial resistance to chloramphenicol develops rapidly in vivo.

Antagonism with Cell-Wall-Active Antibiotics   Chloramphenicol inhibits the production of cell wall proteins by bacteria, and thus retards the incorporation of cell-wall-active antibiotics into the cell wall, antagonizing their effect.[95] Although this antagonism has not been shown in vivo, it theoretically occurs with penicillin, penicillin derivatives, cephalosporins, and vancomycin. In cases where the simultaneous administration of chloramphenicol and a cell-wall-active antibiotic is necessary (e.g., undiagnosed meningitis in children), an unproven but frequently used method to avoid this antagonism, at least for the first dose, is to delay the chloramphenicol for about 2 hours after the first dose of the cell-wall-active antibiotic, to allow incorporation into the cell wall.[95]

Bone Marrow Suppression   The well-known idiosyncratic aplastic anemia seen with chloramphenicol has severely limited the use of the drug. This form of bone marrow depression is usually irreversible, is frequently fatal, and is not dose related. It may appear during or after discontinuation of chloramphenicol therapy; thus, the risk is run by the starting of a course of the drug and is not substantially modified by the later dosage; of course, prompt discontinuation is mandatory if bone marrow suppression appears. The theory that this form of bone marrow suppression is only associated with orally administered chloramphenicol has not been substantiated. The risk of irreversible bone marrow suppression is about 1 in 20,000 to 40,000 courses of therapy. Complete aplastic anemia (pancytopenia) is most common, but isolated suppression of specific cell types is also observed.[92]

Dose-related bone marrow suppression represents a different type of hemotoxicity which is generally reversible. It will occur in about one-half of patients receiving 3 gm chloramphenicol per day for 21 days, and in a greater proportion of those receiving a higher dosage.[96]

The Gray Syndrome   This is seen in premature and in newborn infants receiving chloramphenicol. It is characterized by pallid cyanosis, abdominal distension, and vasomotor collapse, frequently reversible by discontinuing the drug.[97]

DOSAGE

The usual dosage of chloramphenicol is 4 gm per day, given as 1 gm every 6 hours, for severe infections in adults. For more serious or life-threatening infections, up to 6 gm/day may be given initially, with rapid reduction of dose to 4 gm/day. Pediatric dosage is 50 mg/kg/day divided into four doses given at 6-hour intervals. In newborns or premature infants, dosage should be limited to 24 mg/kg/day to avoid the gray syndrome. Oral and intravenous dosages are identical. Chloramphenicol should not be given intramuscularly due to poor absorption.[98] In renal failure no dose modification is necessary except in cases of combined severe renal failure and severe hepatic dysfunction, in which cases the dosage is reduced to one-half or one-fourth.

CLINDAMYCIN

Major advantage	Broad-spectrum activity against major anaerobic pathogens including *Bacteroides fragilis*
Major disadvantage	Pseudomembranous colitis
Primary indication	Infection due to or presumed due to *Bacteroides fragilis,* originating from intestinal microflora
Caveats	Patients receiving this drug must be monitored carefully for diarrhea and the drug discontinued if it occurs. Clindamycin is not active against enterococci, a major pathogen originating from intestinal microflora.

Clindamycin (Cleocin) is one of a group of antibiotics which also includes lincomycin, erythromycin, and tri-acetyl oleandomycin. All have similar pharmacology and antimicrobial spectrum. The other members of the group are of little use in an intensive care unit, although erythromycin has recently been used for treatment of presumptive Legionnaires' disease.

ADVANTAGES

Drug of Choice Clindamycin is the drug of choice for treatment of infections due to the following:

GRAM-POSITIVE AEROBES

None.

GRAM-NEGATIVE AEROBES

None.

ANAEROBES

Bacteroides fragilis must be presumed to be resistant to penicillin. In a routine clinical laboratory, antimicrobial susceptibility testing of anaerobes is not available since well-standardized methods have not been developed. The clinician must presume that a given isolate will have the susceptibility pattern that is characteristic of its species.

Drug of Alternate Choice

GRAM-POSITIVE AEROBES

Staphylococcus aureus—penicillinase-resistant; semisynthetic penicillins or cephalosporins are the drugs of choice
Streptococcus pneumoniae—penicillin is the drug of choice
Streptococcus pyogenes (group A, β-hemolytic)—penicillin is the drug of choice

GRAM-NEGATIVE AEROBES

None.

ANAEROBES

Clindamycin is a drug of alternate choice for most anaerobes, penicillin being the drug of first choice for essentially all except *B. fragilis*

Use in Synergistic Combinations None.

Lack of Cross-allergenicity with Penicillin This makes clindamycin an alternative for some infections for which penicillin or penicillin derivatives would otherwise be used in the patient with a history of penicillin allergy.

Wide Distribution in the Body Clindamycin appears in bone[99] and joint fluid[100] in adequate levels, and has been associated with good clinical antimicrobial effect in various soft tissue infections.[101] However, it is not useful in meningitis.

DISADVANTAGES

Lack of Activity Against Important Pathogens Although clindamycin is active against most anaerobic bacteria, it is less active against several species of *Clostridium*.[102] It also is notably inactive against enterococci[103] which can be important pathogens in infections resulting from intestinal microflora, for which clindamycin is often used due to its anaerobic spectrum.

Pseudomembranous Colitis This is a specific colonic lesion which appears during or after administration of clindamycin.[102] It is not dose related. Reported incidence varies greatly in different hospitals, with clusters also occurring within a single hospital.[104] One study reported an incidence of 20 percent.[105] In half of these cases of diarrhea, true ulcerations were seen on colonoscopy. More typical series show incidences of 1 to 2 percent. Pseudomembranous colitis presents clinically as persistent diarrhea with abdominal cramps; fever is not characteristic. The stools often contain blood and mucus and may contain neutrophils. A characteristic ulceration with pseudomembrane formation is seen by endoscopy. Antiperistaltic medications, such as Lomotil, may aggravate the lesion. Recent observations have implicated strains of *Clostridium* resistant to clindamycin as possible etiologic agents; this, if confirmed, could explain the tendency of this reaction to occur in clusters. If diarrhea occurs in a patient receiving clindamycin, the drug should be stopped and sigmoidoscopy performed. This same syndrome has been observed with many other drugs with broad antianaerobic spectra, including ampicillin, carbenicillin, tetracycline, erythromycin, and lincomycin.[102] Thus, in cases of clindamycin diarrhea, another antianaerobic drug should be substituted with much caution and only if absolutely necessary. There is some evidence that oral administration of vancomycin may have a beneficial effect in cases which do not respond to discontinuation of the antianaerobic drug.

Ineffectiveness in Meningitis   Clindamycin does not diffuse across the blood-brain barrier sufficiently to be useful in the treatment of central nervous system infections.[106]

Bacteriostatic Effect Against Aerobic Organisms   This makes clindamycin inferior to penicillin derivatives or cephalosporins in infections susceptible to the latter bactericidal agents and also makes clindamycin ineffective in bacterial endocarditis.

Hepatoxicity   Elevation of serum liver enzymes has been reported, with serum glutamic oxalacetic transaminase 20 times normal, alkaline phosphatase 2 times normal, bilirubin of 3.5 mg/100 ml, and pathologic changes seen on liver biopsy.[107] This warrants discontinuation of the drug.

DOSAGE

Severe Infections   Dosage is 1800 to 2400 mg per day divided into doses every 6 to 8 hours (may go as high as 4800 mg per day).

Pediatric Dosage   Dosage is 25 to 40 mg/kg/day.

Usage in Renal Failure   Clearance of clindamycin is mainly hepatic. Thus, dosage need not be modified in renal failure. Clindamycin is not dialyzed, so the same dosage should be continued during dialysis.[63]

VANCOMYCIN

Major advantage	A bactericidal antibiotic active against staphylococci and streptococci, with no known bacterial resistance in clinical cases of infection
Major disadvantage	Ototoxicity and difficulty of administration
Primary indication	Serious or life-threatening infection by *Staphylococcus* sp. when penicillins or cephalosporins are not useful due to bacterial resistance or patient allergy
Secondary indications	Treatment of staphylococcal or streptococcal infection in the patient receiving chronic hemodialysis; oral treatment of pseudomembranous colitis associated with antianaerobic antibiotics
Caveats	This drug has a long serum half-life and low therapeutic index (ratio of toxic level to therapeutic level). It must be given intravenously for systemic infection, with close monitoring of renal function. Allergy is common.

Vancomycin (Vancocin) has been available for a considerable period of time, but has seen little use because of difficulty in administration and its toxicity. Recently, there has been a resurgence of interest in this antibiotic.[108] It has some resemblance to the aminoglycosides in its pharmacology and toxicity, but it is a cell-wall-active, bactericidal antibiotic, active primarily against gram-positive bacteria. It has several definite but special uses.

ADVANTAGES

Drug of Choice Vancomycin is not the drug of first choice for any systemic infections but is used orally for two types of colitis.

STAPHYLOCOCCAL ENTEROCOLITIS

Oral vancomycin has been shown effective against this condition which is an overwhelming intraluminal infection with *Staphylococcus aureus* seen in patients receiving antibiotics to which the staphylococci are resistant. It is characterized by severe diarrhea, with presence of a nearly pure culture of *Staphylococcus aureus* in the stools; this is best demonstrated by a stool Gram stain showing sheets of gram-positive cocci. This condition has become rare in recent years.

PSEUDOMEMBRANOUS ENTEROCOLITIS
ASSOCIATED WITH ANTIANAEROBIC ANTIBIOTICS

There is some evidence that oral vancomycin is useful in this condition.[108,109]

Drug of Alternate Choice

GRAM-POSITIVE AEROBES

Staphylococcus aureus and *Staphylococcus epidermidis*—Penicillinase-resistant semisynthetic penicillins or cephalosporins are the drugs of choice for infections due to these organisms. Vancomycin is used in cases of penicillin allergy, especially of the anaphylactoid type and in serious infections due to oxacillin-resistant (methicillin-resistant) *Staphylococcus* sp.

Enterococci (*Streptococcus faecalis* and *S. faecium;* most group D streptococci)—Ampicillin (for minor infections) or the combination of penicillin and gentamicin (for serious infections) are the drugs of choice for infections due to these organisms. Vancomycin is used in cases of penicillin allergy.

Corynebacterium sp.—Various species of *Corynebacterium* (diphtheroids) occasionally cause endocarditis, infections of vascular access sites for hemodialysis, cerebrospinal fluid shunt sites, or infections in immunocompromised hosts. Penicillin is the drug of choice for these infections in most cases; vancomycin is used if the organism is resistant to penicillin or if the patient has a history of allergy to penicillin.

Infections in Patients with Renal Failure—In infections caused by *Staphylococcus* sp., *Streptococcus* sp., or occasionally other gram-positive organisms in patients with renal failure or requiring dialysis, vancomycin is sometimes used because of ease of dosage (see dosage).

Use in Synergistic Combinations Gentamicin is sometimes used as an adjunct with vancomycin for treatment of serious infections, particularly endocarditis, due to enterococci; care must be taken because of the additive toxicity of these two drugs.[110]

Bactericidal Effect Vancomycin has a definite advantage over chloramphenicol, aminoglycosides, tetracyclines, and erythromycin for treatment of staphylococcal infections because it is rapidly bactericidal.[111] Vancomycin is bactericidal also against other gram-positive organisms with the exception of enterococci, against which it is bacteriostatic.[108]

Lack of Resistance Development Infections due to staphylococci resistant to vancomycin have yet to be reported, although development of in vitro resistance has occurred.[111]

DISADVANTAGES

Allergic Reactions   These are seen fairly commonly with vancomycin, particularly exfoliative erythroderm. However, vancomycin is not cross-reactive with penicillin or cephalosporins in allergic patients.

Ototoxicity and Nephrotoxicity   These reactions are dose related and very similar to those observed with aminoglycosides; they seriously restrict the therapeutic index of vancomycin. Serum creatinine must be followed and dosage adjusted for any change.[108,111]

Infusion-Related Toxicity   Fever and vein irritation occurring with infusion of vancomycin appear to be related to impurities more than to the drug itself. Although less troublesome now than at the time of the drug's introduction, they still may occur.[108] If vancomycin is given intramuscularly, necrosis of injection sites may occur. Thus, vancomycin must be given intravenously for systemic infections. Vein irritation can be minimized by diluting the vancomycin in at least 100 ml of 5 percent dextrose in water or 200 ml of normal saline solution. The methods used to diminish vein irritation with amphotericin B can be used with vancomycin (see p. 126).

Inability to Cross the Blood-Brain Barrier   Vancomycin will not penetrate into the central nervous system in useful concentrations when given systemically, although some entry of drug into the cerebrospinal fluid can be demonstrated in the presence of inflamed meninges. If it is necessary to treat meningitis with this drug, it generally must be given intrathecally.[108,112]

DOSAGE

For Severe Infections   Dosage is 2 gm/day, intravenously, divided into doses every 6 to 12 hours. Peak levels postdose should be 25 to 40 μg/ml and trough levels predose should be 3 to 10 μg/ml. Serum half-life in individuals with normal renal function is 6 hours,[108] so more frequent doses are unnecessary.

Pediatric Dosage   Dosage is 40 mg/kg/day, intravenously, divided into doses every 6 to 12 hours.

Oral Dosage   For treatment of pseudomembranous colitis associated with antibiotics, or of staphylococcal enterocolitis, 500 mg orally every 6 hours. Unfortunately, an oral preparation is not available, so that it is necessary to give the intravenous preparation by mouth, which is very expensive.

Intrathecal Dosage Dosage is 20 mg/day. Intravenous vancomycin in usual dosage should be given concurrently.[108]

Usage in Renal Failure In mild renal failure (creatinine clearance 30 to 50 ml/min, serum creatinine 1.8 to 2.6 mg/100 ml), the dosage should be reduced to 1 gm/day. In severe renal failure, a single dose of 1 gm weekly is usually sufficient. Vancomycin is only slightly dialyzed, so the same weekly schedule can be followed for dialysis patients.[113,114] Serum levels should be monitored in renal failure; levels greater than 30 μg/ml should be avoided.

AMPHOTERICIN B

Major advantage	The only agent available with broad-spectrum antifungal activity; for many fungi it is the only agent available
Major disadvantage	Administration is difficult, with severe adverse effects related to the infusion and to the drug itself
Primary indication	Invasive (systemic) fungal disease
Caveats	Must be given with extreme care, starting with a very low test dose. There are many technical problems with the infusion which may be unknown to the hospital nursing or pharmacy staff. Review of the prescribing information should be mandatory since the practicing clinician employs this agent so rarely.

Amphotericin B (Fungizone) is the only dependable active agent available for treatment of many of the fungal infections becoming increasingly prevalent in intensive care units. For yeasts (*Candida* sp., *Torulopsis glabrata,* and *Cryptococcus neoformans*), another agent, flucytosine (5-fluorocytosine, 5-FC, Oncobon), is available; however, it is not recommended as a single drug treatment of serious fungus infections because of a high incidence of fungal resistance to this agent[115] and the development of resistance in vivo.[116,117] Also, flucytosine is only available for oral administration.

ADVANTAGES

Drug of Choice Amphotericin B is the drug of choice for invasive infection due to the following fungi:

YEASTS

Candida sp.
Torulopsis glabrata
Cryptococcus neoformans

DIMORPHIC FUNGI

Histoplasma capsulatum
Coccidioides immitis
Blastomyces dermatiditis
Paracoccidioides brasiliensis (South American blastomycosis)
Sporotrichum schenkii

Some rarer fungal infections may also be included when susceptibility is shown to the agent (e.g., mucormycosis, aspergillosis).

Note that the infection must be truly invasive to warrant the use of amphotericin B. Frequently, these fungi are grown in cultures from various sites without evidence of actual invasion. Differentiation between surface colonization and invasion by *Candida albicans* and allied yeasts is discussed in Part 1 (pp. 69–72). In cases of dimorphic fungi, rising serologic titers or demonstration of fungal elements in tissue pathologically are frequently used criteria for confirming invasive infection. Positive cultures of cerebrospinal fluid, or presence of antigen in cerebrospinal fluid in the case of *Cryptococcus,* indicate the need for treatment.[118]

Drug of Alternate Choice This situation does not occur. For systemic infections due to susceptible fungi, amphotericin B continues to be the drug of first choice.

Use in Synergistic Combinations Flucytosine is frequently used as an adjunct drug with amphotericin B for treatment of yeast infections.[117,119] Although in vitro testing for synergism is suggested, this testing is beyond the reach of a routine hospital microbiologic laboratory. In addition, in rare cases, other agents such as rifampin show synergism with amphotericin B, but laboratory confirmation of this should be available before starting the adjunct drug.[117,120]

Lack of Resistance Development Development of resistance to amphotericin B during a course of therapy rarely, if ever, occurs.[116]

DISADVANTAGES

Side Effects Related to the Solubilizing Agent in Parenteral Amphotericin B Amphotericin B is an extremely water-insoluble compound; in order to administer it parenterally, bile salts are added to the preparation to form a colloidal suspension. The solubilizing agents cause a number of untoward effects which are observed during the time of actual infusion.[121] These include fever, nausea, vomiting, pruritus, headache, and at times, hypotension. The severity of these effects varies greatly with individuals, sometimes with severe side effects occurring with a low dose of 1 mg of amphotericin B. The effects tend to become milder with continued administration of the drug at the same dosage level. Premedication may avoid or alleviate some of these symptoms (see dosage).

Lack of Oral Absorption   Intravenous administration is absolutely necessary except for treatment of fungal infections confined to the gut lumen.

Renal Toxicity   This is the dose-limiting toxicity of amphotericin B; it is partially reversible, but has a cumulative, nonreversible component as well. It is manifested by rising creatinine in serum and abnormal urinary sediment. Renal tubular dysfunction also appear (see below). Serum creatinine rising toward 3 mg/100 ml requires suspension of amphotericin B administration. With return of creatinine to baseline, treatment can be resumed at a lower dose.[117,121,122]

Potassium Wasting   The renal tubular effects of amphotericin B include losses of potassium and magnesium which can result in hypokalemia or hypomagnesemia. Electrolyte supplementation may become necessary. It is important to avoid administering the electrolytes through the same intravenous line simultaneously with amphotericin B, since these may precipitate the colloidal suspension of the drug.

Hepatotoxicity   This is relatively uncommon, and is not dose related; however, severe liver failure can occur.[116] Liver function studies should be monitored during amphotericin B administration.

Anemia   Amphotericin B regularly induces a normocytic normochromic anemia which corrects after discontinuation of the drug.[123]

Specific Difficulties with Administration of the Drug   Amphotericin B is irritating to veins. It must be administered in dextrose in water solution, not in saline solution, since the latter precipitates a colloidal suspension. If a filter is used in the intravenous medication administration, it should have a pore size of no smaller than 1.0 μm in order not to filter out the amphotericin B colloidal suspension.[124]

DOSAGE

General Method of Administration   For most fungal infections, amphotericin B is given intravenously, starting with a test dose of 1 mg dissolved in 250 ml of 5 percent dextrose in water given over approximately 3 to 4 hours. Subsequently, daily doses are given, starting with 5 mg in 250 to 1000 ml of 5 percent dextrose in water and increasing by increments of 5 mg daily. Optimal concentration of amphotericin B in the infusion is 0.1 mg/ml. Infusions can be given over 3 to 8 hours. Final daily dosage is 1 mg/kg body weight. After this maintanence dose is reached, the dosage interval can be lengthened to three times per week, using the same dose. It is not necessary to shield the infusion bottle from light, despite earlier admonitions to this effect.[125]

Monitoring for Side Effects   The following determinations should be made during therapy with amphotericin B: hematocrit, serum potassium, serum magnesium, liver function studies, and serum creatinine (see disadvantages).

Suppression of Infusion-Related Untoward Effects   The following agents have been used to suppress untoward effects occurring during infusion of amphotericin B:

PREMEDICATIONS

Aspirin: 600 mg, or acetaminophen: 600 mg, for fever, pruritus, headache
Diphenhydramine (Benadryl): 50 to 100 mg I.V., I.M., or P.O. (or other antihistamine) for pruritus, nausea
Prochlorperazine (Compazine): 5 to 10 mg I.M. or P.O., or trimethobenzamide (Tigan), 250 mg P.O. or 200 mg I.M., for nausea and vomiting

CONCURRENT MEDICATIONS

Heparin: 1000 units, added to the infusion bottle to control phlebitis and possibly other infusion-related symptoms
Hydrocortisone (Solu-Cortef): 25 mg, injected into the infusion appartus to control phlebitis

POSTMEDICATIONS

Heparin: 1000 units, injected into the infusion apparatus to control phlebitis
Hydrocortisone (Solu-Cortef): 25 mg, injected into the infusion apparatus to control phlebitis

These medications should be used only if adverse effects appear and only to relieve the adverse effects. The premedications may also be repeated at appropriate intervals during the infusion period. The possibilities of adverse drug reactions or interactions from these medications should be kept in mind.

TOTAL DOSAGE OF AMPHOTERICIN B

For *Candida albicans* and Allied Yeasts   Dosage is 1.0 to 1.5 gm. In some cases of candidiasis confined to the skin or gastrointestinal tract, or of uncomplicated catheter-related *Candida* fungemia, a "minidose" regimen of 20 mg daily for 5 days (after appropriate test dose and dosage buildup as outlined above) has been used successfully.[126]

For Other Fungal Infections   Larger total doses, up to 3 to 3.5 gm are frequently necessary. In some cases, e.g., *Coccidioides* meningitis, lifelong maintenance therapy may be necessary.[127]

Intrathecal Dosage   Intrathecal dosage is 0.5 mg two to three times a week to a total dosage of 15 mg. Before injection, 25 mg of hydrocortisone is administered and allowed to diffuse a few minutes. Five ml of spinal fluid is then removed, mixed with the amphotericin solution, and reinjected.[116,121] Amphotericin B has been given intraventricularly via a subcutaneous cerebrospinal fluid reservoir, but a high risk of complications is encountered.[127]

Usage in Renal Failure   In severe renal failure, amphotericin B dosage should be cut in half; very little amphotericin B is excreted by the kidneys.[128] Amphotericin B is not dialyzable.

CONCLUSION

Antimicrobial agents have provided a needed weapon but clearly can act as a double-edged sword. Intensive care staffs must mount an effective guard to prevent misuse, misguided use, and most especially, overuse.

Peculiarities of bacteria, antibiotics, and the environment require a careful and cautious application of this most useful and prevalent form of therapy. The principles developed here transcend any single antibiotic and can thus be formulated into a matrix to incorporate newer antibiotics.

Reliance upon antibiotics alone will never suffice to cure infection in the intensive care unit: lost resistance, nutrition, immune response, environmental conditions, resistance patterns, the hazards of invasive devices, and other considerations must be given constant attention if we wish to achieve the ultimate goal of survival rather than concentrate upon infection and microorganisms alone.

REFERENCES—PART 2

1. Whelton A: Tetracyclines in renal insufficiency: resolution of a therapeutic dilemma. Bull N Y Acad Med 54:223, 1978

2. Kirby BD, Snyder KM, Meyer RD et al: Legionnaires' disease: clinical features of 24 cases. Ann Intern Med 89:297, 1978
3. Tsai TF, Fraser DW: The diagnosis of Legionnaires' disease (editorial). Ann Intern Med 89:413, 1978
4. Elkyn S, Phillips I: Metronidazole and anaerobic sepsis. Br Med J 2:1418, 1976
5. Applebaum PC, Scragg JN, Bowen AJ et al: *Streptococcus pneumoniae* resistant to penicillin and chloramphenicol. Lancet 2:995, 1977
6. Finegold SM, Bartlett J, Chow AW et al: Management of anaerobic infections (UCLA conference). Ann Intern Med 83:375, 1975
7. Moellering RC Jr, Wennersten C, Weinberg AN: Synergy of penicillin and gentamicin against enterococci. J Infect Dis 124:S207, 1971
8. Gutschik E, Jepsen OB, Mortensen I: Effect of combinations of penicillin and aminoglycosides on *Streptococcus faecalis:* A comparative study of seven aminoglycoside antibiotics. J Infect Dis 135:832, 1977
9. Smith JW, Johnson JE III, Cluff LE: Studies on the epidemiology of adverse drug reactions. II. An evaluation of penicillin allergy. N Engl J Med 274:998, 1966
10. Brown BC, Price EV, Moore MB: Penicilloyl-polylysine as an intradermal test of penicillin sensitivity. JAMA 189:599, 1964
11. Adkinson NF, Thompson WL, Maddrey WC et al: Routine use of penicillin skin testing on an in-patient service. N Engl J Med 285:22, 1971
12. Handbook of Antimicrobial Therapy, rev ed. New York: Medical Letter, Inc, 1976
13. Ries CA, Rosenbaum TJ, Garratty G et al: Penicillin-induced immune hemolytic anemia. Occurrence of massive muscular hemolysis. JAMA 233:432, 1975
14. Bloomer HA, Barton LJ, Maddock RK: Penicillin-induced encephalopathy in uremic patients. JAMA 200:131, 1967
15. Kurzman HA, Rogers PW, Harter HR: Neurotoxic reactions to penicillin and carbenicillin. JAMA 214:1320, 1970
16. Louria DB, Kaminsky T: The effects of four antimicrobial drug regimens on sputum super-infection in hospitalized patients. Am Rev Respir Dis 85:649, 1962
17. Bennett WM, Inger I, Golper T: Guidelines for drug therapy in renal failure. Ann Intern Med 86:754, 1977
18. Handbook of Antimicrobial Therapy, rev ed. New York: The Medical Letter, Inc, 1976, p 36
19. Sande MA, Johnson ML: Antimicrobial therapy of experimental endocarditis caused by *Staphylococcus aureus.* J Infect Dis 131:367, 1975
20. Sklaver AR, Hoffman TA, Greenman RL: Staphylococcal endocarditis in addicts. South Med J 71:638, 1978
21. Finland M: Perspective. Hospital-acquired infections: The problems of methicillin-resistant *Staphylococcus aureus* and infection with *Klebsiella pneumoniae.* Am J Med Sci 264:207, 1972
22. Klimek JJ, Marsik FJ, Bartlett RC et al: Clinical, epidemiologic, and bacteriologic observations of an outbreak of methicillin-resistant *Staphylococcus aureus* at a large community hospital. Am J Med 61:340, 1976
23. Plorde JJ, Sherris JC: Staphylococcal resistance to antibiotics: origin, measurement, and epidemiology. Ann N Y Acad Sci 236:413, 1974
24. Laverdiere M, Peterson PK, Verhoef J et al: *In vitro* activity of cephalosporins against methicillin-resistant, coagulase-negative staphylococci. J Infect Dis 137:245, 1978

25. Manufacturer's package literature: Bactocill (Beecham), Prostaphlin (Bristol)
26. Border WA, Lehman DH, Egan JD et al: Antitubular basement membrane antibodies in methicillin-associated interstitial nephritis. N Engl J Med 291:381, 1974
27. Burton JR, Lichtenstein NS, Calvin RB et al: Acute interstitial nephritis from oxacillin. Johns Hopkins Med J 134:38, 1974
28. Parry MF, Ball WD, Conte JE Jr et al: Nafcillin nephritis (letter). JAMA 225:178, 1973
29. Lee WS: Disc sensitivity as a diagnostic aid in the identification of Group D enterococci. Am. J Med Technol 38:496, 1972
30. Bennett WM, Singer I, Golpen T et al: Guidelines for drug therapy in renal failure. Ann Intern Med 86:754, 1977
31. Nelson JD: Should ampicillin be abandoned for treatment of *Haemophilus influenzae* disease? (editorial) JAMA 229:322, 1974
32. Ward JI, Tsai TF, Filice GA et al: Prevalence of ampicillin- and chloramphenicol-resistant strains of *Haemophilus influenzae* causing meningitis and bacteremia: national survey of hospital laboratories. J Infect Dis 138:421, 1978
33. Mitchell AAB: Incidence and isolation of *Bacteroides* species from clinical material and their sensitivity to antibiotics. J Clin Pathol 26:738, 1973
34. Roy I, Bach V, Thadepalli H: *In vitro* activity of ticarcillin against anaerobic bacteria compared with that of carbenicillin and penicillin. Antimicrob Agents Chemother 11:258, 1977
35. Kluge RM, Standiford HC, Tatem B et al: The carbenicillin-gentamicin combination against *Pseudomonas aeruginosa*. Correlation of effect with gentamicin sensitivity. Ann Intern Med 81:584, 1974
36. Anderson EL, Gramling PR, Vestal PR et al: Susceptibility of *Pseudomonas aeruginosa* to tobramycin or gentamicin alone and combined with carbenicillin. Antimicrob Agents Chemother 8:300, 1975
37. Schimpff S, Satterlee W, Yound VM, et al: Therapy with carbenicillin and gentamicin for febrile cancer patients. N Engl J Med 284:1061, 1971
38. Hoffman TA, Bullock WE: Carbenicillin therapy of *Pseudomonas* and other Gram-negative bacillary infections. Ann Intern Med 73:165, 1970
39. Parry MF, Neu HC: Ticarcillin for treatment of serious infections with Gram-negative bacteria. J Infect Dis 134:476, 1976
40. Ueo K, Fukuoka Y, Hayashi T et al. *In vitro* and *in vivo* antibacterial activity of T-1220, a new semisynthetic penicillin. Antimicrob Agents Chemother 12:455, 1977
41. Brown CH, Natelson EA, Bradshaw MW et al: The hemostatic defect produced by carbenicillin. N Engl J Med 291:265, 1974
42. Ticarcillin. Med Lett Drugs Ther 19:17, 1977
43. Manufacturer's package literature: Amcill (Parke-Davis), Omnipen (Wyeth), Penbritin (Ayerst), others
44. Maxwell D, Szwed JJ, Wahle W et al: Ampicillin nephropathy. JAMA 230:586, 1974
45. Keating JP, Frank AL, Barton LL et al: Pseudomembranous colitis associated with ampicillin therapy. Am J Dis Child 128:369, 1974
46. Bennett WM, Singer I, Golpen T et al: Guidelines for drug therapy in renal failure. Ann Intern Med 86:754, 1977
47. The cephalosporins. Med Lett Drugs Ther 18:33, 1976
48. Washington JA II: Differences between cephalothin and newer parenterally

absorbed cephalosporins *in vitro:* a justification for separate discs. J Infect Dis 137:S32, 1978

49. Moellering RC Jr: Cefamandole—A status report based on the symposium on cefamandole. J Infect Dis 137:S190, 1978

50. Steinberg EA, Overturf GD, Wilkins J et al: Failure of cefamandole in treatment of meningitis due to *Haemophilus influenzae* type b. J Infect Dis 137:S180, 1978

51. Tally, FP, Jacobus NV, Bartlett JG et al: Susceptibility of anaerobes to cefoxitin and other cephalosporins. Antimicrob Agents Chemother 7:128, 1975

52. Regamey C, Libke RD, Engelking ER et al: Inactivation of cefazolin, cephaloridine, and cephalothin by methicillin-sensitive and methicillin-resistant strains of *Staphylococcus aureus.* J Infect Dis 131:291, 1975

53. Hoeprich PD: Antimicrobics and antihelminthics for systemic therapy. In Hoeprich PD (ed): Infectious Diseases, 2nd ed. Hagerstown, Md: Harper & Row, 1977

54. Mangi RJ, Kandargi RS, Quintiliani R et al: Development of meningitis during cephalothin therapy. Ann Intern Med 78:347, 1973

55. Parker MT, Hewitt JH: Methicillin resistance in *Staphylococcus aureus.* Lancet 1:800, 1970

56. Molthon L, Reidenberg MM, Eichman MF: Positive direct Coomb's tests due to cephalothin. N Engl J Med 277:123, 1967

57. Mandell GL: Cephaloridine. Ann Intern Med 79:561, 1973

58. Engle JE, Drugo J, Carlin B et al: Reversible acute renal failure after cephalothin (letter). Ann Intern Med 83:232, 1975

59. Pastervak DP, Stephens BG: Reversible nephrotoxicity associated with cephalothin therapy. Arch Intern Med 135:599, 1975

60. Manufacturer's package literature: Keflin (Lilly)

61. Tures JF, Townsend WF, Rose HD: Cephalosporin-associated pseudomembranous colitis JAMA 236:948, 1976

62. Gralnick HR, McGinness M, Halterman R: Thrombocytopenia with sodium cephalothin. Ann Intern Med 77:401, 1972

63. Bennett WM, Singer L, Golper T et al: Guidelines for drug therapy in renal failure. Ann Intern Med 86:754, 1977

64. Finland M: Changing patterns of susceptibility of common bacterial pathogens to antimicrobial agents. Ann Intern Med 76:1009, 1972

65. Meyer RD, Halter J, Lewis RP et al: Gentamicin-resistant *Pseudomonas aeruginosa* and *Serratia marcescens* in a general hospital. Lancet 1:580, 1976

66. Moellering RC, Wennersten C, Kunz LJ et al: Resistance to gentamicin, tobramycin, and amikacin among clinical isolates of bacteria. Am J Med 62:873, 1977

67. Appel GB, Neu HC: Gentamicin in 1978. Ann Intern Med 89:528, 1978

68. Finland M, Garner C, Wilcox C et al: Susceptibility of recently isolated bacteria to amikacin *in vitro:* comparisons with four other aminoglycoside antibiotics. J Infect Dis 134:S297, 1976

69. Standiford HD, deMaine JB, Kirby WMM: Antibiotic synergism of enterococci. Arch Intern Med 126:255, 1970

70. Mandell GL, Lindsey E, Hook EW: Synergism of vancomycin and streptomycin for enterococci. Am J Med Sci 259:346, 1970

71. Sande MA, Johnson ML: Antimicrobial therapy of experimental endocarditis caused by *Staphylococcus aureus.* J Infect Dis 131:367, 1975

72. Kunin CM: Detection, Prevention, and Treatment of Urinary Tract Infections, 2nd ed. Philadelphia: Lea and Febiger, 1974

73. Smith DH, Gardner P: The ecology of R factors (editorial). N Engl J Med 282:161, 1970

74. Davies J, Courvalin P: Mechanism of resistance to aminoglycosides. Am J Med 62:868, 1977

75. Lerner SA, Seligsohn R, Matz GJ: Comparative clinical studies of ototoxicity and nephrotoxicity of amikacin and gentamicin. Am J Med 62:919, 1977

76. Weinstein L: Antimicrobial agents. Streptomycin, gentamicin, and other aminoglycosides. In Goodman LS, Gilman A (eds): The Pharmacologic Basis of Therapeutics, 5th ed. New York: Macmillan, 1975

77. Babrow SN, Jaffe E, Young RC: Anuria and acute tubular necrosis associated with gentamicin and cephalothin. JAMA 222:1546, 1972

78. Fillastre JP, Laumoneir R, Humbert G et al: Acute renal failure associated with combined gentamicin and cephalothin therapy. Br Med J 2:396, 1973

79. Cabanillas F, Burgos RC, Rodriguez RC et al: Nephrotoxicity of combined cephalothin-gentamicin regimen. Arch Intern Med 135:850, 1975

80. Bryand RE, Hammond D. Interaction of purulent material with antibiotics used to treat *Pseudomonas* infections. Antimicrob Agents Chemother 6:702, 1974

81. Intralumbar and intraventricular therapy of bacterial meningitis. Med Lett Drugs Ther 19:94, 1977

82. Loirat P, Rohan J, Baillet A et al: Increased glomerular filtration rate in patients with major burns. N Engl J Med 299:915, 1978

83. Smithivas T, Hyams PJ, Matalon R et al: The use of gentamicin in peritoneal dialysis. I. Pharmacologic results. J Infect Dis 124:S77, 1971

84. Orme BM, Culter RE: The relationship between kanamycin kinetics, distribution, and renal function. Clin Pharmacol Ther 10:543, 1969

85. Jackson, GG: Present status of aminoglycoside antibiotics and their safe, effective use. Clin Pharmacol Ther 1:200, 1977

86. Neu HC: Tobramycin: an overview. J Infect Dis 134:S3, 1976

87. Tobramycin sulfate (Nebcin). Med Lett Drugs Ther 17:85, 1975

88. Amikacin. Med Lett Drugs Ther 18:97, 1976

89. Finegold SM, Rosenblatt JE: Practical aspects of anaerobic sepsis. Medicine (Baltimore) 52:311, 1973

90. Finegold SM, Bartlett J, Chow AW, et al: Management of anaerobic infections (UCLA conference). Ann Intern Med 83:375, 1975

91. Gleckman RA: Warning—Chloramphenicol may be good for your health (editorial). Arch Intern Med 135:1125, 1975

92. Weinstein L: Chloramphenicol. In Goodman LS, Gilman A (eds): The Pharmacologic Basis of Therapeutics, 5th ed. New York: Macmillan, 1975

93. Kunin CM, Glazko AJ, Finland M: Persistance of antibiotics in blood of patients with acute renal failure. II. Chloramphenicol and its metabolic products in the blood of patients with severe renal disease or hepatic cirrhosis. J Clin Invest 38:1498, 1959

94. Suhrland LF, Weisberger AS: Chloramphenicol toxicity in liver and renal disease. Arch Intern Med 112:747, 1963

95. Hansten PD: Drug Interactions, 3rd ed. Philadelphia: Lea and Febiger, 1975, p 95

96. Gussoff BD, Lee SL: Chloramphenicol-induced hematopoietic depression: A controlled comparison with tetracycline. Am J Med Sci 251:8, 1966

97. Burns JE, Hoggman JE, Cass AB: Fatal circulatory collapse in premature infants receiving chloramphenicol. N Engl J Med 261:1318, 1959

98. Dupont HL, Hornick RB, Weiss CF et al: Evaluation of chloramphenicol acid succinate therapy of induced typhoid fever and Rocky Mountain spotted fever. N Engl J Med 282:53, 1970

99. Nicholas P, Meyers BR, Levy R et al: Concentration of clindamycin in human bone. Antimicrob Agents Chemother 8:220, 1975

100. Plott MA, Roth A: Penetration of clindamycin into synovial fluid. Clin Pharmacol Ther 11:577, 1970

101. Fass RJ, Scholand JF, Hodges GR et al: Clindamycin in the treatment of serious anaerobic infections. Ann Intern Med 78:853, 1973

102. George WL, Sutter VL, Finegold SM: Antimicrobial agent induced diarrhea— a bacterial disease (editorial). J Infect Dis 136:822, 1977

103. McGehee RF Jr: Comparative studies of antibacterial activity *in vitro* and absorption and excretion of lincomycin and clindamycin. Am J Med Sci 256:279, 1968

104. Kabins SA, Spira TJ: Outbreak of clindamycin-associated colitis (letter). Ann Intern Med 83:830, 1975

105. Tedesco FJ, Barton RW, Alpers DH: Clindamycin-associated colitis: a prospective study. Ann Intern Med 81:429, 1974

106. Hoeprich PD: Antimicrobics and antihelminthics for systemic therapy. In Hoeprich PD (ed): Infectious Diseases, 2nd ed. Hagerstown, Md: Harper & Row, 1977

107. Elmore M, Rissing JP, Rink L: Clindamycin-associated hepatotoxicity. Am J Med 57:627, 1974

108. Cook FV, Farrar WE Jr: Vancomycin revisited. Ann Intern Med 88:813, 1978

109. Bartlett JG, Chang TW, Onderdonk AB: Comparison of five regimens for treatment of experimental clindamycin-associated colitis. J Infect Dis 138:81, 1978

110. Watanakunakorn C, Bakie C: Synergism of vancomycin-gentamicin and vancomycin-streptomycin against enterococci. Antimicrob Agents Chemother 4:120, 1973

111. Weinstein L: Vancomycin. In Goodman LS, Gilman A (eds): The Pharmacologic Basis of Therapeutics, 5th ed. New York: Macmillan, 1975

112. Bayer AS, Seidel JS, Yoshikawa TT et al: Group D enterococcal meningitis. Clinical and therapeutic considerations with report of three cases and review of the literature. Arch Intern Med 136:883, 1976

113. Eykyn S, Phillips J, Evans J: Vancomycin for staphylococcal shunt site infections in patients on regular hemodialysis. Br Med J 3:80, 1970

114. Barcenas CG, Fuller TJ, Elms J et al: Staphylococcal sepsis in patients on chronic hemodialysis regimens. Intravenous treatment with vancomycin given once weekly. Arch Intern Med 136:1131, 1976.

115. Utz CJ, Shadomy S: Antifungal activity of 5-fluorocytosine as measured by disc diffusion susceptibility testing. J Infect Dis 135:970, 1977

116. Weinstein L: Flucytosine. In Goodman LS, Gilman A (eds): The Pharmacologic Basis of Therapeutics, 5th ed. New York: Macmillan, 1975

117. Drugs for the treatment of systemic fungal infections. Med Lett Drugs Ther 20:66, 1978

118. Abernathy RS: Treatment of systemic mycoses. Medicine (Baltimore) 52:385, 1973

119. Rabinovich S, Shaw BD, Bryant T et al: Effect of 5-fluorocytosine and amphotericin B on *Candida albicans* infections in mice. J Infect Dis 13:28, 1974

120. Smith JW: Synergism of amphotericin B with other antimicrobial agents (editorial note). Ann Intern Med 78:450, 1978

121. Bennett JE: Chemotherapy of systemic mycoses (part I). N Engl J Med 290:30, 1974
122. Miller RP, Bates JH: Amphotericin B toxicity. A followup report of 53 patients. Ann Intern Med 71:1089, 1969
123. Utz JP, Bennett JE, Brandriss MW et al: Amphotericin B toxicity. Ann Intern Med 61:334, 1964
124. Huber RD, Rifkin, C: In line final filters for removing particles from amphotericin B infusions. Am J Hosp Pharmacol 32:173, 1975
125. Tipple M, Shadomy S, Espinel-Ingroff A: Stability of amphotericin B in polyvinyl chloride intravenous infusion bags. Am Rev Respir Dis 112:145, 1975
126. Medoff G, Dismukes WE, Mead PH III et al: Therapeutic program for *Candida* infection. In Hobby GL (ed): Antimicrobial Agents and Chemotherapy—1970. Bethesda, Md: American Society for Microbiology, 1971
127. Diamond, RD, Bennett JE: A subcutaneous reservoir for intrathecal therapy of fungal meningitis. N Engl J Med 288:186, 1973
128. Feldman HA, Hamilton JD, Gutman RA: Amphotericin B in an anephric patient. Antimicrob Agents Chemother 4:302, 1973

THREE

Bleeding and Clotting Problems in the Critically Ill Patient

George H. Rodman, Jr.

Disorders of the clotting mechanisms and bleeding present some of the most perplexing problems in intensive care. Our present level of understanding of their pathophysiologic mechanisms is far from clear. What is known is quite complex; diagnostic tests are technically difficult to perform and not always available; and therapy is often of limited efficacy. Notwithstanding this somewhat pessimistic assessment, advances in the past few years in our understanding of pathophysiology, diagnosis, and therapeutic modalities have been impressive and encouraging. Although many of the problems in this area represent catastrophic complications in the critically ill—pulmonary embolism, stress gastrointestinal bleeding, and bleeding diatheses—preventive and therapeutic measures for many specific entities are now sufficiently effective to reverse previously hopeless outcomes. Overcoming the limitations we still face requires greater emphasis on knowledge of the fundamental mechanisms of disease rather than employing "cookbook" therapeutic plans because of the complex interactions among organ system functions that are common in such patients.

The general development of surgical practice in the last 20 years has been marked by a trend toward more ambitious goals (more extensive operative procedures on higher risk patients), and as such, has created problems largely unknown in the early years of surgery. Both the frequency and magnitude of bleeding problems has compelled the surgeon to develop a thorough understanding of basic coagulation mechanisms and disorders. Two perceptive quotations underscore the importance of the surgeon's constant striving to fully understand and control hemorrhage: "The only weapon with which the unconscious patient can immediately retaliate upon the incompetent surgeon is hemorrhage"—*W. S. Halstead;* "The confidence gradually acquired from masterfulness in controlling hemorrhage gives to the surgeon the calm which is so essential for clear thinking and orderly procedure at the operating table"—*Harvey.*

This chapter will not deal with surgical procedures and techniques for achieving primary hemostasis. Rather, it will be concerned with the most common disorders of the body's hemostatic mechanisms. Included in this review will be mechanisms of clotting, mechanisms of lysis, the causes of hemostatic failure, the methods of diagnosing hemostatic failure accurately, and guidelines for approaching common clinical crises associated with defects in hemostasis.

HISTORY

Both philosophical and practical reasons justify beginning a discussion of hemostasis with a brief review of the historical aspects of blood clotting. First, our present understanding of hemostasis is based on its historical development which, like many medical advances, exhibits a curious circular pattern. Second, Santayana may be right when he said, "Those who do not study history are condemned to repeat it." Third, since we do not yet possess complete understanding or agreement concerning the clotting process, we must maintain knowledge of both the presently accepted concepts as well as those that have been abandoned throughout history.

HISTORY OF SURGICAL HEMOSTASIS

When considering evolutionary priority, it is reasonable to assume the primacy of hemostasis: the organism could not develop a method for pumping, aerating, and detoxifying (cardiovascular, pulmonary, and renal systems) the body fluids before evolving a mechanism for preventing the external loss of such fluids (hemostasis).[1] Our current understanding of hemostatic principles is based on six major discoveries: direct pressure, cautery, tourniquet, ligature, blood fractions, and absorbable hemostatics.

The control of hemorrhage probably originated in primordial times when the first human applied digital pressure to a bleeding wound. Local remedies in the form of poultices (leaves, herbs, mud) were the next stage of hemostasis. The ancients—Hippocrates, Celsus, and Galen—advocated the use of the fire rod (cautery) and developed a plan for hemorrhage control: (1) pressure, (2) styptics, (3) stringents, (4) ligature, and (5) cautery, as a last resort.

During the Dark Ages, prior knowledge was often lost or disregarded. Hemostasis was no exception, and the hot iron reigned as the primary hemostatic method. Attempts to abandon the Arabian practice of using boiling oil were largely frustrated until the Renaissance era brought the genius of Ambroise Paré. A serendipitous finding supplied the spark; boiling oil ran out in the midst of battle. Paré noticed that the neglected wounds of casualties healed better than those that received boiling oil therapy. Later, using the anatomic studies of Leonardo and Vesalius, Paré insisted on direct vessel ligation and the abandonment of the heat principle.

Morel discovered the benefit of a tourniquet in aiding hemostasis. Harvey's description of the circulation, the application of the tourniquet, and carbolized cat gut enabled Joseph Lister to extol the virtues of operating in a bloodless field. Carnot's introduction of gelatin around 1900 led to the hemostatic utility of oxidized cellulose in 1942. Cushing introduced the silver slip for direct vessel control and then, working with Bovie in 1928, reintroduced the ancient principle of cautery. By so doing he completed a curious circular pattern common to many areas of achievement. Perhaps the application of the newest topical hemostatic aid (microcrystalline collagen)* could even be construed as modernization of the ancient poultice therapy.

* Avicon, Inc, Forth Worth, Texas: Avitene-MCH (microfibrillar collagen hemostat)

HISTORY OF COAGULATION SCHEMES

Hippocrates ascribed clotting of blood to temperature changes, i.e., cooling. Hewson, in 1771, observed that cooling in fact prolonged the clotting time.[2] He directed attention to the plasma rather than the red blood cell as the domicile of coagulation factors. He identified an insoluble plasma substance, which today we know as *fibrin*, as the end point of clotting and so introduced the modern era of the study of coagulation. This era reached maturity in the early 1900s when Morowitz[3] applied the knowledge gained from early protein chemistry to formulate the so-called "classical theory of coagulation." Morowitz suggested that thromboplastins (phase 1) were responsible for converting prothrombin to thrombin (phase 2) and that thrombin stimulated the conversion of fibrinogen to fibrin (phase 3). He also knew that the reaction required calcium. It was left to Armand Quick in 1935[4] to provide a method for measuring prothrombin, thereby adding *quantifiable* data to *qualitative* coagulation chemistry for the first time. Morowitz's theory is generally accepted as a clear definition of the later phases of coagulation (phase 2 and phase 3). However, it is phase 1, dealing with *thromboplastin generation*, that defies accurate description (Fig. 3-1).

Understanding the important role of platelets in clotting did not come easily. The identification of a platelet dependent bleeding disease, purpura hemorrhagica, antedated Bizzozeros' discovery of the platelet in peripheral blood by 150 years. Bizzozeros' observations in 1881[5] are amazingly accurate, even today. He noted that the clotting of blood occurred only after initial hemostatic control had been achieved by platelet accumulation at the site of vessel injury. Duke's[6] introduction of the *bleeding time test* in 1912 clearly confirmed the prime importance of platelets in the initiation of the clotting scheme.

Owren's[7] identification of Factor V in 1947 initiated a new era of discovery which has resulted in the identification and characterization of 13 coagulation factors. This knowledge "explosion" resulted in a chaotic profusion of terminologies. The International Committee on Nomenclature achieved some semblance of order in the early 1960s by assigning Roman numerals to each clotting factor, eliminating the confusing eponyms. Table 3-1 lists the known clotting factors and their synonyms; to aid in description, activated factors are identified, for example, as Va.

SCHEME OF COAGULATION

Comprehensive reviews of coagulation are available for in-depth study.[8-11] The following description will, we hope, provide operational knowledge for accurate diagnosis and treatment.

The normal mechanism of clotting requires participation of (1) vasculature, (2) platelets, and (3) coagulation factors. Capillary injury is resolved by coaptation of the severed ends due to the low intravascular

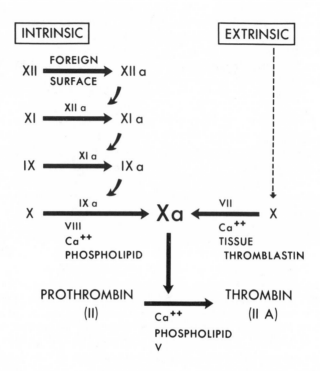

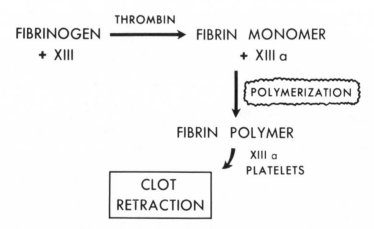

Fig. 3-1. (Top) The two pathways resulting in activation of Factor X (intrinsic & extrinsic) necessary for thrombin formation (Phase II). (Bottom) Fibrin formation from fibrinogen (Phase III).

TABLE 3-1
Known Clotting Factors and Synonyms

Factor	Synonym
I	Fibrinogen
II	Prothrombin
III	Tissue thromboplastin
IV	Calcium
V	Proaccelerin
VI	Not assigned
VII	Proconvertin
VIII	Antihemophilic factor A (AHF)
IX	Christmas factor
X	Stuart-Prower factor
XI	Plasma thromboplastin antecedent (PTA)
XII	Hageman factor
XIII	Fibrin stabilizing factor

pressure. Injured *arterioles* and *venules,* on the other hand, undergo active constriction due to the presence of smooth muscle in the vessel wall. Simultaneously platelets adhere to the damaged endothelial vessel lining. The key to this whole process of *platelet adherence* seems to be some as yet poorly understood ability of collagen or damaged cells to attract platelets. Platelets then undergo a "release reaction," whereby substances such as adenosine diphosphate (ADP), serotonin, catecholamines, and other intracellular products are extruded into the plasma. Some are potent platelet adhesive factors which attract and bind additional free platelets. ADP seems to be the most important of these adhesive substances, while catecholamines play an important role by inducing the further release of ADP. The resultant hemostatic plug formed by platelets will stop bleeding only if the following conditions are met: (1) the injury to the vessel wall is small; (2) vascular constriction or coaptation by pressure has occurred; and (3) intravascular pressure does not blow out the friable platelet plug. If these conditions are not met, bleeding would continue or restart if it were not for the formation of fibrin strands by the coagulation protein interactions which reinforce the platelet plug and add the strength necessary to resist intravascular hydrostatic pressure (Fig. 3-2).

The coagulation proteins produce a fibrin clot (i.e., an *insoluble* gel derived from the *soluble* protein called *fibrinogen*) by two pathways: *intrinsic* and *extrinsic* (Fig. 3-3). The distinction relates to the formation of *thrombin,* the catalyst for the fibrinogen-fibrin reaction. The intrinsic pathway uses factors present only in the plasma while the extrinsic pathway incorporates certain extraplasma (tissue) factors as well. Both seem to function simultaneously in vivo, although their separation in the test tube is quite clear. If platelet-rich plasma is placed in a glass

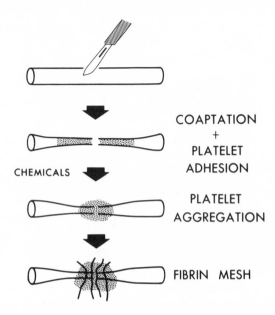

Fig. 3-2. Series of key platelet reactions initiated by trauma to a blood vessel resulting in clot at site of injury. Fibrin strands reinforce weak platelet plug.

test tube and incubated at body temperature, a visible fibrin clot will develop in about 5 to 15 minutes. However, when a trace amount of tissue extract from organs such as lung or brain is added to the same plasma, clot formation occurs very rapidly, within 10 to 12 seconds. In test tube no. 1, intrinsic Hageman Factor (XII) activated the clotting system utilizing substances present in plasma. In test tube no. 2, "tissue factor," an extrinsic substance, initiated the clotting by reacting with Factor VII. Thus the tissue factor pathway is a short cut bypassing many of the reactions found in the intrinsic system. The process whereby the activation of one coagulation factor catalyzes the activation of the next in sequence, culminating in the formation of thrombin, is the basis for the cascade or "waterfall" theory of the mechanism of clotting introduced by MacFarlane[12] and Davie and Ratnoff.[13]

The obvious difference in the two systems (intrinsic and extrinsic) resides in the potency of tissue factor. This substance has been found in a large number of different tissues (brain, lung, placenta, liver, spleen, kidney, caval and aortic intima, small vessel walls, leukocytes, and plasma membranes of endothelial cells). The highest concentrations in humans are found in brain and the intima of both arteries and veins. Most people call this tissue substance *thromboplastin*. The intrinsic system contains Factors VIII, IX, XI, XII, and platelet factor 3, all of which interact to result in the activation of Factor X. It is initiated by the

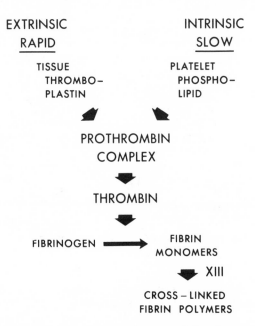

Fig. 3-3.   Both the rapid "extrinsic" pathway and the slower "intrinsic" pathway result in thrombin formation. What actually initiates the in vivo "intrinsic" pathway is unknown.

activation of Factor XII, in vitro by glass and in vivo by exposed collagen (therefore, any foreign substance works), or by other components of blood as yet unidentified. The extrinsic system requires the addition of tissue thromboplastin. The reaction with Factor VII (unique to the extrinsic system) and calcium forms a Factor X activator. Subsequent reactions in both groups are the same. Factor Xa combines with Factor V and the phospholipid present in either platelets or tissue thromboplastin, forming a prothrombin activator which rapidly converts prothrombin to thrombin. Once thrombin is formed, it catalyzes the conversion of fibrinogen to the insoluble gel fibrin. The conversion of fibrinogen to fibrin seems to be a two-step reaction. The first reaction, leading to the formation of fibrin monomer, demands thrombin action on fibrinogen; the second step, however, the polymerization of fibrin strands, is vital and occurs independent of thrombin. Once the fibrin monomers have aligned themselves to form fibrin strands (polymerization), another coagulation factor is necessary to add strength to these bonds—fibrin stabilizing factor, Factor XIII. Conveniently, this strengthening factor is activated by the direct action of thrombin. Factor XIII induces durable covalent bonding between the fibrin monomers. These tough fibrin strands then intertwine within the initially weak, but still hemostatic, platelet plug, providing the necessary reinforcement (Fig. 3-4).

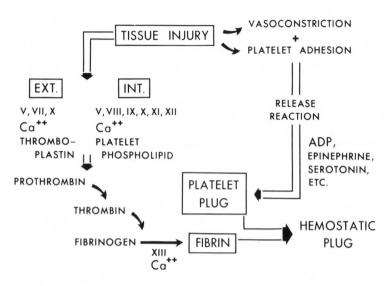

Fig. 3-4. Summary diagram illustrating the interplay of platelets and coagulation protein leading to hemostatic plug formation.

The extrinsic clotting system activated by the release of thromboplastin from damaged tissues is well understood, including the sequence of the activated factors. Unfortunately, the same agreement cannot be reached about the activation of the intrinsic system. While the in vitro trigger of the intrinsic pathway is the activation of Hageman (Factor XII) by contact with glass producing XIIa, the in vivo trigger still is unknown. Nevertheless, in both the extrinsic and intrinsic system the crucial step is the formation of active prothrombin by Factor X. Areas of present agreement are that four factors are required to activate Factor X (Factor IXa, VIII, phospholipid, and calcium) and that Factor Xa, V, calcium, and phospholipid are required to activate prothrombin. The exact sequence and nature of the reactions between these factors is still controversial.

In summary, phase 1 is the activation phase or the generation of thromboplastin; in phase 2 thrombin is formed from prothrombin by reaction with previously formed thromboplastin; and in phase 3, thrombin's action on fibrinogen results in fibrin formation. Polymerized fibrin then forms the visible end point of the coagulation scheme—the tough fibrin clot. This fibrin clot is not only an efficient sealant for hemostatic purposes but also a medium for tissue repair. Thus, the last step in hemostasis serves as the first step in wound healing, an obvious biologic convenience.

Several additional biologic conveniences of the clotting system are worth mentioning. (1) The platelet release reaction contributes directly to the coagulation mechanism by exposing lipoproteins (phospholipid and platelet factor 3) at the platelet surface which accelerates the clotting mechanism. (2) Thrombin, once formed, enhances the aggregation of platelets by inducing the release of ADP and other platelet constituents. (3) The whole process has a built-in amplification system since a few molecules of Factor XIIa can activate hundreds of molecules of Factor XI which in turn will activate thousands of Factor IX molecules. (4) The hemostatic process overlaps the inflammatory process via Factor XII activation which seems to be important in states such as sepsis induced disseminated intravascular coagulation (DIC).

Factor XIIa can activate prekallikrein-forming kallikrein which is important in the inflammatory response. Furthermore, this system is capable of internal amplification resulting in increased production of both Factor XII and kallekrin. In 1970, McKay[14] found that epinephrine activates Factor XII in vivo. This discovery has led to the postulation that clotting activation might occur in any stress state (high catecholamine levels), such as shock or sepsis. Even the chronic stress of intense economic and social pressures has been suggested as a cause of the tendency toward spontaneous clotting and myocardial infarction in well-developed countries.

The activation of Factor XII has been shown to stimulate the fibrinolytic system, increase vascular permeability and vascular dilatation, induce smooth muscle contraction, aid leukocyte migration through vessel walls, and induce pain. Although an appreciation of the full physiologic significance of these interactions still eludes us, it is obvious that Factor XII may play an important part in clotting, in clot lysis, in the complement systems, and in the kinin and inflammatory reaction.[15] Despite the obvious importance of Factor XII, its congenital absence in humans produces only a laboratory abnormality, i.e., an increase in the partial thromboplastin time, and is not associated with pathologic bleeding.[16]

FIBRINOLYTIC SYSTEM

If the finely tuned chemical reactions leading to clot formation were not appropriately balanced by a clot removal (lysis) system, widespread vascular thrombosis might occur. Several mechanisms allow the biochemical processes previously described to be tempered by physiologic control: (1) rapidly flowing blood greatly reduces the concentration of *any* activated coagulation factor by simple dilution; (2) activated clotting factors are rapidly removed by the liver; (3) naturally occurring inhibitors of Factor Xa and thrombin are abundant in plasma; and (4) activation of the fibrinolytic system allows clot lysis to limit the extent of coagulation. In pathologic states where rapidly flowing blood is absent (shock), or liver dysfunction is present, the coagulation system is inadequately controlled and excesses do occur. These clinical states will be discussed following a description of the fibrinolytic scheme.

Plasmin is the active proteolytic enzyme of the fibrolytic system (Fig. 3-5). Plasmin is formed from plasminogen, a protein residing

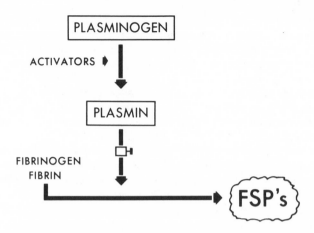

Fig. 3-5. Plasmin "splits" fibrin and fibrinogen forming "split products." Regulatory control (screw clamp) of plasmin activity occurs via naturally occurring plasmin inhibitors.

within the thrombus. The factor that activates plasminogen to form plasmin is unknown, but it may well be present within the wall of the vessel in which clotting occurs and diffuses into the thrombus. Such "tissue activators" have been found in urine (urokinases), tears, and saliva; they are also abundant in injured tissues. Stress (exercise) and catecholamines, known clotting activators, also activate the fibrinolytic system. In addition, naturally occurring plasmin inhibitors exist to modulate the activity of the lytic system (Fig. 3-6).

Plasminogen is always available for conversion to plasmin because of its strong affinity for fibrinogen. In other words, where fibrinogen goes (clot) so goes plasminogen (lysis). Naturally occurring plasmin is neutralized by plasmin inhibitors. However, plasminogen activators in the fibrin clot form plasmin which can lyse the clot from within while its external integrity is still preserved. What else activates plasminogen to form plasmin? Factor XII and thrombin—biologic convenience reigns supreme! Even fibrinopeptides, those breakdown products of thrombins, are felt to activate plasminogen through their effect on fibrinogen. Finally, the mere presence of fibrin itself activates plasminogen.

Fibrin is composed of fibrinogen molecules (fibrin monomers). Plasmin can digest not only fibrin (fibrinolysis) but also fibrinogen (fibrinogenolysis). Thus, the digestive process of fibrin yields a number of fragments termed "fibrin and fibrinogen degradation products" or fibrinogen and fibrin split products (FSPs).

Routine laboratory procedures do not distinguish between fibrinogen and fibrin degradation products. These fragments may exert strong anticoagulant action by competitively inhibiting thrombin and disturbing the fibrin polymerization phase of fibrin formation. In addition, these

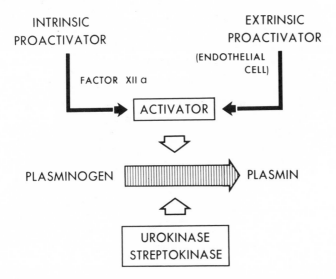

Fig. 3-6. Activation and modulation (urokinase) of the fibrinolytic system. Factor XIIa important in the "intrinsic" pathway also activates plasmin.

"split products" inhibit platelet aggregation thus affecting secondary hemostasis as well as primary hemostasis. Therefore, the physiologic role of the fibrinolytic system seems to be the removal of fibrin, the end product of coagulation, once it has served its purpose. The patency of blood vessels is either (1) *maintained,* since deposited fibrin is removed from the walls of vessels or (2) *re-established,* if thrombosis has occurred (recanalization).

In summary, the coagulation scheme has evolved into a system of complex interactions whose precision is assured by numerous inherent safeguards. These safeguards are in the form of rate control with the ability to bring the whole coagulation system to a screeching halt. This correlates with internal adjustments which allow the re-establishment of vascular integrity.

CLINICAL APPLICATION

DIAGNOSIS

Methods initiated to control hemorrhage which persists after initial anatomic hemostatic procedures frequently carry into the postoperative period. The list of possible reasons for the symptoms of primary hemostatic failure—oozing from all cut surfaces, absence of fresh clot, and disappearance of old clot—is long and complex. To unravel and correct these disorders, one must (1) have a good understanding of coagulation, (2) select and interpret the various diagnostic tests to pinpoint the cause, and (3) select appropriate therapy to combat the defect. Within the scope of this chapter we will assume surgical bleeding has been controlled. Nonsurgical bleeding may result from (1) a deficiency of platelets, (2) a disorder of the coagulation system, (3) excess fibrinolysis, or (4) presence of an anticoagulant. These defects may be congenital or acquired. *Time permitting, a searching history and physical examination are the most valuable guides in detecting hemorrhagic disorders.* However, for the crisis state which often confronts those caring for the critically ill patient, specific lab tests may be the only means of establishing the diagnosis (Table 3-2).

TABLE 3-2

Clotting Factors, Minimum Level Required for Hemostasis,
and Clinical Manifestation of Deficiency State

Factor	Minimum Level Hemostasis	Clinical Importance
I	100 mg%	Rare as isolated defect
II	20–40%	Liver disease coumadin $R_x \downarrow$ vitamin K
V	< 25%	Labile factor in stored blood
VII	10–20%	Rare as isolated defect
VIII	> 30% Major surgery < 30% Minor surgery	Classical hemophilia von Willebrand's disease
IX	25–30%	Acts like hemoph. A
X	10–20%	Rare
XI	15–25%	Rare
XII	No bleeding if level ↓	—
XIII	< 5%	—

History and Physical Examination The history should include directed questions. Remember, most patients usually don't volunteer a bleeding tendency history since it is "normal" for them. Questions searching for specific medications (aspirin, coumadin, etc.) may avoid disasterous complications. The physical examination may reveal multiple bruises, hematomas, telangiectasis, or a large spleen or liver. As a general rule, a large liver usually doesn't function well, either in the manufacturing or clearing of coagulation factors. If the history or physical exam suggests a defect in hemostasis, then a minimum battery of tests should include bleeding time, platelet count, peripheral smear, PT, PTT, and thrombin time.

Laboratory Tests The standard Lee-White whole blood clotting time enjoys historical prestige but not clinical usefulness. It may fail to detect all but the most severe clotting factor deficiencies. Evaluation of clot retraction, if excessive fibrinolysis is suspected, may be the most important use of the whole blood clotting test.

The bleeding time tests primary hemostatic plug (platelet) formation. *This test will be abnormal in any quantitative or qualitative platelet defect.* The platelet count should be known in order to properly interpret abnormalities of the bleeding time. The bleeding time is rarely prolonged until the platelet count drops below 100,000 per cubic millimeter. Prolongation of the bleeding time in the presence of a normal platelet count suggests that a *qualitative* platelet abnormality exists and further platelet testing may be indicated. Several reviews on the different systems employed to test qualitative platelet function have been published.[17-19] The modified Ivy method of determining bleeding time utilizes a blood pressure cuff around the upper arm inflated to 40 mm of mercury followed by a calibrated skin incision in the forearm measuring 1 mm in depth and 10 mm in length. The end point of the test is cessation of bleeding. The mechanics of the test clearly limit its usefulness as a repetitive test in the critically ill patient.

History	Bleeding gums, bruising, epistaxis; "normal" may be abnormal
Physical exam	Hepatosplenomegaly, hematomas, multiple bruises, telangiectasias
Lee-White clotting time	Nonspecific; evaluation of clot lysis
Bleeding time	Qualitative or quantitative (<100,000) platelet abnormality; modified Ivy method; limited application in ICU

Several observations made by investigators during the attempt to elucidate the clotting mechanism form the basis for the modern laboratory workup of bleeding disorders. If plasma is extracted from whole blood anticoagulated with a calcium chelating material, such as oxalate or citrate, a fibrin clot will form 2 to 3 minutes after the addition of calcium. If the plasma is exposed to glass during collection, clotting will occur even faster after the addition of calcium (60 to 90 seconds). If tissue factor (thromboplastin) and calcium are added, a solid fibrin clot usually forms in about 12 seconds—the one-stage prothrombin time (PT) test. This PT test devised by Quick is the most sensitive test for measuring the efficiency of the extrinsic pathway leading to thrombin formation. Prolongation of the PT will occur if any of the coagulation factors of the extrinsic or intrinsic pathways (Factors I, II, V, VII, X) are deficient or inhibited.

The clotting time of a mixture of citrated plasma, calcium ions, and crude phospholipid (derived from brain tissue or soybeans) is called the partial thromboplastin time (PTT). The PTT test is the best screening test for defects in the intrinsic clotting system. Prolongation of the PTT suggests a missing factor or circulating anticoagulant. Thus, a deficiency, absence, or inhibition of Factors I, II, V, VIII, IX, X, XI, or XII results in an elevated PTT.

The conversion of fibrinogen to fibrin is measured by the *thrombin time*. The control test is performed by adding a dilute solution of bovine thrombin to a pure solution containing fibrinogen (patient's plasma) and observing the time for formation of visible fibrin clots. Thrombin is normally undetectable in circulating blood. Prolongation of the thrombin time occurs if the concentration of fibrinogen is very low or high, or if inhibitors of fibrin formation are present. These inhibitors may be intrinsic, such as the degradation products of fibrinogen, or extrinsic, such as heparin.

By combining these three tests (PT, PTT, thrombin time), proper diagnosis can be approached. A prolonged PTT in association with a normal PT and thrombin time points to the intrinsic system and suggests a deficiency or inhibition of those factors peculiar to the intrinsic system (Factors VIII, IX, XI, and XII). The specific defect will require further testing using a known factor-deficient plasma. Clinically, the most common causes of an isolated elevation of PTT are classic hemophilia and von Willibrand's disease. An isolated increase in PT with normal PTT and thrombin times suggest Factor VII deficiency—a factor found solely in the extrinsic system. These two combinations, isolated PT or isolated PTT, are relatively rare findings in the bleeding patient. Most common is an increased PT and increased PTT with normal thrombin time, suggesting defects in both intrinsic and extrinsic system prior to the reaction of thrombin with fibrinogen.

Both tests (PT and PTT) are prolonged if an affected factor is less than 30 percent of the normal circulating blood level. Prolongation of both the PT and PTT are common abnormalities in liver disease when hepatic production of coagulation factors (Factors II, V, VII, IX, X) is impaired. Likewise, vitamin K deficiency or coumadin therapy will cause decreased production of vitamin K dependent factors by the liver (Factors II, VII, IX, X). Prolongation of all three tests (PT, PTT, and thrombin time) occurs most commonly in disastrous states or diffuse hemorrhage secondary to circulating thrombin inhibitors, either heparin or products of fibrin digestion found in secondary fibrinolysis, i.e., DIC. True hypofibrinogenemia may result in prolongation of clotting in all three test systems, but rarely does any clinical situation produce the required low levels (50 to 100 mg%). Thus, the thrombin time may serve as a screening test for secondary fibrinolysis; other, more specific tests are available—latex agglutination, staphylococcal clumping test, and immunologic determinations for fibrin split products.

Test	System Tested	Factors Tested
PT	Extrinsic	I, II, V, VII, X
PTT	Intrinsic	I, II, V, VIII, IX, X, XI, XII
TT	Fibrinogen; fibrin	Fibrinogen, FSPs, heparin

Occasionally, it is important to identify the specific isolated defect of coagulation prompting the bleeding state. Single factor deficiency is characteristic of congenital bleeding while the bulk of acquired defects are due to multiple factor deficiencies. When necessary, factor assay is accomplished by establishing a test system in which all coagulation factors are present in abundance save one: the absent factor then is rate limiting. Standard curves are constructed by adding various dilutions of normal plasma to deficient (e.g., Factor VIII) plasma and measuring the clotting time based on the PTT. The plasma to be tested is evaluated in a similar manner. The amount of factor deficiency in the test plasma is then deducted by comparing clotting time in the test plasma versus that in normal plasma.

Test	Mechanism	Frequency	Disease States
↑ PT	↓ VII	Rare	
↑ PTT	↓ VIII,IX	Rare	Classical hemophilia; von Willebrand's disease
↑ PT, PTT	Intrinsic, extrinsic	Common	Liver disease, vitamin K deficiency, coumadin therapy
↑ PT, ↑ PTT, ↑ TT	Intrinsic, extrinsic, fibrin formation	Disastrous clinical situations	DIC, FSPs, heparin, hypofibrinogenemia (<100 mg%)

CONGENITAL DEFECTS

A hereditary deficiency of any of the clotting factors (except Factor XII) is associated with a bleeding disorder. An in-depth discussion of all congenital coagulopathies is not within the scope of this chapter. However, the two most frequent disorders, classical hemophilia and von Willebrand's disease, will illustrate the importance of sophisticated laboratory analysis and directed therapy in the correction of these coagulopathies.

Hemophilia A   The most common congenital disorder of bleeding is hemophilia A (Factor VIII deficiency), which occurs once in 10,000 male births and is transmitted by sex-linked recessive inheritance. Although hemophilia B (Factor IX deficiency) is clinically similar to hemophilia A, it is far less frequent. Factor VIII is actually present in normal amounts in hemophiliac plasma but is functionally inert. A level of 5 percent seems to be sufficient to avoid spontaneous hemorrhage, but bleeding will occur at this level after trauma or surgery. Spontaneous hemorrhage occurs commonly inside the cranium, in the bowel wall and bowel mesentery and in the urinary tract. Indeed, critically placed hematomas are the real danger to patients since congenital disorders, including hemophilia, seldom cause death by blood loss. Thus, the therapy is directed toward correcting the coagulation deficit primarily to avoid the risk of a critically positioned spontaneous bleed.

Several good reviews exist which discuss the management of hemophilia in detail.[20,21] One must remember that the maintenance of adequate Factor VIII levels in the hemophiliac in the perioperative period requires large quantities of replacement products to achieve a factor level at least 30 percent of normal. At this level, hemostasis should be complete. Even less complex procedures, such as Penrose drain removal or tracheal intubation, demand a level of at least 5 percent. Factor VIII replacement, due to its lability even at refrigerated temperatures, can only be accomplished by administering fresh warm blood (less than 4 hours old), fresh frozen plasma, cryoprecipitates, or AHF (antihemophiliac factor) concentrates. By administering 10 to 14 bags of cryoprecipitate or its equivalent in concentrated AHF, as a loading dose followed by 8 to 10 bags every 8 to 12 hours, one can expect adequate hemostasis to occur in a 70-kg man about to undergo a laparotomy. Because of its short biologic half-life, Factor VIII may have to be administered every 8 to 12 hours for 1 to 2 weeks during the recovery period. Although formulae are available for Factor VIII replacement dosage, undue reliance on such guidelines when treating the ICU patient may not accomplish adequate hemostasis. Estimates of the required dose should be made from the following formula:

Units administered =
(desired concentration − initial concentration) × plasma volume

where a unit of Factor VIII is its average content in 1 ml of normal fresh plasma. For the ICU patient with substantial alteration and fluxes of plasma volume, as well as fever, sepsis, and varying degrees of coagulation factor consumption, distribution and degradation of administered Factor VIII may be unpredictable. Therefore, the above formula, although serving as an initial guideline, should not replace careful monitoring of the actual state of coagulation by PTT testing performed several times daily.

Von Willebrand's Disease   Von Willebrand's disease occurs with about the same frequency as classical hemophilia. Unlike hemophilia, it is transmitted as an autosomal dominant trait which is associated with the true absence of Factor VIII. In fact, the addition of hemophiliac plasma to von Willebrand plasma will correct the coagulation deficit. Increased PTT as in hemophilia indicates a disorder of the intrinsic clotting system. The increased bleeding time associated with von Willebrand's disease is due to an additional qualitative dysfunction of platelet adhesion. Conveniently, infusions of fresh frozen plasma or cryoprecipitate correct both the Factor VIII deficiency *and* the platelet abnormality with normalization of the PTT as well as the bleeding time.

The PTT in both diseases is very useful since values less than twice the normal will allow surgical procedures to occur safely without excess bleeding secondary to hemostatic failure. Therapy usually requires much larger quantities of replacement products for hemophiliacs than for von Willebrand's disease. Patients with von Willebrand's disease may continue to synthesize Factor VIII from precursors contained in the infusate.

GUIDELINES FOR RX: HEMOPHILIA A AND VON WILLEBRAND'S DISEASE

1. Maintain PTT ≤ twice normal
2. Factor VIII level ≥ 30% for major surgery
3. Factor VIII level ≥ 5% for minor surgery
4. Use FFP if no volume restrictions
5. Use cryoprecipitates or AHF concentrate if only small volume infusion desired. AHF concentrate *does not* correct platelet dysfunction of von Willebrand's disease

Other congenital disorders infrequently result in significant bleeding and are much rarer. However, once identified, appropriate replacement therapy should precede surgical procedures and continue in the postoperative period with monitoring by the PT and PTT. The goal should be to maintain the partial thromboplastin time less than twice normal.

ACQUIRED DISORDERS

Hemorrhagic disorders due to acquired coagulation deficiencies are usually secondary to an underlying disease process which commonly affects multiple phases of coagulation; they are also frequently difficult to separate, thus making specifically directed therapy difficult. Acquired bleeding disorders may arise from (1) deficiency or abnormality of any clotting factor; (2) an inhibition of any reaction; (3) platelet defects, both quantitative and qualitative; and (4) inappropriate fibrinolysis activation. A discussion of common coagulation disturbances and a review of difficult clinical problems with hemorrhagic components should provide a perspective for attacking the multifaceted problem of acquired hemostatic disorders.

Platelet Abnormalities   Although platelets play a key role in hemostasis, their full spectrum of activity is not fully understood. For proper function in primary hemostasis, they must stick to the vessel wall and to each other. Platelets do not, however, stick to intact endothelium, blood cells, or other undamaged cells. ADP appears to be the major physiologic stimulus to platelet aggregation. Platelets also plug holes, activate the intrinsic clotting mechanism via platelet factor 3, and induce clot retraction which generates the recovery of thrombin for more coagulum formation. Platelets, derived from megakaryocytes formed in bone marrow, undergo retraction due to the presence of *thrombasthenin*—a contractile protein resembling the muscle protein actomyosin. This enzyme, an ATP-ase, may provide the energy required for retraction.

Deficits in platelet number and/or defects in function are frequent causes of disordered hemostasis. Congenital defects in platelet number or function are very rare but can be found in newborns of thrombocytopenic mothers. In this situation, maternal thombocytopenia is most commonly caused by drugs (heroin) or ITP. Other abnormalities include erythroblastosis fetalis and isoimmunization thrombocytopenia as a result of maternal sensitization by fetal platelets.[22] The isolated abnormality of platelet dysfunction as a cause of bleeding can occur as an effect of many different drugs, viral infections, and leukemias. In addition, accelerated destruction of platelets is often found in giant cavernous hemangioma and idiopathic thrombocytopenia purpura (ITP).

ITP has been well studied and seems to represent a platelet autoimmune phenomenon resulting in shortened life span of platelets. Steroid therapy (prednisone 5 to 80 mg/day) will provide temporary control of the tendency toward the thrombocytopenic state of ITP in about 90 percent of patients, but remission is only temporary. Splenectomy results in an immediate response in about three-fourths of those patients and two-thirds of them will have a permanent remission. The necessity for platelet transfusion prior to splenectomy for ITP is still debated. Since splenectomy may be performed safely with platelet counts of 10,000 to 50,000 if careful attention is paid to surgical hemostasis, preoperative platelet transfusion may not be necessary. Those surgeons and anesthesiologists who desire platelet counts of 50,000 to 100,000/cu mm during the operative procedure should give platelet transfusions in the operating room just prior to operation—*not* the night before. In general, platelets from a single unit of fresh blood will raise the circulating platelet count of a 70-kg adult to 10,000 to 12,000/cu mm. Therefore, for patients requiring preoperative platelet transfusion, a "platelet-8-pack" will most likely result in the elevation of platelet count 50,000 to 100,000/cu mm. A platelet-8-pack may be prepared from the platelet fractions of 8 units of whole blood.

Thrombocytopenic patients characteristically bleed continuously from surgical wounds and from all raw surfaces. However, rebleeding is rarely a problem once direct hemostatic control has been achieved. Rebleeding will occur if the hemostatic disorder includes a defect in the coagulation mechanism as well. Rebleeding can be traced to the failure of the coagulation mechanism to reinforce the hemostatic plug with fibrin strands. Hours after wounding, when vasoconstriction abates, arteriolar pressure overcomes the weak platelet plug and rebleeding occurs. The severity of bleeding in thrombocytopenic states correlates fairly well with the platelet count. The normal count is 150,000 to 400,000/cu mm. Platelet counts greater than 100,000 are rarely associated with bleeding signs and symptoms directly related to platelet problems.

Platelet counts of 30,000 to 100,000 will provide excess oozing after wounding. Spontaneous hemorrhage without trauma is usually seen only if the count is below 30,000/cu mm, although some hematologists feel that a count of less than 10,000 represents the only true emergency—the risk of intracranial bleeding—and is the only indication for platelet infusions.

NORMAL AND ABNORMAL PLATELET COUNTS

Normal	150,000–400,000/cu mm
Rare cause of bleeding	≥100,000/cu mm
Minimum level after trauma	50,000–100,000/cu mm
Rare *spontaneous* bleeding	≥30,000/cu mm
True emergency	<10,000/cu mm

Thrombocytosis can also induce bleeding, although the reasons are unclear. Perhaps it is related to the consumption of coagulation factors in a hypercoagulable system, i.e., these platelets may not function normally. Transient thrombocytosis occurs most commonly after splenectomy but only rarely causes bleeding. Reactive thrombocytosis may reach counts of 1,000,000/cu mm by the second postoperative week. Spontaneous mesenteric vascular infarctions have been reported in splenectomized patients.[23]

Platelets may be present in sufficient number but function abnormally. Many drugs (e.g., including aspirin, indomethacin, and phenylbutazone) affect the platelet release reaction. The blockage of ADP released from aggregate platelets results in increased bleeding time. Clinical oozing can occur after only two aspirin tablets and may last for 5 to 7 days. If a drug effect is added to existing thrombocytopenia or another coagulation disorder (liver disease), the results may be disastrous. No specific antidote for the defect in platelet function secondary to the aspirin effect is known. Although aspirin-affected platelets probably never regain intrinsic release functions, they still can respond to exogenous ADP released from transfused platelets. Replacement therapy is limited to platelet concentrates and can be given before the aspirin disappears from the circulation, i.e., 5 to 7 days if clinical bleeding occurs.

SOME CLINICAL PLATELET AFFECTORS

Rx	*Action*	*Result*
ASA, indomethacin, phenylbutazone	Inhibits platelet release reaction	Prolongs bleeding time; clinical oozing
Platelet transfusion (1 pack)	↑ Platelet count	Short half-life; platelet survival curve
Splenectomy	↑ Platelet count	>1,000,000/cu mm; mesenteric thrombosis

The short life span of the ex vivo platelet significantly reduces the efficiency of therapy. Only about 20 percent of platelets will circulate after 24 hours of storage in ACD at 4 C. Few, if any, transfused platelets can be expected to survive after 48 hours of storage. Freezing techniques are ingenious but need more investigation. Frozen platelets function less well immediately upon transfusion but regain function within 24 hours. A convenient rule of thumb is that one unit of platelet concentrate should raise the total platelet count 10,000/cu mm in a normal person. A platelet survival curve (platelet count done at 1, 4, and 12 hours after platelet transfusion) can aid in detection of increased destruction of platelets. If the 1-hour post-transfusion platelet count responds as predicted (i.e., platelet count increases 10,000 platelets per cubic millimeter per unit) but the 4-hour value is the same as the value prior to therapy, destruction is probably occurring.

RX FOR THROMBOCYTOPENIA

Rx	*Effect on Platelet Count*
One unit fresh whole blood	↑ 10,000/cu mm
"Platelet-8-pack"	↑ 50,000–100,000/cu mm
Steroids	Temporary remission ITP
Splenectomy	75% immediate remission, 50% permanent remission

Defibrination/Hyperfibrinolysis In vitro blood clotting results in serum deficiency of certain coagulation factors (I, II, V, VIII). If this occurs in vivo the blood might be pictured as a mixture of plasma and serum. With such coagulation factor deficiencies, severe *defibrination* results causing a prolongation of the PT and PTT; in fact, fibrinogen may be so low that clot never forms.

For many years it has been known that fibrinogen and fibrin left at room temperature for several days will demonstrate fibrin clot lysis, i.e., fibrinolytic activity. Fibrinolytic activity is now known to occur in blood under a wide variety of physiologic and pathologic conditions, i.e., stress, exercise, fear, abruptio placenta, amniotic fluid embolism, liver disease, prostatic carcinoma, and shock. The fibrin breakdown (split) products (FSPs) attract the most interest since increased amounts occur in many human disease states. There are indications that these products affect platelet function and potentiate the effect of biologically active peptides (bradykinins) which in turn increase capillary permeability). If these products are injected into animals, diffuse hemorrhage from experimental operative wounds will result.

FSPs interfere with the polymerization of fibrin monomers. Thus, if test plasma containing FSPs is added to a fibrinogen solution, the thrombin induced clotting of fibrinogen will be retarded, i.e., a prolonged thrombin time. Fibrinolysis is confirmed by demonstrating the presence of fibrin split products in the test serum by immunochemical means.[24] Excess fibrinolysis occurs when an imbalance of plasmin and plasmin inhibitors results in excessive circulating plasmin. This excess of plasmin results in the dissolution of fibrin, fibrinogen, and other plasma proteins, especially the coagulation factors. In this manner the lysis of well-formed clots in the absence of sufficient circulating coagulation factors leads to widespread bleeding: spontaneous from mucous membranes or rebleeding from previously dry wounds and venipuncture sites. The initiating factor in this process may not be apparent in every case. Activators are known to be abundant in the endothelial lining of veins and arteries. Massive release of activators can occur in electrical shock, carcinoma of the prostate, cirrhosis, abruptio placenta, and amniotic fluid embolus.

Primary fibrinolysis is rarely seen as the major cause of a coagulopathy. However, fibrinolysis occurring secondary to widespread intravascular coagulation always accompanies DIC. Therapy should, therefore, be limited to treating the initiating event and not the secondary fibrinolysis.

If fibrinolysis is the primary problem, then therapeutic inhibition of the fibrinolytic system may significantly control hemorrhage. Such therapy is available in the form of episolonaminocaproic acid (Amicar) introduced in 1954. Four to five grams of Amicar should be given intravenously as a loading dose over the first hour followed by continuous infusion at the rate of 1 gm per hour. Antifibrinolytic drugs, with rare exception, should not be given in defibrination syndrome unless heparin therapy has also been started. Blunting the active fibrinolytic response with Amicar enhances the stability of the fibrin clot at the bleeding site, but does so at the risk of increasing fibrin deposition in some areas of the microcirculation, i.e., glomerular capillaries. Primary fibrinolysis may result in postoperative bleeding after prostatic surgery. Urine contains a high concentration of urokinase which can break down fibrin clots as soon as they are formed by activating plasminogen to form the thrombolytic enzyme plasmin. Amicar will arrest this bleeding by blocking the activation of plasminogen. Since Amicar is concentrated in the urine, 1 gm every 3 hours intravenously should control bleeding by blocking the activation of plasminogen by urokinase.[25]

However, if the active fibrinolytic system is a secondary physiologic response to a pathologic diffuse intravascular coagulation, then inhibition of the "protective fibrinolysis" may result in a fatal widespread intravascular coagulation (thrombosis). The guiding principle must be that bleeding directly attributable to primary fibrinolysis is rare. Secondary hyperfibrinolysis associated with hemorrhage is much more common than it is a primary disorder; it usually is *not* the basic coagulation defect and therefore should not be treated. The basic coagulation defect associated with demonstrable fibrinolysis in the majority of cases is DIC.

FIBRINOLYSIS

Primary	*Secondary*
Rare	Common (associated with DIC)
Prostatic surgery, cirrhosis	Sepsis, shock, OB complications
Normal platelet count	*Low* platelet count
↑ PT, PTT	↑↑ PT, PTT
↑↑↑ FSPs	↑ FSPs (variable amounts)
Rx: Amicar (heparin?)	Correct underlying disorder

The bleeding tendency in hyperfibrinolysis is due to the products of fibrinolytic digestion of fibrin. Fibrin degradation products (or fibrin split products) consist of four fragments, cleaved by plasmin from fibrin, ranging in molecular weight from 50,000 to 270,000. These fragments, designated X, Y, D, and E, are themselves potent anticoagulants. They inhibit (1) the generation of prothrombin converting activity, (2) the interaction of fibrinogen with thrombin, (3) the polymerization of fibrin, and (4) platelet function.

Disseminated Intravascular Coagulation (DIC) The term "consumptive coagulopathy" originally described a variety of poorly characterized bleeding disorders caused by the transformation of circulating plasma to serum. Serum is plasma minus clotting substances; and the in vivo lack of clotting substances was ascribed to consumption. The hemorrhagic diathesis of DIC results when widespread activation of the clotting mechanism has consumed the plasma clotting factors (I, II, V, VIII, and platelets). DIC has many synonyms (defibrination syndrome, consumptive coagulopathy, disseminated intravascular thrombosis), but the most popular is simply DIC. DIC, as described by McKay,[26] is not a distinct pathologic entity but rather an intermediary mechanism of disease. It is both a bleeding disease state and a thrombotic disorder. As a disease of the microcirculation, however, it should be distinguished from disease states in which thrombosis is the main problem, i.e., major vessel thromboembolism. Since some consumption of coagulation factors occurs physiologically, the whole DIC phenomenon represents a broad spectrum of events, with the extreme pathologic endpoint being diffuse hemorrhage that occurs when coagulation factors have been used up.

The initiation of the DIC syndrome proceeds through the physiologic hemostatic process. Thromboplastin entering the circulation or spontaneous clotting on damaged endothelial surfaces initiates clotting via the intrinsic and extrinsic pathways. Fibrin so formed is dissolved by the fibrinolytic system. The pathologic nature of the process is to be found in the degree of this normally physiologic sequence. Widespread intravascular activation of the clotting system consumes coagulation factors; widespread activation of the fibrinolytic system destroys clots. These two processes working together in excess produce a widespread hemorrhagic diathesis. Furthermore, the presence of DIC implies that the defense mechanisms which normally prevent this runaway phenomenon of the coagulation system have failed. First, the reticuloendothelial system normally removes fibrin, activated clotting factors and thromboplastin from the circulation so that the capacity for pathologic widespread clotting cannot proceed. Second, hepatic efficiency in removing the activated clotting factors left over after physiologic coagulation (particularly Factors X and XII) must be impaired. Third, the circulating inhibitors of the fibrinolytic system must be significantly deficient or blocked to allow the initiation of widespread clotting.

McKay's description of DIC as an intermediary mechanism directs our attention to the factors predisposing to DIC because, to be ultimately effective, therapy must be directed at the cause. In some patients many predisposing factors must be operative, creating several possible combinations of clinical events predisposing to DIC (shock, trauma, sepsis, acidosis, pregnancy).

DIC and Sepsis   Gram-negative sepsis may be the most important cause of clinical and subclinical DIC. Although the pathophysiology is not well worked out, the interplay of white blood cells, platelets, clotting factors, and vascular endothelium is widely appreciated. Gram-negative sepsis may also include sluggish blood flow, stagnation, impaired liver and kidney function, and reticuloendothelial system blockade; thus, the primary defense mechanisms that normally prevent widespread clotting are inactivated.

The Schwartzman reaction in the laboratory animal is perhaps the best experimental model to describe the relationship of DIC and sepsis. Two intravenous injections of purified gram-negative bacterial endotoxin given 24 hours apart result in massive DIC. The first injection produces little noticeable coagulation disturbance but saturates the reticuloendothelial system, neutralizing its ability to control excess clotting. Endotoxin injected 24 hours later is then free to activate clotting through Factor XII (Hageman Factor), increasing platelet aggregation and damaging endothelial cells. Other experimental methods confirm the regulatory importance of the reticuloendothelial system. Thorotrast injected initially to blockade the reticuloendothelial system will allow a single injection of endotoxin to cause DIC in the animal. Interestingly, the pregnant rabbit also will develop DIC after only one injection of endotoxin. The clinical correlate to this latter model may be represented by the hypercoagulable state of pregnancy.

Other experimental situations also produce DIC: thromboplastin infusions or pit viper venom acting through the extrinsic clotting system, stasis in large capillary hemangiomas (Kasabach-Meritt Syndrome), fat emboli initiating phase 1 of the coagulation system by activating Factor XI and XII, mismatched transfusions which liberate lipids and ADP, and necrotic material circulating in certain obstetrical and cancer patients. The obvious implication of these experimental findings is that any clinical state, or perhaps therapy, known to impair reticuloendothelial system may set the stage for DIC: chemotherapy, steroids, pregnancy, snake bite, and massive tissue trauma.

Clinical Features of DIC Diffuse bleeding from all wounds, puncture sites, urinary tract, and other mucous membranes is the most common clinical manifestation of DIC. The severity of bleeding seems to correlate inversely with the levels of fibrinogen and circulating platelets. The thrombotic manifestations may not be as obvious for they occur primarily in the microcirculation. If DIC is severe, cutaneous thrombosis may cause acrocyanosis particularly visible in the hands and feet, but the most vital organ damaged by the thrombotic process is the kidney. The deposition of fibrin microthrombi in the glomerular capillaries can be presumed when hematuria and oliguria develop. Other organs commonly involved in the bleeding-clotting process are the brain, the heart, the adrenals, the entire gastrointestinal tract, particularly the pancreas, and the lung. Even red blood cells are damaged when traversing the difficult passage through the fibrin laden capillaries. Schistocytes (helmet cells) seen in the peripheral smear reflect damaged red blood cells in transit through the circulation.

The clinical syndrome of DIC can range from a transient drop in the platelet count to life threatening hemorrhage and renal shutdown associated with worsening sepsis, prostatic carcinoma, or obstetric complications. Regardless, the therapy must be directed primarily at the underlying disorder and only secondarily toward correction of the coagulation disturbance. In fact, significant salvage rates have only come when the primary disease process which caused the immediate disorder has been brought under control, i.e., shock resuscitated and acidosis corrected, sepsis controlled by debridement and/or drainage and appropriate antibiotics, or dilatation and curettage performed for retained fetus. The paramount importance of this primary therapy is highlighted when one considers that *the only therapy available for direct control of the coagulation disturbance of DIC is heparin.* The potential pitfalls of heparinizing the bleeding patient with DIC are obvious.

CLINICAL CAUSES OF DIC

Infections	*Tissue Injury*
Gram-negative sepsis	Crush
Rickettsia	Fat emboli
Obstetric	*Vascular*
Septic abortion	Local—aortic aneurysm,
Abruptio placenta	hemangioma
Retained fetus	Systemic—shock,
Amniotic fluid embolus	vasculitis
Malignancy	*Miscellaneous*
Prostate, pancreas, lung,	Snake bite
kidney, colon, ovary	Heat stroke
	Incompatible transfusion

Laboratory Diagnosis of DIC The suspicion that DIC is the cause of clinical hemorrhage requires laboratory confirmation. Acute DIC massive enough to cause diffuse hemorrhage is not hard to recognize. Routine tests usually provide enough information for a provisional diagnosis. The presence of fibrin degradation products (FSPs) will cause prolongation of the PT and PTT since they inhibit coagulation through the intrinsic and extrinsic pathways. In addition, since FSPs block the conversion of fibrinogen to fibrin, the thrombin time will be prolonged. Thrombocytopenia develops due to consumption of platelets in the forming microthrombi. Thrombocytopenia alone, however, must not be interpreted as indicating DIC. Even though sepsis and DIC are associated, about three-fourths of septic patients with positive blood cultures can have isolated thrombocytopenia with no clinical signs suggesting DIC. Many tests will detect fibrin split products, i.e., staphylococcal clumping tests, the FI test, latex agglutination, and the paracoagulation tests. The paracoagulation tests such as ethanol gelation and protamine sulfate are so named because they are able to detect fibrin strand formation (gel) from larger FSP fragments when these chemicals are added to plasma. However, in primary fibrinolysis, the breakdown products of fibrinogen do not undergo paracoagulation, so the ethanol gelation and protamine sulfate tests will be negative. The paracoagulation tests are simple to perform but much less specific than tests for fibrin degradation products (FSPs). Classically then, primary fibrinolysis is distinguished from secondary fibrinolysis by (1) the absence of red blood cell fragmentation, (2) slight decrease in fibrinogen, (3) increased lytic activity, (4) negative paracoagulation tests. No test is pathognomonic of DIC; and since DIC may appear as massive diffuse hemorrhage, initial criteria should be based on fairly routine laboratory tests. The PT, PTT, thrombin time, platelet count, and fibrinogen levels are most useful. If the results of these tests are abnormal, DIC can then be confirmed by any of the series of tests mentioned above to detect fibrinolysis.

DIC VERSUS PRIMARY FIBRINOLYSIS

	DIC	*Fibrinolysis*
Platelet count	↓	Normal
Bleeding time	↑	Normal
RBC fragments	Present	None
PT	↑↑	Slight ↑
PTT	↑↑	Slight ↑
Fibrinogen	↓↓	↓
FSPs	↑	↑
Thrombin time	↑	↑
Paracoagulation tests		
Ethanol gelation	Positive	Negative
Protamine sulfate	High titer	Low titer

Therapy for DIC Treatment considerations must be two-fold in DIC. First, control of the underlying process that initiated DIC is mandatory. Second, coagulation intervention can only be considered as symptomatic care for the bleeding problem. Frequently, massive efforts directed at the first obviates the potentially dangerous therapy for the second. Four therapeutic choices are available for coagulation manipulation as secondary therapy: (1) *Do nothing:* this may be the best choice if the underlying disease process seems to be correcting itself. The risk inherent in this approach is obviously the extent of continuing defibrination during the correction process. (2) *Heparin:* this will stop the abnormal accelerating clotting problem of DIC, but in addition it may potentiate bleeding. (3) *Replacement therapy:* platelet transfusion or clotting factors in the form of fresh frozen plasma (FFP) may buy time in replacing the deficiencies produced by massive consumption. Theoretically, this could add fuel to the fire, but there is no evidence that this has, indeed, ever occurred. Replacement can be considered after heparinization. (4) *Amicar:* directed specifically at active fibrinolysis as a way to control the bleeding. The disadvantage is that fibrin deposition may then assume critical proportions in critical locations. This is rarely indicated and must be done in association with heparin. Combinations of these choices are popular, particularly heparin and replacement therapy.

RX FOR DIC

Do nothing	Appropriate if underlying cause corrected
Heparin	Biochemically sound; clinically potentiates bleeding
Replacement products	Platelets, FFP; "fuel to fire"
Amicar	Stops fibrinolysis; abnormal clotting continues

Heparin Therapy for DIC DIC has two important consequences: (1) impaired microcirculation due to microthrombosis, and (2) consumption of the hemostatic control functions caused by an increased utilization of platelets and clotting factors. The essential pathogenetic factor is intravascular generation of thrombin. Therefore, logic suggests that neutralization of thrombin activity would be the most effective means of preventing consumptive coagulopathy. Since heparin does not influence the fate of the already established microthrombosis, its main effect is the prevention of further consumption of hemostatic factors. Although animal experiments support the use of heparin in sepsis-associated DIC, no such efficacy has been proven to date in critically ill patients.

While documentation of improvement in clotting factors exists with heparin and blood component therapy, the mortality has not been significantly altered compared to nonheparinized groups of patients.[27] Heparin interrupts the cycle of thrombin release, fibrin deposition, clotting factor activation, and further thrombin release which characterizes DIC. In the therapy of DIC, heparin is *adjunctive* therapy in a multifaceted therapeutic approach and should *not* be relied upon as a single specific drug for this disorder. Extreme caution must be taken in heparin use. The persistence of FSPs exerts a strong anticoagulant effect. If diffuse vasculitis is present or a local defect in the vasculature exists, heparin should not be used.

Heparin therapy for DIC consists of a loading dose of 2000 to 5000 units with continuous infusion of approximately 500 to 1000 units per hour. The guidelines listed below should be used in association with platelet counts and fibrinogen levels. Clinically, however, the control of bleeding is the index of effective therapy. Heparin should be discontinued as soon as the underlying disease trigger has been effectively treated.

GUIDELINES: HEPARIN RX FOR DIC

Laboratory Dx DIC (no bleeding)	No bleeding, no heparin
Correcting underlying cause	No heparin
Open wounds	Heparin?; extreme caution
Lab Dx DIC (significant bleeding, no contraindications)	Heparin 2000 to 5000 units loading dose; 500 to 1000 units/hr maintenance
DIC (amniotic fluid embolus)	No heparin; replacement Rx only

Liver Disease and Vitamin K Deficiency

Liver All the identified coagulation proteins except Factor VIII are made solely in the liver. Parenchymal liver disease thus may lead to a deficiency of any or all the factors creating many common clinical disorders of hemostasis. In addition, advanced liver disease (cirrhosis) causing portal hypertension may be associated with thrombocytopenia secondary to hypersplenism. (Bleeding from varices seems to be related to portal pressure not to thrombocytopenia per se.) In addition, cirrhotic livers release plasminogen activators and the diseased liver cannot clear activated clotting factors efficiently. If lytic activators are not cleared, the resultant FSPs may interfere with platelet function. Thus, many factors in liver disease contribute to deregulate the normally well-balanced process of coagulation. Therapy for coagulation disorders in case of severe liver disease is basically supportive since no specific therapy is available for the primary process, i.e., liver disease. Fresh frozen plasma, cryoprecipitate, and platelets (or fresh whole blood) seem to be the best therapy, but such therapy is frequently futile and certainly an expensive exercise. Vitamin K should be administered in a dose of 10 to 20 mg daily for three consecutive days. But even vitamin K therapy will not be effective in primary liver failure. Exchange transfusions in hepatic failure and extra corporeal liver perfusion have been advocated, but presently are not generally available for safe use.

Vitamin K Deficiency Prothrombin, Factors VII, IX, and X all require vitamin K for synthesis in the liver. Vitamin K is a fat soluble constituent of normal diet. Vitamin K dietary deficiency is extremely rare and occurs only in patients malnourished for a long time. The body absorbs vitamin K manufactured by the gut flora. Thus, biliary fistulae or biliary ductal obstruction which results in deficient micelle formation of fats in the gut may lead to inadequate vitamin K absorption. Antibiotics which eliminate the gut flora and starvation (NPO) can lower vitamin K levels. Therefore, a prolonged PT may imply a defect in gut flora production of vitamin K, an inability to absorb vitamin K, or a hepatocyte dysfunction in manufacturing Factors II, V, VII, and X. This latter condition will respond poorly if at all to vitamin K administration.

LIVER DISEASE/VITAMIN K DEFICIENCY

Clinical Problem	Factors Deficient	Lab Abnormality	Treatment
Liver Disease portal hypertension	II, V, VII, IX, X	↑ PT; ↑ PTT; ↓ platelets; ↓ fibrinogen	Vitamin K; FFP: platelets
Vitamin K Deficiency biliary fistula, biliary obstruction, NPO (>5 days), antibiotics	II, VII, IX, X	↑ PT	Vitamin K 10– 20 mg/day for 3 days

Uremia   Riesman[28] suggested in 1907 that the bleeding of uremia was associated with circulating toxins. Further study has elucidated some of the mechanisms, but the major advances have been the control of the cause of uremia through dialysis. It also appears that qualitative platelet defects can be reversed by dialysis. Platelet factor 3, a phospholipid with thromboplastic activity, is essential for the conversion of prothrombin to thrombin by the intrinsic system. Guanidino-succinic acid (GSA) and phenolic acids which are elevated in uremic plasma decrease platelet aggregation induced by ADP, epinephrine, and collagen. In addition, GSA and phenolic acids are known effectors of anaerobic glycolysis (enzyme inhibitors), but how they affect platelet function is unknown. Dialysis removes GSA and phenol acid levels, thereby tending to normalize the platelet aggregation response. It is the platelet aggregation response which determines the level of platelet factor 3, the phospholipid necessary for induction of further phases of coagulation.

UREMIA

Problem	Mechanism	Treatment
Uremic bleeding	Qualitative platelet defect (GSA, phenolic acid)	Dialysis

Shock and Trauma   Patients with severe shock have shown decreases in all the coagulation factors and platelets through many pathogenetic pathways: inadequate tissue perfusion, stagnant flow, endothelial damage, and decreased liver perfusion with diminished production of Factors II, V, VII, IX, X, and XIII. Decreased hepatic clearance, particularly of Factor Xa also occurs. Microthrombi can be found in the liver, kidneys, lung, heart of patients dying in shock caused by hemorrhage, sepsis, or myocardial infarction. Despite this, hemorrhagic shock is not felt to produce clinically significant DIC, even in the presence of substantial hypoperfusion and acidosis. As far as septic shock is concerned, a multitude of studies describing the association of septic shock with coagulation changes have still failed to elucidate the cause of these mechanisms. Endotoxin is known to activate the kinin system which contains known activators of Factor XII (Hageman). Parenthetically, a great deal of misleading information has come from experiments in nonprimate animals which are known now to exhibit marked species differences in the hemodynamic response and coagulation changes attendant to the shock state.

Cardiopulmonary Bypass Bleeding   Roughly 50 percent of postoperative bleeding after cardiopulmonary bypass will be due to a bleeding vessel—failure of surgical hemostasis. However, before returning the patient to surgery, all efforts must be made to correct the coagulation disturbances that may be coexistent. Indeed, the presence of the bleeding site may be suggested by continued hemorrhage after correction of coagulation problems. Heparin must be added to prevent the ex vivo clotting which occurs when citrated blood is circulated through a pump oxygenator. Blood contacting foreign surfaces in the pump oxygenator causes mechanical damage to red blood cells and platelets and also activates Factor XII. In addition, destroyed platelets release platelet Factor IV, a potent heparin inhibitor. Some clotting factor consumption occurs when blood collecting in the operative field is aspirated and returned to the pump. This aspirated material contains abundant quantities of tissue thromboplastin. Heparin therapy during cardiopulmonary bypass is therefore mandatory. The most important therapeutic consideration, since heparin must be used to avoid the activation of the clotting process secondary to extracorporal circulation of blood, is that the previously administered heparin dose has been appropriately neutralized. Usually, protamine is given in the operating room after the patient is disconnected from the bypass equipment. However, in the postoperative period previously neutralized heparin, due to rapid inactivation of the protamine portion of the heparin-protamine salt complex, may cause a heparin rebound phenomenon. Thus, the causes of postcardiopulmonary bypass bleeding may be (1) too little heparin intraoperatively resulting in a failure to block thrombin generation, (2) unneutralized heparin, i.e., too little protamine, (3) decreased number of platelets due to the type and time of bypass (bubble oxygenators seem harsher than the membrane type), and (4) fibrinolysis, as a primary event (extremely rare).

As in liver disease, an isolated abnormality is usually not enough to cause significant clinical hemorrhage after cardiopulmonary bypass: multiple defects must exist in the coagulation system. If the cause of postoperative bleeding is due to excess heparin effect, then abnormalities of the PT and PTT and thrombin time will be manifest. Severe thrombocytopenia, less than 30,000 to 50,000 platelets per cubic millimeter, in a situation where coagulation factors may be deficient contributes to the coagulopathy and deserves platelet transfusion therapy. Heparin excess should be treated specifically with protamine sulfate. Protamine reverses the anticoagulant effect of heparin, but protamine has a weak anticoagulant effect itself. Approximately one mg protamine sulfate binds 100 units of heparin in vitro. However, for clinical use, calculations for total protamine dosage are made at the ratio of 1.5 mg per 100 units of heparin. One-half the dose (maximum 50 mg) is given intravenously over 10 to 15 minutes. Hypotension has been associated with more rapid administration. Heparin rebound or recurrent bleeding may occur after adequate initial neutralization due to the rapid metabolism of the protamine portion of the bound heparin-protamine salt, releasing further free heparin. Such a situation is controlled by giving more protamine.

BLEEDING AND CP BYPASS

Problem	Treatment
Failure of surgical hemostasis	Correct coagulation disturbances; reoperation
Intraoperative consumption	More heparin intraoperatively
Thrombocytopenia	Platelet transfusion
Unneutralized heparin (heparin rebound)	More protamine; 1.5 mg/100 units heparin, give ½ dose over 15–20 min

TRANSFUSIONS: COMPONENT THERAPY AND COMPLICATIONS

With the availability of the multiple bag collection and separation system, preparation of the various blood components has become simple and relatively inexpensive. From a single unit of whole blood one can obtain red blood cells, platelets, plasma, cryoprecipitate (Factor VIII), gamma globulin, and albumin. Because few patients require all of these blood constituents, the transfusion of whole blood should be the exception rather than the rule. The increased demand for non-red blood cell fractions has made the need for component banking more pressing.

The physiologic rationale for avoiding whole blood transfusions as a primary method of treating coagulation disturbances is sound. In fact, resuscitation of patients in hemorrhagic shock can be readily accomplished by "component" therapy—packed red cells, extracellular fluid volume expansion with balanced electrolyte solutions, and fresh frozen plasma, cryoprecipitates and platelets as needed to correct coagulation protein deficiencies. But the realities of blood banking supply and demand factors cast a shadow on the ideal therapy of hemorrhage and coagulopathies which are particularly limiting, for example, at 4 o'clock A.M. on a Sunday, when no recently drawn blood is available and mobilization of technicians and donors may be difficult, although major blood replacement is commonly required because of Saturday night trauma. If laboratory factor analysis and ample quantities of components were available 24 hours a day, 7 days a week, then treatment of coagulation disturbances arising in the ICU patient could approach the ideal. Such availability is the exception rather than the rule. Guidelines for therapy, therefore, must strike some balance with reality.

The plasma fraction contains all factors essential for coagulation except platelets. Thirty percent of an essential factor is necessary for hemostasis. An international unit of a given factor is contained in 1 ml of plasma. For example, a 70-kg adult with a plasma volume of 40 ml/kg will have 2800 units of each factor. Fresh frozen plasma retains all essential factors at about 1 unit per milliliter and, because of widespread availability, remains the mainstay of component therapy for coagulation disturbances in the ICU patient. Factor concentrates should be considered in cases in which large volumes cannot be given. Concentrates are available containing Factor II, VII, IX, and X, but not V [Konyne (Cutter) and Proplex (Hyland)]. The major problems with these concentrates are: (1) hepatitis (perhaps 50 percent incidence per unit), (2) the induction of clotting since these factors are present as activated factors, and (3) anaphylaxis. Replacement of coagulation proteins lost by dilution when massive blood transfusion is required can be easily accomplished with 500 ml of fresh frozen plasma. The adequacy of fresh frozen plasma replacement is confirmed by normalization of the PT and PTT.

Transfusion of banked whole blood in large quantities (> 8 units) can alter hemostasis. The coagulation changes of massive blood transfusion may be in the form of transfusion reaction or of a primary coagulation change. Hemolysis liberates erythrokinase from the stroma of the red blood cell. The enzyme is a potent thromboplastic agent; free hemoglobin, also liberated, is not thromboplastic. The majority of transfusion reactions manifested by fever, chills, or urticaria represent minor incompatibilities (mostly between donor and host WBCs) and respond to cessation of transfusion and symptomatic therapy (Benadryl 50 mg I.M.).

Stored blood is an imperfect clotting package, being deficient in platelets, calcium, and Factors V and VIII. However, it must be noted that calcium deficits will cause hemodynamic disturbances, even cardiac standstill, before interfering with the coagulation mechanism. Thus, guidelines for calcium replacement during massive transfusion are directed at improving cardiovascular performance and *not* at correcting existing coagulation disturbances. A transfusion rate greater than 5 units of whole blood in 1 hour, or 10 units in 24 hours, will usually cause a defect in primary hemostasis by dilution of platelets and a decrease in labile Factors V and VIII. By contrast, fibrinogen and prothrombin, well preserved in banked blood, usually remain stable. Thus, the abnormalities of coagulation detected by standard coagulation tests usually include prolongation of the PT and PTT with thrombocytopenia noted following massive blood transfusion. Disorders of the extrinsic (PT) and intrinsic (PTT) clotting systems are present due to the dilutional loss of the labile Factors V and VIII.

Thrombocytopenia after massive transfusion is a result of using platelet-poor stored banked blood. Following restoration of red cell volume and plasma volume, specific therapy directed at normalizing the dilutional coagulation change will consist primarily of fresh frozen plasma; and for the occasional patient with severe thrombocytopenia, i.e., less than 30,000 to 50,000/cu mm, platelet transfusion therapy as previously described may be indicated. Most patients, however, do not demonstrate a coagulopathy secondary to thrombocytopenia at these levels of circulating platelets, and correction of the coagulation factor deficit with fresh frozen plasma will cause clinical bleeding to cease. But if platelet transfusion is necessary, standard blood filters (175 microns) or special platelet filters should be used when administering platelets. Either type will retain large platelet aggregates without effecting the viability of platelets reaching the recipient. If components are unavailable, the use of fresh whole blood (less than 6 hours old) may provide platelets in sufficient numbers as well as levels of Factors V and VIII sufficient to correct all aspects of the coagulation disorder. If fresh whole blood is transfused for this purpose, a filter with a pore size of 175 or more microns should be used to ensure the benefits of viable platelets. Attempts to establish rigid criteria for platelet transfusions have been unsuccessful. Rather, each patient must be treated as an individual in terms of the clinical bleeding problem.

Bicarbonate infusions have been suggested as required therapy when large volumes of banked blood are transfused. True, stored blood is acidotic. This is a lactic acidosis combined with a major respiratory component (Pco_2 may exceed 150 torr but is removed with the first passage of the transfused blood through the lungs). Alkalinazation of blood, however, is not necessary during transfusion. In fact, controlling the hemorrhage along with adequate volume replacement achieving complete resuscitation will usually result in an alkalosis. This alkalosis usually has both a spontaneous respiratory component and a metabolic component due to bicarbonate excess produced by citrate metabolism. Even though potassium is extruded from stored red blood cells, studies of massive transfusion have shown that hypokalemia rather than hyperkalemia is the rule. The red blood cells gradually take potassium back after they have been transfused into the body, a phenomenon actually hastened by postresuscitation alkalosis. In fact, hyperkalemia after transfusion is usually associated with acidosis secondary to "undertransfusion" or incomplete resuscitation. Thus, adequate resuscitation avoids the complications attributed to blood transfusions (acidosis and hyperkalemia). These are the results of too little blood, not too much.

MASSIVE TRANSFUSION

Transfusion	Coagulation Defect	Lab Abnormality	Therapy
5 units/hr or 10 units/24 hr	Factors V, VIII	↑ PT, ↑ PTT	Fresh whole blood, fresh frozen plasma
	Platelets	↓ platelets	Platelet transfusion

COMPONENT THERAPY

Component Rx	Defect Corrected	Monitor	Clinical
FFP	*All* coagulation proteins (1 unit/ml), 30% activity required	PT, PTT	250–500 cc FFP per 8 units whole blood
Concentrates	II, VII, IX, X (*not* V)	PTT	Small volume required; high risk of hepatitis
Platelets	Thrombocytopenia (<50,000/cu mm)	Platelet count	Special filter needed

There are additional advantages to the component therapy concept. When packed red cells are used to replace red cell deficiency with appropriate crystalloid solutions used to maintain intravascular volume, the risk of massive antibody infusion and allergic complications is reduced since less plasma is employed. Frozen O group red cells can be used for all different ABO groups. Oxygen transport function is well maintained since 2, 3-DPG remains at high levels if blood is frozen soon after harvesting. Furthermore, white cells and platelets are removed. Since antibodies to these formed elements are responsible for a significant number of febrile transfusion reactions, especially in patients who have had large numbers of transfusions in the past, frozen blood can decrease febrile reactions. The use of blood free of white cells may also be desirable for potential transplant recipients to avoid isosensitization.

BLEEDING IN THE CRITICALLY ILL PATIENT—AN APPROACH

Coagulation tests are probably not necessary for every preoperative patient if a good history is obtained and a thorough physical examination is performed unless one is considering the use of prophylactic anticoagulation to prevent deep vein thrombosis. Remember the most common bleeding tendency encountered in patients today is not hemophilia or any of the more serious acquired disorders of hemostasis, but rather is an abnormality in platelet function resulting from self-administration of aspirin. This can only be detected by a careful history and documented by a bleeding time. For evaluation of bleeding problems in the critically ill patient, a reasonable screen should include PT, PTT, platelet count, and thrombin time. For the patient with severe underlying disorders known to be associated with secondary coagulation disturbances, sequential determinations of PT, PTT, platelet count, and fibrinogen levels should be made. Should hemostatic failure occur, the clinical situation may provide an important clue to the underlying cause. Vaginal bleeding suggests retained abortus; hematuria is associated with carcinoma of the prostate; spiking fever suggests an undrained abscess.

A consideration of several categories of bleeding disorders and determination of patterns of abnormal coagulation should lead one to a correct diagnosis and therapy. The most common disorders confronting the clinician may be categorized as congenital or acquired, with congenital disorders subdivided into disorders of coagulation proteins (hemophilia) and rarer platelet disorders (isosensitization), or disorders of both coagulation proteins and platelets (von Willebrand's). Acquired disorders of coagulation proteins are most commonly due to liver disease and vitamin K deficiency. Platelet disorders can be caused by drug effects (aspirin, indomethacin, phenylbutazone), immunologic defects (ITP), or the more severe coagulopathies affecting both protein and platelets as in DIC, dilutional defects of massive blood transfusion, or excess heparin. Each of these categories has a particular pattern of abnormal clotting tests.

A normal PT and PTT rules out hemophilia, von Willebrand's disease, liver dysfunction, and vitamin K deficiency. If, on the other hand, PT and PTT are abnormal, any of the major categories of disorders may exist. A normal platelet count suggests that all but ITP, dilutional effect, or consumptive coagulopathy states may be present. A combination of prolonged PT, prolonged PTT, decreased platelets, and prolonged thrombin time suggests global disruption of the coagulation scheme (DIC, dilution, or heparin excess). A low fibrinogen and demonstration of FSPs in such a situation confirms DIC. Heparin excess or dilutional coagulopathies are characterized by the absence of FSPs. In addition, a thrombin time returning to normal after protamine infusion means heparin excess was the basic problem.

BLEEDING PROBLEMS IN ICU

Lab Abnormality	Mechanism	Clinical Appearance
↑ PT	↓ II, VII, IX, X	Liver disease, coumadin therapy, vitamin K deficiency

Lab Abnormality	Mechanism	Clinical Appearance
↑ PT, ↑ PTT, normal platelets	Intrinsic/extrinsic	Congenital disorders, liver disease, vitamin K deficiency
↑ PT, ↑ PTT, ↓ platelets,	Intrinsic/extrinsic platelets	DIC, cardiopulmonary by-pass, cirrhosis, dilutional
↑ PT, ↑ PTT, ↓ platelets, FSPs present	Global disruption	DIC
Qualitative or quantitative platelet defect	Number, aggregation, adhesion	ITP, drugs, consumption

In summary, bleeding problems arising in otherwise critically ill patients when due to a failure of hemostatic mechanisms are rarely the patient's primary problem. An awareness of coagulation disturbances as an associated problem should lead easily to a coagulation surveillance scheme based on serial determinations of routinely available coagulation tests. Providing appropriate supplemental therapy before a chemical coagulation abnormality becomes a hemorrhagic clinical catastrophe follows the dictum that prevention of complications occurs with greater ease and more favorable results than even the most heroic therapy when complications are established. Should hemorrhagic complications ensue, all efforts should be directed toward:

1. Identifying and correcting predisposing causes
2. Identifying the specific coagulation phase disrupted through the rational application of lab tests
3. Choosing therapy aimed specifically at the defective mechanism

GASTROINTESTINAL BLEEDING

One must differentiate between massive gastrointestinal bleeding from an independent etiology, such as an active duodenal ulcer, gastric ulcer, or Mallory Weiss tear and the hemorrhagic gastritis, or stress ulceration, seen in critical illness. The former are best treated with early operative intervention yielding good results; the latter carries a high mortality rate no matter how it is treated—but may well be preventable. This discussion will deal only with prevention and treatment of erosive stress gastritis.

Acute stress ulceration probably begins as tiny superficial erosions, usually multiple, in the fundus and body of the stomach. Very little submucosal scarring, typical of chronic peptic ulcer disease, is present. Early routine endoscopy performed in multiple injury patients has demonstrated superficial erosions within hours after injury. The etiology of stress ulceration should be considered to be multifactorial: (1) gastric mucosal ischemia, (2) bile reflux, (3) decrease in gastric mucosal ATP content, and (4) increased back diffusion of hydrogen ion—secreted hydrogen ion can traverse the gastric mucosa. Recently attention has been called to the stress-induced "energy crisis" of the gastric mucosa which may allow back diffusion of hydrogen ion even though the mucosa remains grossly intact. In addition, certain factors, such as bile salts, aspirin, and alcohol, increase the permeability of gastric mucosa to hydrogen ions.

Treatment of Stress Bleeding   As a general rule, the risk of stress bleeding correlates with the severity of the underlying illness; the highest incidence is found among septic patients. Management must be based upon prevention of stress bleeding in high-risk surgical patients since surgical intervention is so hazardous. Antacids are the mainstay of therapy both for prevention and treatment of stress bleeding. Experimental evidence suggests that stress ulcers *do not* form in the absence of acid. In addition, all pepsin activity ceases at a pH of 5. For treating active bleeding, several clinical studies report cessation of hemorrhage when large quantities of antacids are given to achieve and maintain pH around 7. This range (pH 5–7) then appears to be a goal of preventive therapy.[29] Furthermore, in terms of reducing the acidity of the stomach, the use of cimetidine (Tagamet), which is now available in parenteral and enteral forms, has been reported to prevent hemorrhage in stress patients. Cimetidine is an H_2-receptor antagonist of histamine-induced gastric acid secretion.

Since bile salts reflux into the stomach and increase the back diffusion of hydrogen ions, the intragastric installation of cholestyramine, which binds bile salts, would seem to be a reasonable preventive maneuver. Hydrogen ion permeability is related to the cell membrane energy-dependent transport functions. This may be clinically translated to the goal of providing adequate substrates to the gastric mucosa. This energy boost for the stress patient involves (1) assuring adequate gastric perfusion, i.e., adequate cardiac output, (2) intragastric installation of dextrose for direct absorption, i.e., 50 ml of 50 percent dextrose every 2 to 4 hours, and (3) adequate total calories and protein via parenteral alimentation.

Vitamin A (50,000 to 100,000 units daily), in a double blind study in Vietnam among burn patients, cut the incidence of stress ulceration from 60 percent to 18 percent.[31] Although the control incidence of 60 percent in this study of burn patients exceeds common ICU prevalence, vitamin A as adjunctive therapy in prevention of stress ulceration in the high risk burn patient seems reasonable. Vitamin A is important in promoting normal mucous cell function in the stomach.

Since the primary therapy for massive hemorrhage secondary to stress gastric ulceration in the critically ill patient is prevention, these measures must be instituted as soon as the patient arrives in the intensive care unit.

Most such patients already have a nasogastric (NG) tube in place, so all medications may be directly administered. Suction is discontinued for 15 to 30 minutes. Antacid therapy, to be effective, must be titrated to a pH of 5.0 of gastric contents; this may require hourly instillation of as much as 60 ml of antacid solution (e.g., Maalox, Mylanta, Amphogel), and 50 ml of a 50 percent glucose solution and 1 gm of cholestyramine may also be added every 2 to 4 hours. Three hundred mg of cimetidine may be given intravenously every 6 hours. Should massive stress bleeding occur, attempts should then be made to titrate the gastric pH to 7.0 by increasing the hourly antacid regimen and measuring gastric aspirate with pH paper 15 minutes after instillation.

PREVENTION OF STRESS GASTRITIS

Drug	Mechanism	Dose
Antacids	↓ Acid	Titrate to pH 5–7; keep pH 7 if bleeding
Cholestyramine	Binds bile salts	1 gm q 4 hr
Cimetidine	H_2 antagonist, ↓ acid	300 mg q 6 hr I.V.
Glucose (50%)	↑ Membrane energy	50 ml q 2–4 hr
Vitamin A	↑ Mucous protection	50,000–100,000 units daily
Total parenteral nutrition	Maintains mucosal "energy" balance	2000–3000 calories; 70 gm protein

Further steps may be taken should stress gastric bleeding become massive. Iced saline lavage and blood replacement as the sole therapy for stress induced gastric bleeding have proven to be inadequate. This failure to control massive gastric bleeding from hemorrhagic gastritis by nonoperative means places the patient at the worst possible risk for surgery, particularly after multiple system failure has ensued. Many ingenious methods of nonsurgical therapy have been proposed for treating this problem: (1) intragastric norepinephrine (Levophed), (2) endoscopic electrocoagulation, (3) intra-arterial pitressin.

Enthusiasts of topical norepinephrine have reported about a 50 percent success rate in temporarily stopping gastric mucosal bleeding.[32] The success of topical Levophed results from its potent vasoconstrictive effects on the gastric mucosa and has no systemic effect since it is absorbed directly into the portal system and metabolized in the liver. The recommended dose is 8 mg of Levophed mixed in 100 ml of saline. The gastric contents are aspirated 30 minutes later, and if bright red bleeding is still present this procedure is repeated every 30 minutes.

The endoscopic electrical coagulation of superficial erosions of the stomach is limited by the availability of specialized equipment and personnel. Great care and skill must be applied to cause coagulation of open blood vessels by heat without destroying normal tissue. Technical failures can lead to either increased bleeding or perforation. Thus far, rebleeding rates have been 25 to 50 percent.[33]

In 1963 Nusbaum and Baum[34] reported the technique of selective angiography for the diagnosis of the site of G. I. bleeding. Five years later they reported on the selective visceral arterial infusion of vasopressin.[35] Vasopressin (Pitressin) is a potent vasoconstrictor that acts directly on the contractile elements of capillaries and arterioles. The smooth muscle of larger veins is less responsive. The recommended initial dose is 0.2 units per minute. A convenient method of administration uses 100 units of Pitressin (20 units per vial) mixed in 500 ml of normal saline infused at 1 ml per minute. *Selective infusion is the key to control.* Nonselective infusion (celiac artery) is usually not successful in controlling bleeding gastric vessels. Infusion can achieve an 85 percent success rate if direct left gastric or gastroduodenal vessels can be catheterized.

NONOPERATIVE RX FOR STRESS GASTRITIS BLEEDING

Iced saline lavage; transfusions	Initial Rx, but frequently inadequate
Intragastric norepinephrine	8 mg/100 ml per N-G tube, repeat q 30 min
Endoscopic cautery	Technical limitations
Vasopressin-left gastric artery	Good success rate, 0.2–0.4 units/min

Massive Gastric Hemorrhage Secondary to Esophageal Varices   Massive variceal hemorrhage secondary to portal hypertension requires a dual therapeutic approach:

1. Mechanical and pharmacologic control of the ruptured varix at the esophagogastric junction
2. Correction of the coagulation disturbances secondary to the liver disease

The coagulation disturbances secondary to liver disease involve defects in the intrinsic and extrinsic pathway as well as thrombocytopenia secondary to hypersplenism from the portal hypertension. Although thrombocytopenia secondary to hypersplenism may be severe, i.e., less than 50,000/cu mm, bleeding from varices is more directly related to portal pressure than it is to the severity of the coagulation disturbance. Both intravascular volume restoration and correction of coagulation disturbances must be considered initial therapy. Replacement therapy—fresh frozen plasma, cryoprecipitates, and platelet transfusions (if the platelet count is less than 30,000/cu mm)—should be instituted quickly. However, therapy must be simultaneously directed at mechanical and/or pharmacologic control of the actual bleeding site at the esophagogastric junction.

Vasopressin Therapy   Portal pressure can be reduced by 50 percent after vasopressin therapy—either systemically administered or selectively infused into the superior mesenteric artery—through its effect upon splanchnic blood flow. The recommended initial dose is 0.2 units per minute with a maximal safe dose of 0.4 units per minute. Approximately 80 percent of the patients can be well controlled initially by vasopressin infusions. Rebleeding may not occur, even though cessation of therapy is accompanied by the expected return to higher portal pressure. Peripheral venous infusion seems to be just as effective in lowering portal pressure and controlling variceal hemorrhage as selective superior mesenteric artery infusion but with fewer technical problems such as catheter placement and infection.[36] If bleeding is well controlled with peripheral vasopressin infusions, then the infusion rate should be left at the controlling dosage for 12 hours. If no further bleeding ensues, then the dose may be tapered (each dimunition of the infusion rate should be followed by an 8- to 12-hour observation period for further bleeding). Close observation should be maintained for at least 24 hours after cessation of vasopressin infusion.

Sengstaken-Blakemore Tube   The   Sengstaken-Blakemore   (SB) tube can be used to treat endoscopically proven variceal hemorrhage with a high success rate and low complication rate,[37] if care is taken to ensure proper placement and function. Guidelines, which should be rigidly adhered to, include:

1. Assure the patency of all the lumens and test the balloons before insertion.
2. Empty the stomach completely with an Ewalt tube.
3. Have tracheal suction on stand by.
4. Do not anesthetize the pharnyx.
5. Lubricate the tube well.
6. Pass the tube through the nose to the 50 cm mark on the tube.
7. Fill the gastric balloon with 200 ml of air and clamp.
8. Use gentle traction in pulling the tube out until the resistance created by positioning the balloon at the C-E junction is felt.
9. Attach a helmet-type traction apparatus to the patient and secure the tube to the frame of the helmet.
10. Irrigate the distal tube in the stomach; if there is no blood return the esophageal balloon is not inflated.
11. If bleeding continues, then the esophageal balloon should be inflated to 40 torr using continuous monitoring.
12. A small (10 or 12 F) nasogastric tube should be placed through the other nostril until it meets the resistance near the esophageal balloon. This allows "sumping" of the blind segment of the esophagus to avoid aspiration of esophageal secretion.
13. Leave the gastric and/or esophageal balloon inflated for 24 hours; deflate the esophageal balloon first and observe for bleeding. If no bleeding occurs in 24 hours the gastric balloon is then deflated. If no bleeding occurs in another 24 to 36 hours, the tube may be removed. The most serious complication associated with the SB tube is esophageal rupture due to initial malposition or inadvertent dis-

lodgment of the gastric balloon. Pulmonary complications due to aspiration of blood, gastric content, or saliva are so frequent that endotracheal intubation must be considered imperative if any disorder of consciousness or shock-like state persists. Chest X-ray is mandatory to assure proper SB tube placement.

RX FOR VARICEAL HEMORRHAGE

Therapy	Mechanism	Clinical
Blood, fresh frozen plasma, platelets	Resuscitation, pancoagulopathy, of liver disease	May require large quantities FFP; keep platelets 50,000/cu mm
Vasopressin Arterial Venous (peripheral)	↓ Splanchnic flow in SMA	0.2–0.4 units/min 0.2–0.4 units/min
SB tube	Tamponade C-E junction	Rigid guidelines

PELVIC TRAUMA

The frequency of associated injuries, complications, and mortality secondary to massive hemorrhage from pelvic fracture is markedly increased in those patients with posterior pelvic ring fractures, i.e., involving the ilium, sacroiliac joint, and sacrum. Proper management of patients with extensive pelvic fracture demands an appreciation of the extent to which the retroperitoneum may accommodate extravascular collections of blood. Disruption of large venous channels can result in the loss of as much as 4000 ml of blood before tamponade is achieved. It has been common practice to transfuse 8 to 10 units of blood before laparotomy in such patients who have no free intraperitoneal blood documented by peritoneal lavage, since failure to achieve operative control of pelvic hemorrhage occurs in approximately 75 percent of the cases. However, large volume blood transfusion therapy antedates the use of external compression devices ("G-suit" or MAST)* which have been employed to control the bleeding of fractures. The efficacy of external counterpressure, both for extremity bleeding and for intra-abdominal bleeding, has been quite well documented. Gardner et al.[38,39] described the clinical use of external counterpressure by means of a G-suit in the treatment of massive abdominal hemorrhage secondary to gynecologic catastrophes, ruptured aortic aneurysm, and other large vessel injuries. Hemorrhage from massive trauma was controlled by the G-suit in Vietnam casualties;[40] MAST have also been used in civilian trauma.[41]

The MAST may be inflated to a maximum pressure of 105 torr, which can exceed mean intra-arterial pressure and prevent further arterial

* Military Anti-Shock Trousers (MAST), David Clark Co., Worcester, Mass.

bleeding. Once hemodynamic stability is achieved, the MAST pressure is lowered by 10 torr increments to 40 torr over a 6- to 10-hour period. This pressure is maintained for an additional 24 hours before continued deflation. Early application, i.e., before major hematoma has collected, appears more efficacious than late application. If hemodynamic stability is not achieved, angiographic studies and/or surgery must be contemplated before the coagulopathy of massive transfusion therapy occurs.

Reports of the nonoperative control of pelvic hemorrhage by angiographic identification of a single vessel bleeding and clot embolization of that vessel and/or vasopressin infusion have met with some success.[42] Although usually ascribed to venous bleeding, the massive bleeding from pelvic fracture is often from an arterial source, commonly the obturator artery. Thus selective catheterization of the bleeding vessel with subsequent embolization via the catheter may control hemorrhage and avoid the hazards of surgical exploration. If all other mechanisms have failed to control bleeding, then surgical exploration must be undertaken, although the associated mortality rate is 75 percent. Bilateral internal iliac artery ligation may not be successful since collateral flow is so plentiful; it may only exacerbate bleeding when the posterior peritoneum's tamponade effect is released.

RX FOR HEMORRHAGE FROM MAJOR PELVIC FRACTURE

Rule out intra-abdominal bleeding	Peritoneal lavage
Apply MAST early	Maintain 40 torr inflation pressure for 24 hr
Monitor and correct coagulopathy	FFP, platelets
Angiography/embolization	Bleeding despite MAST
Surgery	High mortality

MISCELLANEOUS CAUSES OF NON-COAGULOPATHY BLEEDING IN CRITICALLY ILL PATIENTS

Postoperative patients admitted to the ICU must have careful monitoring to assure the competence of the cardiovascular system as well as to detect continued hemorrhage from the operative site. Rebleeding rates following certain massive injuries or particular types of operations (liver and pancreas) demand constant attention to blood volume as estimated by serial hematocrits and hemodynamic profiles (blood pressure, urine output, cardiac filling pressures, and cardiac output). Certain disorders of surgical bleeding occur frequently enough to justify an organized approach to permit early detection and therapy.

Bleeding from pleural or mediastinal chest tubes occurs frequently after operation. Patency of these drainage tubes must be maintained to permit evacuation of blood from the chest cavity and to monitor the bleeding rate. Persistent bleeding of 50 ml/hr requires careful observation, and if the rate exceeds 100 ml/hr for 4 to 5 hours, reexploration is probably indicated if coagulation studies are normal. The bleeding may originate from the chest tube insertion site (intercostal vessels) as well as the operative area (pleural, pericardial, pulmonary parenchyma, or mediastinum).

Bleeding from the urinary tract after surgery is also a common clinical problem. The tendency for bleeding to continue in the operative site (prostatic bed) following transuretheral resection of the prostate is perpetuated by urokinase activation of the fibrinolytic mechanism. The therapeutic mainstay for postoperative hematuria is irrigation with sterile saline solution through a large Foley catheter (22 F). The purpose is to remove all clots so that bladder decompression and contraction may be assured to achieve mechanical pressure control. Occasionally, Amicar therapy may be indicated. In routine clinical practice, this may be the only real indication for the use of Amicar. If repeated irrigation results in "clearing" of the saline solution, continuous traction may be applied to the Foley catheter by taping the external portion of the catheter to the inner aspect of the patient's thigh. This provides a tamponade effect similar to Sengstaken-Blakemore tube treatment of esophagogastric varices. Should bleeding continue, reoperation will be necessary.

In general, the decision to reoperate for direct attack upon persistent bleeding is based on (1) recognition of continued bleeding, and (2) rapid correction of any predisposing factor disrupting normal coagulation. Serial hematocrits done every 2 to 4 hours are useful in decision making. If the diagnosis can be established, reoperation should be performed before the hazards of massive transfusion (dilutional coagulopathy) have accumulated. Early hemodynamic instability (blood pressure dropping 20 to 30 mm Hg from a previously normal level) is not uncommon after major prolonged operative procedures. This problem reflects continued extracellular fluid losses and is best treated with crystalloid infusions. If red cell volume is also needed, as evidenced by a decreasing hematocrit, continuing blood loss should be suspected, particularly if this becomes a repetitive cycle. *Waiting for abdominal distention to suggest large accumulations of blood at the operative site constitutes unnecessary delay in the appropriate correction of surgical bleeding.*

POSTOPERATIVE BLEEDING GUIDELINES

Site	Signs	Treatment
Chest tubes	100 ml/hr for 4 hr	Keep tubes patent; correct coagulation disturbances; reoperation
Postoperative hematuria	Clot occlusion; Foley catheter	Irrigate clear; traction tamponade; Amicar(?); reoperation
Intra-abdominal hemorrhage	Repeated cycles of hypotension/fluid bolus; ↓ Hct	Reoperation; correct coagulation disturbances

THROMBOTIC DISORDERS

DEEP VEIN THROMBOSIS AND PULMONARY EMBOLISM

Present Status of Deep Vein Thrombosis Our understanding of the pathogenesis of spontaneous intravascular thrombus formation, particularly in the venous circulation, has not progressed much beyond Virchow's description of more than 100 years ago. The classic triad of intravascular stasis, alteration in the intimal lining of veins, and some tendency toward a hypercoagulable state are cited, although the exact mechanism and initiating sequence are not fully understood. Thrombin accumulation in areas of venous stasis can initiate platelet aggregation and fibrin production. This platelet aggregation may result in the release of platelet factor 3 which can further increase the rate of thrombin production. In a similar manner, intimal damage may initiate thrombosis through the extrinsic coagulation mechanism by the release of thromboplastic substances and through the intrinsic coagulation cascade by activating Factor XII. Hypercoagulability is difficult to quantitate because reliable tests are not available. Furthermore, failure to detect systemic hypercoagulability would not eliminate the possibility of local hypercoagulability, particularly in the areas of highest risk—the lower extremity.

It is clear that the seriously injured or critically ill patient is at high risk of deep venous thrombosis. Phlebographic and I[125]-labeled fibrinogen studies provide convincing evidence that venous stasis and thrombosis occur in any supine patient at bed rest; although what actually occurs at the intima-blood interface to promote thrombosis is not yet known. Although the process is called "thrombophlebitis," there is little evidence confirming that the initiating event in the intimal lining is true inflammation. Direct endothelial damage exposes raw collagen which activates the clotting process, but this does not explain thrombosis in uninjured extremities. One current theory suggests that during stress or injury, a circulating chemotactic substance attracts white cells to capillary endothelium at the basement membrane junction. This process may lead to the formation of a nidus of erythrocytes, platelets, and fibrin—the scaffolding for a continued process of coagulation.

Although I[125]-labeled fibrinogen and venography studies show that thrombosis of the lower extremity begins in the calf veins, the natural history of the formed clot in an individual patient is largely unpredictable. About one-third of these thrombi lyse without clinical manifestation. Another third remain confined to the calf, may be symptomatic locally, and occasionally give rise to small, nonfatal emboli. The remaining third of the thrombi will pose a serious risk because they propagate proximally into larger veins of the lower extremity.

The trauma patient is at particular risk of thromboembolism. Although many abnormalities have been identified in platelet adhesiveness and survival times and in fibrinolysis, the entire mechanism is unclear. The available evidence suggests that the key reaction in the control of thrombin formation is the activation of Factor X by the small platelet nidus. In the early postoperative period, spontaneous thrombosis seems to be related to depressed fibrinolytic activity. In addition, increased levels of α-1-antitrypsin, an antiplasmin and fibrinolytic inhibitor, have been found in the plasma of postoperative patients. This would tend to shift the balance toward thrombosis. In massively injured patients or patients developing early systemic complications, continued enhancement of the fibrinolytic response may explain the seemingly rare occurrence of clinically significant deep vein thrombosis or pulmonary embolism among these groups in the surgical intensive care unit.

Diagnosis of Deep Vein Thrombosis Two cardinal principles described our difficulty in detecting venous thrombosis of the lower extremity reliably: (1) the bedside clinical evaluation of the patient is not good enough by itself to detect deep vein thrombosis; even the "most reliable" physical finding, i.e., unilateral leg swelling, has been found to be unreliable. (2) Contrast venography is the single best method of establishing the presence of venous thrombosis. Yet, because of discomfort to the patient, difficulty in obtaining sequential studies, safety (hazard of induced chemical phlebitis), and interpretation, venography is *not* a feasible routine diagnostic test. As a result, three noninvasive diagnostic methods have been extensively examined: (1) I^{125} fibrinogen scanning, (2) ultrasonography, and (3) plethysmography.

I^{125}-Labeled Fibrinogen Scan The ability to detect thrombi externally by the uptake of isotopically tagged fibrinogen provided great impetus to study the problem of venous thrombosis prospectively. The procedure is relatively simple to perform, leaving only its interpretation and accuracy open to discussion.[1] The fibrinogen scan becomes positive only if the labeled fibrinogen is deposited on an existing or extending thrombus. Its major limitation for clinical use is its inability to detect thrombus formation in the most important area, i.e., above the upper third of the thigh. The scan technique cannot be used in the vicinity of large wounds, such as those found in reconstructive hip procedures, or near major fractures, since fibrinogen deposition is expected as part of the healing process. Approximately one-third of patients over 40 years of age will have a scan-detectable calf venous thrombosis after major abdominal surgery. This incidence increases to 50 percent in patients following abdominal prostatectomy or in the paretic extremity of patients with completed strokes. Using venography as the standard, fibrinogen scanning has only about 80 percent specificity, i.e., a false positive rate of about 20 percent, combined with a sensitivity of 88 to 90 percent, i.e., 10 to 12 percent false negative rate.

I^{125} FIBRINOGEN SCANNING

Advantages	Limitations
Bedside evaluation	Silent area = pelvic plexus
Safe	10% false positive,
Serial exams	15% false negative
Detection of major vein clots	

Plethysmography Plethysmographic methods measure the rate at which the blood is drained from the leg after a brief period of mechanically induced total venous occlusion. Like ultrasound, plethysmographic methods are not sensitive enough to pick up non-major-vein thrombi since these do not interfere with venous flow in major channels. Its sensitivity to detect thrombosis is 90 percent, while its specificity is less accurate (80 to 85 percent) and potentially more dangerous—undetected significant thrombus.

Ultrasonography Ultrasonography can detect occlusion of the major venous channels of the lower extremity (iliac, femoral, and popliteal). The principle of ultrasonography is based on the analysis of the frequency change which occurs when an emitted sound encounters flowing blood. The frequency of the sound changes in proportion to the velocity of blood flow. Thus, obstruction of a major venous channel (no flow) or continuous flow unaffected by Valsalva or respiratory maneuvers results in a "positive" test. But ultrasonography will not detect obstruction of venous muscular branches in the thigh or calf or of the deep pelvic venous plexus. Inability to detect thrombosis in the calf veins by ultrasonography accounts for most of the false negatives (20 percent) of this examination when compared to venography.

PLETHYSMOGRAPHY / ULTRASONOGRAPHY

Advantages	*Limitations*
Bedside evaluation	Silent area = calf veins, pelvic plexus
Safe	10% false positive
Serial exams	20% false negative
Major vein clots	

In summary, in terms of missed locations, only I^{125} fibrinogen scanning detects thrombi where they most frequently occur (calf veins). However, since the majority of calf vein clots never form lethal emboli, its routine use in critically ill patients does not seem warranted. Ultrasonography and plethysmographic methods, on the other hand, will detect major vein thrombi, which are clinically dangerous; but some are missed. Thus, the advantages of simplicity and safety of noninvasive methods compared to venography must be weighed carefully against their limitations (Table 3-3).

Prophylaxis of Deep Vein Thrombosis The severity of the two major consequences of deep venous thrombosis—pulmonary embolus and the postphlebetic syndrome—have served to direct attention toward prophylaxis. The postphlebetic syndrome results from destruction of the valve system during recanalization and induces significant venous hypertension of the lower extremity. This can lead to ecchymoses, dermatitis, and ultimately, persistent venous ulceration. Fatal pulmonary embolism is the consequence of dislodgement of a major thrombus. Since the supine

TABLE 3-3
Proposed Methods for Diagnosis of Venous Thrombosis

Dx Venous Thrombosis
Clinical
Venography
I^{125}-fibrinogen scanning
Impedance plethysmography
Doppler ultrasound

Note: Each method must be evaluated as to diagnostic specificity, sensitivity, and safety.

position induces thrombosis, ambulation is the best prophylaxis. Antistasis measures commonly used when ambulation is not possible include elastic stockings, leg elevation, and leg exercises. These are not suitable or reliable substitutes. Electrical calf stimulation and intermittent pneumatic compression devices are the only physical measures that bear promise to prevent deep venous thrombosis of the lower extremity. However, further investigation is necessary to prove their efficacy.

Pharmacologic interventions are currently the mainstay of prophylaxis. The administration of any anticoagulant must start *before* operation since the initial stages of thrombosis occur during the procedure. Oral anticoagulants (Coumadin, warfarin) are effective but are difficult to control. These coumarin derivatives block the hepatic synthesis of vitamin K-dependent clotting Factors II, VII, IX, and X. They have a limited direct effect on the clotting mechanism. They create a hypoprothrombinemic state which begins as the vitamin K-dependent clotting factors decrease at a rate consistent with their individual biologic half-lives (Factors II, 60 hours; VII, 6 hours; IX, 24 hours; X, 40 hours). The optimal anticoagulation effect of coumarin derivatives, therefore, requires 3 or more days to develop. Larger doses prolong duration but do not stimulate a faster onset. Coumarin derivatives are absorbed promptly through the gastrointestinal tract, transported in plasma bound to albumin, metabolized in the liver, and excreted in bile at varying rates. Steatorrhea, biliary obstruction, and antibiotics which alter intestinal flora may interfere with vitamin K absorption and production, and, thus, potentiate the effect of these anticoagulants. The anticoagulant effect of coumarin derivatives is measured by the prothrombin time. Clotting curves of normal plasma and test plasma can be compared. Effective anticoagulation is considered to be two times normal, or 22 to 38 percent of the normal activity. Current recommendations are 10 to 15 mg warfarin given preoperatively for 2 days. The anticoagulant effect is regulated by maintaining prothrombin time at 1.5 to 2 times normal controls, remembering that the peak effect of this drug does not occur until 36 hours after ingestion. In patients with fractured hips,[43] deep vein thrombosis was prevented when PT was two times normal, and bleeding complications seemed to occur with higher frequency when the prothrombin time was two and one-half to three times normal. When bleeding complications do occur, vitamin K (10 to 20 mg) is the specific antidote to warfarin. However, coagulation activity may not begin to approach normal following vitamin K therapy until 4 to 6 hours later. Significant bleeding due to warfarin overdosage is usually best treated with infusions of 250 to 500 ml fresh frozen plasma, which restores circulating levels of Factors II, VII, IX, and X.

WARFARIN GUIDELINES

Indications	Dose	Monitor	Overdose
Oral prophylaxis	10–15 mg q day × 2; daily dose adjustment	PT = 2 × normal	Vitamin K, 20 mg; FFP, 500 ml

Low-Dose Heparin for Prophylaxis of Deep Vein Thrombosis   Because of the difficulty in maintaining effective but safe levels of anticoagulation with coumarin-type drugs, low-dose heparin has been investigated as an alternate means of interfering with the coagulation scheme. The availability of the I^{125} fibrinogen test has confirmed the effectiveness of low-dose heparin in preventing the development of deep vein thrombosis (DVT). A review of Hirsch[44] in 1975 showed that low-dose heparin reduced the incidence of DVT from 42 percent in untreated patients to 15 percent in those receiving low-dose heparin as demonstrated by I^{125} scan. But does low-dose heparin decrease the incidence of fatal pulmonary embolism? Kakkar[45] reported that in a randomized multicenter trial involving over 4000 surgical patients, the incidence of thrombosis and pulmonary embolism were significantly reduced; however, less than 50 percent of the entire group had deep vein thrombosis detected. To date, more than two dozen clinical trials have been reported attesting to the efficacy and safety of low-dose heparin. The original concern over its use in surgical patients—inducing bleeding in operative areas—therefore, does not seem warranted. Due to the exceptionally low incidence of fatal pulmonary embolism in the normal population of postoperative general surgical patients, much larger studies involving many thousands of patients must be conducted in order to provide convincing evidence that low-dose heparin reduces the risk of fatal pulmonary embolism as well as preventing deep vein thrombosis.

Five thousand units of heparin are administered subcutaneously every 12 hours. This regimen results in blood concentrations approximately one-fifth of those required to prolong the PTT or the Lee White clotting time to accepted therapeutic levels. Yet this dose is sufficient to enhance the activity of anti-thrombin-3, the main plasmin inhibitor of the activated coagulation enzymes, especially Factor Xa. The inactivation of Factor Xa stops conversion of prothrombin to thrombin. At this heparin dose level, there is enough heparin-mediated anti-thrombin-3 activity to block the new generation of thrombin but not enough to turn off the thrombin activity already present at the site of required thrombosis in healing wounds.

Patients undergoing intracranial operations are potentially excluded from this therapy since the smallest amount of postoperative intracranial bleeding might be catastrophic. Coe, in 1977,[46] found external pneumatic calf compression to be more effective than low-dose heparin in patients undergoing prostatectomy, cystectomy, and other open urologic procedures. It is conceivable, therefore, that the same may apply to other "noncandidates" for low-dose heparin, i.e., CNS operations, eye operations, peptic ulcer and severe hypertension. At the present time, the following groups of patients may be considered candidates for low-dose heparin prophylaxis: (1) patients over 40 years of age undergoing abdominal, gynecologic, or thoracic surgical procedures, (2) those with other risk factors (obesity, varicose veins, previous thrombophlebitis or pulmonary embolism, estrogen, or anovulatory therapy), and (3) hospitalized patients with chronic debilitating disease, congestive heart failure, and strokes (Table 3-4).

TABLE 3-4
Factors in Selection of Patients for "Low-Dose"
Heparin Prophylaxis

High Risk Group
Elderly (> 65 yr)
Lower extremity fracture
Hip surgery
Pelvic surgery—extensive dissection
Past Hx of thromboembolism
CHF
Cancer surgery
Obesity
Vein surgery

For surgical patients, after a screen of the coagulation system for preexisting disorders (PT, PTT, and platelet count) has been made, low-dose heparin is given as 5000 units subcutaneously 2 hours before surgery and 5000 units every 8 or 12 hours postoperatively for 5 days. No monitoring of coagulation by serial testing is necessary unless unexplained bleeding occurs. Prophylaxis must continue until full ambulation is attained since a direct correlation has been demonstrated between the duration of bed rest and the development of deep vein thrombosis.

GUIDELINES FOR HEPARIN PROPHYLAXIS

Indication	Dose	Monitor
DVT prophylaxis	5000 units SC preoperatively, 5000 units q 8–12 hr × 5 days	No test necessary

Antiplatelet Drugs as Prophylaxis for DVT   Recent studies demonstrating that the platelet nidus may initiate venous as well as arterial thrombosis have lead to the use of drugs known to alter platelet function in hopes of preventing venous thromboembolism. Dextran, the most widely studied of antiplatelet drugs, impairs the platelet release reaction and platelet aggregation as well as decreases platelet adhesiveness. It also impairs fibrin polymerization and alleviates stagnant blood flow. These latter effects may be as important in preventing venous thrombosis as the direct platelet inhibitory effects. Dextran was effective in one study in reducing venous thrombosis after hip surgery from 55 percent to 16 percent.[47] However, limitations for general use include increased costs, necessity for intravenous infusion, the risk of possible fluid overload, allergic reactions, and rare instances of renal failure.

The antiplatelet effect of aspirin has been studied extensively as prophylactic therapy for venous thrombosis. Acetylsalicylic acid (300 mg) inhibits platelet aggregation with an onset 1 to 2 hours after ingestion and lasting 2 to 7 days with a single dose. More clinical trials are necessary before recommending acetylsalicylic acid (ASA) as effective DVT prophylaxis. Dipyridamole (Persantin) is ineffective in preventing thrombosis of calf veins, while hydroxychloroquine (Plaquenil) has been shown to be effective in reducing the incidence of venous thrombosis in general surgical patients.[48] Sulfinpyrazone (Anturan) has been suggested for use in reducing the frequency of transient cerebral ischemic attacks but has not been proven to be effective in the prevention of venous thromboembolism in postoperative surgical patients.[49]

ANTIPLATELET DRUGS

Drug	Mode of Action	Dose	Efficacy
ASA	Inhibits platelet function	300 mg b.i.d.	?
Hydroxychloroquine	Inhibits platelet function	200 mg b.i.d.	General surgical patients
Sulfinpyrazone	Inhibits platelet function	200 mg b.i.d.	Arterial thrombosis, venous thrombosis(?)
Dipyridamole	Inhibits platelet function	75 mg b.i.d.	Ineffective

Treatment of Deep Venous Thrombosis   The therapeutic mainstay for established deep venous thrombosis is full and immediate anticoagulation of the patient with intravenous heparin. The diagnosis may be suspected on clinical grounds by examination of the patient, and may be confirmed by the various noninvasive tests described in the previous section or by the appearance of pulmonary embolism.

Heparin plays many roles in altering the coagulation cascade. Its main effect is to markedly potentiate the action of anti-thrombin-3. The half-life of the anticoagulant effect of intravenous heparin is 1.5 hours. Traditionally, a safe effective anticoagulation level is presumed to exist when the whole blood clotting time is 2 to 3 times normal and the activated partial thromboplastin time is 1.5 to 2 times normal as measured before the next dose is administered. There are pitfalls, however, in the use of heparin:

1. Commercial heparin is standardized in International Units according to its ability to prolong the clotting time of sheep plasma. The number of units may vary from 130 to 170 units per mg, so it is prudent to order heparin as *units*, not mg.
2. Samples of plasma collected in citrate (as the test tube anticoagulant) are more sensitive to heparin than oxalated plasma.
3. Various partial thromboplastin tests differ in their sensitivity.
4. Other drugs (ASA, indomethacin) may cause bleeding despite presumably safe heparin dose administration.
5. Patients with acute thrombosis require more heparin to achieve an effective therapeutic effect, presumably from the binding of heparin to fibrinogen instead of anti-thrombin-3.
6. Patients with right-sided heart failure seem to require more heparin; therefore, dosage adjustments must coincide with the improvement of the underlying condition.
7. Many of the hemorrhagic complications reported with the use of heparin have been associated with intramuscular injections rather than intravenous administration.
8. The benefit of heparin in treating venous thrombotic disease is clearly documented; the benefit in arterial thrombotic disease is less well established.
9. No lab test is entirely satisfactory for monitoring the anticoagulant effect of heparin therapy. Although the whole blood clotting time is the time-honored test for monitoring the anticoagulant effect, it is time consuming, difficult to standardize, inadequately sensitive, and poorly reproducible. The activated PTT has been recommended as a substitute, but its critics note that its sensitivity is limited to the midtherapeutic range of heparin anticoagulation.

Basu et al.[50] found that hemorrhagic complications occurred in patients with heparin dosages and activated PTT values similar to those patients who encountered no bleeding. The overall incidence of bleeding was reported as 8 percent, with 13 percent occurring in postoperative patients and 4 percent in nonsurgical patients. Recurrence of thromboemboli was related to low activated PTT values. Salzman, in 1975,[51] compared three groups of patients requiring heparin therapy for deep venous thrombosis: (1) the first group received intermittent heparin therapy with monitoring by the PTT, (2) the second group also received intermittent heparin therapy in the same dose, 5,000 to 10,000 units every 4 hours with *no* control testing done, and (3) the third group received continuous heparin infusion controlled by monitoring the PTT. They found: (1) no difference in mortality, (2) the total incidence of major and minor hemorrhage in each of the three groups was comparable, and (3) the complication of major hemorrhage was greater in the first two groups (intermittent heparin). Continuous intravenous heparin administered significantly decreases major complications by reducing the total daily dose while maintaining effective therapy. Thus, a loading dose of 5,000 to 10,000 units heparin I.V. should be followed by 750 to 1000 units hourly by continuous infusion.

Other monitoring tests including protamine sulfate titration, PRT (plasma recalcification time), thrombin time, and PT have been described but not suited for routine use in monitoring heparin therapy. As techniques for more direct assays are developed, precise adjustments of the coagulation cascade can be envisioned which should separate therapeutic effects from the risk of bleeding complications.

Other complications of heparin therapy include (1) allergic reactions (urticaria, bronchial constriction) usually appearing after 4 to 7 days of heparin therapy, (2) thrombocytopenia, which is rare but may promote bleeding, also 4 to 7 days after therapy; the platelet count should be monitored to avert bleeding complications caused by an unrecognized drop in the platelet count, and (3) hemorrhage, which may be minimal mucosal oozing or life-threatening intracranial hemorrhage, hemothorax, gastrointestinal bleeding, or significant hematuria. Hemorrhage into the iliopsoas or rectus abdominus muscle or retroperitoneal space may even simulate an acute abdomen. Femoral nerve palsy has been reported from hemorrhage and hematoma formation in the iliopsoas muscle (Table 3-5).

The failure rate of heparin anticoagulation therapy (recurrent thromboembolism and serious hemorrhage) is less than 10 percent. Hemorrhage is treated by stopping heparin and giving protamine sulfate 20 to 30

TABLE 3-5

Contraindications to Complete Anticoagulation

Bleeding abnormality—preexisting
GI ulceration (gastric, duodenal, colitis)
CVA—recent
Organ bleeding (pulmonary, GI, GU)
Malignant hypertension
Subacute bacterial endocarditis
Intracranial/ophthalmic surgery
Spinal/regional anesthesia
Pregnancy (heparin probably okay; *not* coumadin)

---

mg if signs of bleeding persist. If therapy is prolonged for 10 days, the
incidence of recurrent pulmonary embolism is less than 5 percent.

HEPARIN FOR DVT

Indication	Mechanism	Dose	Monitor	Complications
Clinical Dx, noninvasive confirmation	Potentiates antithrombin-3 activity	5000–10,000 units loading dose; 750–1000 units hourly for 10 days	None specific; platelet count	Allergic thrombocytopenia; hemorrhage

Oral anticoagulation with a coumarin derivative should overlap intravenous heparin therapy. The suggested duration of oral therapy varies with the site and process: (1) calf vein thrombosis—4 to 6 weeks,
(2) major deep vein thrombosis—3 to 6 months, (3) mild pulmonary embolism with normal venogram—4 to 6 weeks, and (4) major pulmonary
embolism—6 months.

COUMADIN FOR DVT

Indication	Mechanism Action	Dose
After 7–10 days of heparin, overlap Rx	Inhibits vitamin K-dependent factor production	15–30 mg loading dose, after 48–72 hr adjust; 6 weeks–6 months

Role of Surgery in Initial Therapy of DVT   Venous thrombectomy enjoyed
initial enthusiasm as treatment for iliofemoral thrombosis. The results
of subsequent follow-up studies demonstrated greater than 50 percent
reocclusion rate following venous thrombectomy. Nevertheless the procedure is probably indicated for *phlegmasia cerulea dolens,* a severe
form of deep vein thrombosis where stasis and venous hypertension is
so extensive that the arterial circulation becomes impaired. However,
immediate bedrest, elevation of the extremity, and full heparinization
may reverse the physical changes of the lower extremity within 8 to
12 hours, thus obviating the need for early venous thrombectomy.

PULMONARY EMBOLISM

The true incidence of pulmonary embolism is unknown; indeed, most
pulmonary emboli are never detected. About 75 percent of pulmonary
emboli originate from the lower extremity veins and about 25 percent
from the pelvic venous plexus.

Diagnosis   The plain chest X-ray offers little in the way of specific criteria for the diagnosis of pulmonary embolism. The typical wedge-shaped

peripheral density associated with pulmonary infarction occurs in only 10 percent of those patients with a proven pulmonary embolus. Frequently, however, a patchy nonsegmental infiltrate appears in the area of the pulmonary embolus suggesting some reflex changes in ventilation as well. This infiltrate is frequently seen in the lower lung fields (right slightly greater than left) since the lower lobes are the most frequent locations for pulmonary emboli.

Arterial blood gas determinations are the most sensitive tests for diagnosing a pulmonary embolus. No other routine tests, including chest X-ray, electrocardiogram, and biochemical determination of enzymes, are as accurate as the findings of arterial hypoxemia. A Po_2 greater than 80 torr virtually excludes the diagnosis of a significant pulmonary embolus. If the clinical situation suggests that a pulmonary embolus is likely and arterial hypoxemia is present, then a lung scan is indicated. Of course, there are many other reasons for hypoxemia as well.

A normal perfusion lung scan excludes the diagnosis of pulmonary embolus. Radioactive iodine-labeled albumin is injected intravenously and uptake qualitated over the lung fields. A "positive" perfusion scan must be correlated with the plain chest X-ray. The lung scan thus enjoys great sensitivity in documenting areas of poor perfusion but lacks a significant degree of specificity. The nonspecificity of positive perfusion lung scans is chiefly related to the decrease in pulmonary blood flow which may develop in any poorly ventilated area of the lung (bronchial mucous plug, atelectasis). Combination ventilation-perfusion lung scanning evolved as a diagnostic aid for pulmonary embolism to improve upon this lack of specificity of the perfusion scan alone. Pulmonary ventilation scans are done with radioactively labeled inert gases, usually xenon (Xe^{133}), which is injected intravenously in saline solution or inhaled through a specially designed delivery system. Simultaneous ventilation perfusion scans eliminate all lung conditions which cause perfusion defects other than those due to embolism. This test thus provides a specificity level of 80 to 90 percent.

The most specific test available for diagnosing a pulmonary embolus is pulmonary angiography. However, this test is expensive, time consuming, hazardous, and is not readily applicable to critically ill patients. Nevertheless, if heparin therapy is also considered too hazardous to initiate despite strongly suggestive evidence of pulmonary embolism obtained from blood gases, chest X-ray, and scanning techniques, then a pulmonary angiogram is indicated to settle the question (Table 3-6).

Treatment of Pulmonary Embolism For a single documented pulmonary embolus, full anticoagulation with heparin should be started immediately. The only absolute contraindication is the possibility of life-threatening postoperative bleeding and bleeding into the central nervous system. After a loading dose of 5,000 to 10,000 units of heparin given intravenously, full anticoagulation is maintained by the continuous intravenous infusion of 1000 units of heparin per hour (in an average-

TABLE 3-6

Methods Available for Diagnosing Pulmonary Embolus

Diagnosis Pulmonary Embolus	
Clinical	Insensitive/nonspecific
Blood tests	Nonspecific
Chest X-ray	Nonspecific
Lung scan ($\dot{Q}$)	Sensitive/nonspecific
Lung scan ($V/\dot{Q}$)	Sensitive/specific
Angiogram	Sensitive/specific/invasive

sized adult). Heparin therapy for major pulmonary embolism must be continued for a minimum of 10 days. Warfarin therapy should be initiated and overlapped for at least 3 days before discontinuing heparin. An adequate level of warfarin is confirmed when the prothrombin time is twice normal. Anticoagulation therapy for pulmonary embolism should be continued for 3 to 6 months (see pp. 185 and 188).

RX FOR PULMONARY EMBOLISM

Drug	Dose
Heparin	5,000–10,000 units, 750–1000 units/hr
Warfarin	7-day minimum overlapping Rx

Recently, thrombolytic agents (urokinase, streptokinase), used to dissolve pulmonary emboli, have effected significant angiographic and hemodynamic improvement in some patients. Urokinase is derived from human urine and can activate endogenous plasminogen. Streptokinase, also a plasminogen activator, is derived from hemolytic streptococci. Both drugs must be given parenterally and must be administered within 5 days of clot formation or embolization in order to exert an effect. A randomized controlled clinical trial using urokinase and streptokinase was begun at the National Heart and Lung Institute in 1967.[52] Urokinase was administered for 12 to 24 hours, initiated with 2,000 CTA units per pound per hour. Streptokinase dosage was 250,000 units intravenously in 30 minutes followed by 200,000 units/hr for 24 hours. Thrombolytic therapy was effective after a major pulmonary embolus as determined by angiographic resolution, improvement in right heart hemodynamics, and lung scan. However, significant bleeding (49 percent versus 27 percent in heparin-treated controls) during the course of thrombolytic therapy was a serious disadvantage of this approach. In both groups, heparin and oral anticoagulants were administered after the fibrinolytic agent. No significant differences in mortality rates were noted between the urokinase-treated and the heparin-treated groups. Theoretically, thrombolytic therapy could best serve those patients with massive emboli, unstable hemodynamics, arrhythmia, or recurrent emboli through rapid removal of occluding embolic material with the restoration of normal pulmonary artery patency. Such thrombolytic therapy in the form of urokinase and/or streptokinase is not yet available for general use for nonsurgical treatment of pulmonary emboli.

Although the failure rate in terms of recurrent pulmonary emboli with adequate heparin therapy is very low, a more direct attack to prevent further embolization is sometimes indicated. Caval interruption procedures may be employed for specific indications: (1) septic emboli, (2) recurrent embolization while on adequate heparin therapy, and (3) a bleeding complication of heparin therapy. When comparing partial caval interruption (plication, filters) to total ligation, very little difference is seen in the early mortality (8 percent versus 13 percent) or the recurrence rate (8 percent) of pulmonary emboli. However, a significant decrease (16 percent versus 43 percent) in the incidence of venous stasis in the lower extremity favors partial caval interruption procedures.[53] Because of the high mortality incurred by operating on these seriously ill patients, the Mobin-Uddin umbrella, a simpler form of interruption, was devised. Under local anesthesia the internal jugular vein is exposed and the umbrella placed in the cava below the renal veins (third lumbar vertebra) using fluoroscopy. This procedure is accompanied by a mortality rate of less than 1 percent in extremely high risk patients. In a review of 2000 umbrella placements[54] the complication rate due to malpositioning was around 5 percent; recurrent emboli occurred in less than 1 percent. Filter migration, one of the serious hazards of umbrella placement, may be related to the early use of a smaller (23 mm) umbrella as opposed to the currently employed 28-mm model.

ALTERNATIVES TO HEPARIN RX

Method	Mechanism	Clinical
Thrombolytic Rx	Activates lytic	Not for general use
Urokinase	system	
Streptokinase		Reserved for "unstable" patients with pulmonary embolism
Caval interruption	Blocks anatomic	
Ligation/plication	pathway	Mortality, 10–15%
Umbrella		Mortality, 1%

Pulmonary embolectomy as an emergency procedure has been advocated as a heroic measure for treating the patient dying from massive pulmonary embolization. Only 30 percent of patients with ultimately fatal massive emboli survive for one-half hour or longer. Since heparin therapy in conjunction with supportive treatment is so efficacious, it is apparent that there are few clinical situations in which the unstable patient suffering massive pulmonary embolism can be diagnosed and prepared for pulmonary embolectomy in less than 30 minutes. Even in the well-monitored patient in the intensive care unit, perhaps only a few steps from an operating room, this seems to be true. Survival beyond 1 hour suggests that prevention of further embolization by adequate heparinization will be sufficient treatment. Thus, pulmonary embolectomy remains an heroic procedure with rare application.

As an alternative to open pulmonary embolectomy, Greenfield et al.[55] have devised a technique for transvenous removal of major pulmonary emboli using a suction device. A cup device controlled by a steerable mechanism is passed through the femoral vein into the pulmonary artery. After angiographic confirmation of the cup's position adjacent to the occluding clot, suction is applied through the cup to extract the clot. If the procedure is successful, a vena caval umbrella may be positioned through the same femoral venotomy. Initial results in a few patients have been encouraging but, as in open embolectomy, those patients who may benefit most from an operative procedure are those most difficult to stabilize for any therapeutic intervention.

SUMMARY

Venous thromboembolism can be lethal in patients at prolonged bed rest. Recent major advances in preventing the occurrence of deep vein thrombosis by both mechanical and pharmacologic means seem to be the best method of reducing the incidence of fatal pulmonary emboli. The appropriate use of mechanical calf stimulation, oral anticoagulants (coumadin or ASA), or parenteral anticoagulants (low-dose heparin) produces a minimal number of complications from bleeding and a documented decrease in the incidence of calf vein thrombosis. When the diagnosis of deep vein thrombosis is established by one or more of the noninvasive means (I^{25} fibrinogen scanning, ultrasonography, plethysmography), full anticoagulation with heparin maintained by continuous infusion is indicated. The duration of anticoagulation therapy is determined by the severity of the thromboembolic problem, with major pulmonary emboli requiring the longest duration—3 to 6 months. With adequate heparin therapy, the recurrence rate of pulmonary emboli is low (less than 10 percent), but the overall mortality rate is still significant (10 to 20 percent), even when caval interruption procedures are performed. More aggressive attempts to correct the hemodynamic embarrassment secondary to a large clot occluding a major pulmonary artery, i.e., emergency pulmonary embolectomy, transvenous aspiration of the clot with suction apparatus, or thrombolytic therapy using naturally occurring fibrinolytic activators (urokinase and streptokinase), have made no significant improvement in the overall mortality rate of massive pulmonary embolism. Therefore, all efforts must be directed at the prevention of venous thromboembolic disease.

CONCLUSION

This review of bleeding and clotting disorders in I.C.U. patients has emphasized pathophysiologic mechanisms which become manifest as hemorrhagic crises and organ system failures. Such an approach forms the basis for pharmacotherapeutics aimed at both correcting disordered biochemical pathways and preserving organ function. Clearly a crisis-oriented approach in the I.C.U. is a logical therapeutic outgrowth based on the frequency of life-threatening problems. Nevertheless, specific plans must be adopted that are dedicated to the prevention of hemorrhagic complications by laboratory surveillance and early corrective therapy.

Patients with multisystem trauma, liver disease, vitamin K deficiency, and sepsis are a common population in the I.C.U. Chemical evidence of coagulopathy in these patients usually precedes clinical hemorrhage to the extent that frequent determinations of PT, PTT, and platelet count can lead to the early use of supportive therapy in the form of vitamin K, fresh frozen plasma, cryoprecipitates, and platelet infusions. Failure to do so often results in hemorrhage and multiunit blood transfusions which add dilutional changes to an existing coagulopathy.

Similar principles of preventive therapy must be formulated and applied to hemorrhagic gastritis and major pelvic fracture where coagulopathy becomes a secondary phenomenon if primary therapy fails. Direct surgical therapy has not resulted in improved survival for these two entities. Likewise, the prevention of venous thromboembolism yields a more favorable outcome than any form of surgical therapy. Thus, effective therapy for established coagulation disorders is best served by preventive surveillance rather than heroic transfusion and surgical techniques. Monitoring and manipulation of the clotting mechanisms must parallel advanced techniques now routinely applied to cardiopulmonary, microbiologic, and nutritional problems so that maximum therapy can be achieved for critically ill patients.

REFERENCES

1. Schechter DC: The history of the evolution of methods of hemostasis and the study of blood coagulation. In Ulin AW, Gollub SS (eds): Surgical Bleeding—Handbook for Medicine, Surgery & Specialties. New York: McGraw-Hill, 1966

2. Hewson W: Experimental Inquiries into the Properties of the Blood, 2nd ed. London: T Cadell, 1772
3. Morawitz P: Beitrage zur Kenntnisder Blutgerinnung. Beitr Chem Physiol Pathol 5:133, 1904
4. Quick AJ: The prothrombin in hemophilia and in obstructive jaundice. J Biol Chem 109: lxxvii, 1935
5. Bizzozero G: Ulser einen neuen Formbestandteil des Blutes und dessen Rolle bei der Thrombose und der Blut gerinnung. Virchows Arch 90:261, 1882
6. Duke WW: The pathogenesis of purpura hemorrhagia with special reference to the part played by blood platelets. Arch Intern Med 10:445, 1912
7. Owren PA: Parahemophilia: Hemorrhagic diathesis due to absence of a previously unknown clotting factor. Lancet 1:446, 1947
8. Spaet TH: Progress in Hemostasis and Thrombosis. New York: Grune & Stratton, 1972
9. Williams WJ: Hemostasis (Part IV). In Williams WJ et al (eds): Hematology. New York: McGraw-Hill, 1972
10. Biggs R, MacFarlane RG: Treatment of Haemophilia and Other Coagulation Disorders. Philadelphia: Davis, 1966
11. Triantaphy Illopoulos E: Selected topics on blood coagulation. CRC Crit Rev Biochem 1:305, 1973
12. MacFarlane RG: An enzyme cascade in the blood clotting mechanism and its functions as biochemical amplifier. Nature 202:498, 1964
13. Davie EW, Ratnoff OD: Waterfall sequence for intrinsic blood clotting. Science 145:1310, 1964
14. McKay DG, Latour JG, Parrish MH: Activation of Hageman factor by L-adrenergic stimulation. Thrombos Diath Haemorrh 23:417, 1970
15. Austen KF: Hageman factor-dependent coagulation, fibrinolysis and kinin generation. Transplant Proc 6:39, 1974
16. Ratnoff OD, Colopy JE: A familial hemorrhagic trait associated with a deficiency of a clot forming fraction of plasma. J Clin Invest 34:602, 1955
17. Hartman RC: Tests of platelet adhesiveness and their clinical significance. Semin Hematol 5:60, 1968
18. Hellem AJ: Platelet adhesiveness. Ser Haematol 1:99, 1968
19. Meyer D: In vitro platelet adhesiveness. Methods of study: Clinical significance in platelet function and thrombosis. Adv Exp Biol 34:123, 1974
20. Breckenridge RT, Ratnoff OD: Therapy of hereditary disorders of blood coagulation. In Ratnoff OD (ed): Modern Treatment, vol 5. New York: Harper & Row, 1968
21. Salzman EW, Britten AFW: Hemorrhage & Thrombosis. Boston: Little, Brown, 1965
22. Aster RH: Thrombocytopenia due to diminished or defective platelet production. In Williams WJ et al (eds): Hematology. New York: McGraw-Hill, 1972
23. Baly J, Minton JP: Mesenteric thrombosis following splenectomy. Ann Surg 181:126, 1975
24. Merskey C, Kleiner GJ, Johnson AJ: Quantitative estimation of split products of fibrinogen in human serum, relation to diagnosis and rx. Blood 28:1, 1966
25. Vinnicombe J, Shuttleworth, KED: Aminocaproic acid in the control of hemorrhage after prostatectomy. Lancet 1:230, 1966
26. McKay DG, Margaretten W: Disseminated Intravascular Coagulation: An Intermediary Mechanism of Disease. New York: Harper & Row, 1965

27. Lasch HG, Heene DH: Heparin therapy of DIC. Thromb Diath Haemorrh 33:105, 1974
28. Reisman D: Hemorrhages in the course of bright's disease with special reference to the occurrence of hemorrhagic diathesis of nephritic origin. Am J Med Sci 134:709, 1907
29. Simonian SJ, Curtis LE: Treatment of hemorrhagic gastritis by antacid. Ann Surg 184:429, 1976
30. Bodily K, Fischer RF: The prevention of stress ulcers by metiamide, an H_2-Receptor antagonist. J Surg Res 20:203, 1976
31. Chernov MS et al: Stress ulcer: A preventable disease. J Trauma 12:831, 1972
32. LeVeen HH, Falk GS et al: Control of gastrointestinal bleeding. Am J Surg 123:154, 1972
33. Papp JP: Endoscopic electrocoagulation in upper gastrointestinal hemorrhage. JAMA 230:1172, 1974
34. Nusbaum M, Baum, S: Radiographic demonstration of unknown sites of gastrointestinal bleeding. Surg Forum 14:374, 1963
35. Nusbaum M et al: Clinical experience with the diagnosis and management of gastrointestinal hemorrhage by selective mesenteric catheterization. Ann Surg 170:506, 1969
36. Kaufman SL, Maddrey WC et al: Hemodynamic effects of intra-arterial and intravenous vasopressin infusions in patients with portal hypertension (Abstract). Invest Radiol 11:368, 1976
37. Bauer JJ, Kreel I, Kark A: The use of the Sengstaken-Blakemore Tube for immediate control of bleeding esophageal varices. Ann Surg 179:273, 1974
38. Gardner WJ, Taylor HP, Dohn DF: Acute blood loss requiring 58 transfusions. JAMA 167:985, 1958
39. Gardner WJ, Storer J: The use of the G-suit in control of intra-abdominal hemorrhage. Surg Gynecol Obstet 123:792, 1966
40. Cutler BS, Daggett W: Application of the "G-Suit" to the control of hemorrhage in massive trauma. Ann Surg 173:511, 1971
41. Kaplan G, Civetta JM et al: The MAST in civilian pre-hospital emergency care. J Trauma 13:843, 1973
42. Ring EJ, Waltman A et al: Angiography in pelvic trauma. Surg Gynecol Obstet 139:375, 1974
43. Sevitt S, Innes I: Prothrombin time and thrombo test in injured patients on prophylactic anticoagulant therapy. Lancet 1:124, 1964
44. Hirsh J: Venous thromboembolism, diagnosis, treatment and prevention. Hosp Practice 10:53, 1975
45. Kakkar VV: Efficacy of low-dose heparin in preventing postoperative fatal pulmonary embolus; results of an international multicentre trial. Lancet 2:45, 1975
46. Coe N, Collins R, Klein LA et al: Prevention of thromboembolism in postsurgical urology patients. Surgery 83:230, 1978
47. Evarts CM, Feil DJ: Prevention of thromboembolism disease after elective surgery of the hip. J Bone Joint Surg 83:1271, 1971
48. Carter AE, Eban R, Perritt RD: Prevention of postoperative deep vein thrombosis in legs by orally administered hydroxychloroquine sulfato. Br Med J 3:94, 1974
49. Evans G: Effect of drugs that suppress platelet surface interaction on the incidence of amaurosis fugax and transient cerebral ischemia. Surg Forum 23:129, 1972

50. Basu D, Gallus A, Hirsh J et al: A prospective study of the value of monitoring heparin treatment with the activated PTT. N Engl J Med 287:324, 1972

51. Salzman EW, Deykin D et al: Management of heparin therapy—a controlled prospective trial. N Engl J Med 292:1046, 1975

52. Fratantoni JC, Ness P, Simon TL: Thrombolytic therapy. N Engl J Med 293:1073, 1975

53. Couch NP, Baldwin SS, Crane C: Mortality and morbidity rates after inferior vena caval clipping. Surgery 77:106, 1975

54. Bohling C, Auer A, Hershey FB: The Mobin-Uddin Filter for prevention of pulmonary embolism. Am J Surg 128:809, 1974

55. Greenfield LJ, Peyton MD, Brown P, Elkins R: Transvenous management of pulmonary embolic disease. Ann Surg 180:461, 1974

FOUR

Cardiovascular Drugs

D. David Glass

History has amply recorded that drugs with cardiovascular activity have long been part of the healer's armamentarium. Since the time of the ancient Egyptians and Romans, plants containing cardiac glycosides, for example, have been used to treat human diseases. In Witherings' publication of 1785 entitled *An Account of Foxglove and Some of its Medical Uses: With Practical Remarks on Dropsy and Other Diseases,* there is an eloquent discussion of the observed effects of digitalis—although it is apparent that he did not understand the basis of its action on the heart. In 1895, Oliver and Schofer first demonstrated the pressor effects of suprarenal extracts and, in 1910, Barger and Dale coined the term *sympathomimetic amines* describing the adrenal extracts. The cardiac glycosides and sympathomimetic amines, despite their long usage, continue to undergo study and evaluation of their actions and indications. While statements can be made of many pharmacologic agents, few classes have undergone such broad swings in their indications and contraindications as cardiovascular support compounds. Current therapy of the cardiovascular system now must consider the action of a drug not only on the heart, but on the peripheral circulation as well. Further, myocardial function is assessed not just in terms of work produced, but also in terms of energy consumed in the form of oxygen cost of that therapy.

Qualitative and quantitative differences in activity between various vasoactive and cardiotonic compounds make a "cookbook" recipe of therapy impossible for critically ill patients. Further confusion has occurred because of the development and use of a multitude of drugs formulated simply to elevate blood pressure. Fifteen years ago that seemed a viable concept. As our understanding of cardiovascular physiology has evolved, however, this approach has proved to have less and less merit. As our concepts of the regulation of the circulation and treatment of acute cardiac failure grow, one gains a distinct impression that emphasis must shift from agents that stimulate the circulation to depressant compounds which enhance cardiac function by effecting a more appropriate balance of energy supply and demand. This approach is especially salutary to enhance cardiovascular function in the face of a multitude of acute diseases.

Individualizing appropriate therapy for each patient necessitates a basic understanding of the cardiovascular system under normal and abnormal conditions. The effects of specific drugs, their advantages and disadvantages, clinical indications, and hazards will be presented. Finally, an approach to therapy in patients with and without impairment of oxygen delivery to the myocardium will be discussed.

CARDIOVASCULAR FUNCTION AND PHYSIOLOGY OF CIRCULATORY COMPENSATION

The hallmark of patients with circulatory insufficiency is the inability of the heart to respond to stress. The body has a variety of compensating mechanisms to aid the heart's response when its basic function is compromised. Increased sympathic tone to the heart leads to an increase in heart rate and strength of contraction. Increased blood volume from renal sodium retention and contraction of the venous bed further aids the heart by increasing myocardial fiber length and augmenting cardiac output through the Frank-Starling Principle.

In addition, the peripheral vascular bed, mediated by the autonomic nervous system, maintains perfusion pressure by vasoconstriction. While this vasoconstriction maintains pressure, it does so at the expense of an ever-increasing resistance to cardiac ejection and an ultimate diminution of flow. The relationship between flow pressure and resistance is thus illustrated:

$$\text{Flow} = \frac{\text{Pressure}}{\text{Resistance}}$$

When one considers therapy, then, in cardiovascular insufficiency, one must consider the insult produced by the underlying disease process and the potential long-term harmful effects on cardiac function induced by the body's own defense mechanisms to stress.

Without question, the development of the stress response has permitted the organism to transiently maintain vital organ perfusion—if one allows an evolutionary perspective. However, when the stress is excessive or longstanding—or cardiac disease exists—ultimate survival is dependent upon the clinician's ability to rapidly restore the balance between peripheral demands and the heart's ability to meet those demands.

REGULATION OF CARDIAC OUTPUT

Cardiac output, by definition, is the stroke volume times the heart rate. Therefore, regulation of the intact circulation must be dependent upon alterations in either the cardiac rate or the amount of volume ejected. The factors that control rate and stroke volume have a marked influence on intrinsic cardiac performance as well. Ultimately, because of their effects on myocardial oxygen consumption, most of the determinants of cardiac function become the responsibility of the peripheral circulation and the activity of the autonomic nervous system. While each of the factors determining cardiac output—heart rate, preload, afterload, contractile state—cannot be totally separated in vivo, each will be discussed separately.

HEART RATE

At a constant stroke volume, cardiac output is a linear function of heart rate. The importance of rate is most easily appreciated in patients with fixed heart rates—due to implanted pacemakers or intrinsic sinus node disease. These patients have a virtually fixed cardiac output no matter what physiologic demand is presented.

The autonomic nervous system is the most important controller of heart rate. This autonomic nervous system control is mediated by both circulating catecholamines and those liberated within the myocardium. An increase in heart rate, or positive chronotropic effect, is mediated through the β-adrenergic system. This increase in rate occurs by increasing the slope of diastolic repolarization so that the threshold to depolarization is reached more quickly. Parasympathetic innervation, or the cholinergic response of the sinus node, is essentially opposite in effect. We therefore can say that the heart rate is eventually determined by a balance between parasympathetic input and stimulation of the β-adrenergic system. In the normal heart, the parasympathetic system appears to be dominant. However, the parasympathetic nervous system cannot restrain sinus node automaticity in patients with ischemic heart disease, often leading to tachy- and brady-arrhythmias.

The importance of rate in acutely ill patients lies chiefly in achieving a balance between optimum cardiac output and the oxygen cost of increasing heart rate, particulary when rates exceed 100 per minute.

STROKE VOLUME

Three of the four major determinants of myocardial oxygen consumption (MVO_2) are directly related to stroke volume. They are: (1) the amount of the initial stretch of the myocardial fiber on the intrinsic part of the Frank-Starling mechanism termed the *preload,* (2) the pressure against which the myocardium must develop tension to eject the stroke volume or the *afterload,* and (3) the *contractile state* of the myocardium. Their individual effects will now be analyzed further.

Preload In 1871 Bowditch postulated the "all or none law of the heart"— if conditions of the heart muscle remain constant, contractions are equal in strength regardless of the strength of the stimulus applied; that is, the heart either contracts to its fullest extent or not at all. The "all or none law of the heart" depends upon the intrinsic state of contractility at a given moment and the presystolic (end-diastolic) fiber length and ultimately the end-diastolic volume in the ventricle. At any given ventricular compliance, the diastolic volume is related to diastolic pressure. This pressure, not volume, is the clinical parameter most easily measured. It is obvious, then, that in conditions which affect compliance, such as ischemia, the measured end-diastolic pressure may give little indication of the volume the ventricle will be able to eject.

The physiology underlying the heart's ability to eject various volumes at any given inotropic state have been elucidated using electronmicroscopy. As ventricular end-diastolic fiber length increases, the sarcromeres become elongated and the number of active sites for chemical interaction between the adjacent actin and myosin filaments increases.

The particular ventricular response is also related to the action of humoral agents, neurogenic tone, and the metabolic state of the myocardium. Therefore, each ventricle actually can perform on one of a family of ventricular function curves; the particular curve is actually determined by the interrelationship of these many factors. A sample ventricular function curve (Fig. 4-1) representing the relationship between the ventricular end-diastolic fiber length and the ventricular stroke work or cardiac output is illustrated, also showing the effects in changes of contractility on the placement of the ventricular function curve. However, changes in extrinsic forces can result in a shift in performance at a given preload as well. The ultimate therapeutic implication is that many extrinsic factors can be modified to alter ventricular performance at a given fiber length or preload. The clinical task is to attain the maximum stroke volume or fiber length at the best ventricular compliance possible (end-diastolic pressure) and at the same time keep the end-diastolic pressure within the hydrostatic limits tolerated by the lung, i.e., approximately 25 torr. The end-diastolic pressure is also critical in regulating subendocardial blood flow. The higher the end-diastolic pressure, the more subendocardial flow may be compromised.

Afterload Frank's experiments in 1895 showed that ventricular performance on the ejection of volume is influenced by the resistance against which the ventricle contracts. This has been termed the afterload or aortic impedance, which is intimately related to the peripheral vascular resistance. The mass and viscosity of blood also plays a role in the resistance or impedance against which the ventricle is emptying. Studies

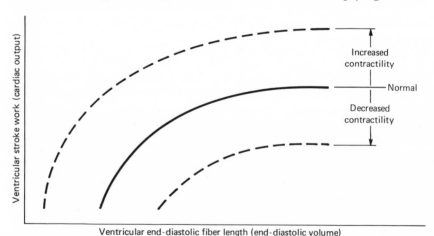

Fig. 4-1. Representation of a "family" of ventricular function curves. An individual filling pressure representing myocardial fiber length may be associated with different stroke work outputs reflecting differences in myocardial contractility.

by Sonnenblick[1] showed that an increase in afterload produced a decrease in muscle shortening when preload and the contractile state were held constant. The afterload, i.e., the resistance the ventricle must overcome or the tension the ventricle must develop, is determined not only by vascular resistance, but by the ventricular radius as well, in accordance with Laplace's law.* (In heart failure, the ventricular radius increases as the heart dilates. The myocardial wall tension necessary to produce the same work thus is increased.) Since this development of wall tension is one of the prime determinants of oxygen consumption, this relationship is most important in the heart in which oxygen delivery is limited by preexisting coronary artery disease.

Contractile State When preload and afterload are held constant, stroke volume is determined by the contractile state. This important property of muscle is determined by the cyclic force-generating processes at the contractile sites of muscle. During diastole, extracellular calcium is concentrated in the region of the sarcolemma or myocardial cell membrane, and its invaginations known as the sarcotubular system. Excitation of the cell and depolarization are accompanied by rapid entry of extracellular calcium into the cell and subsequent binding to troponin C. When this binding occurs, contraction is initiated. Removal of this calcium results in a relaxation of the muscle. The quantity of ionic calcium delivered to the heart contractile proteins, therefore, determines the extent and force of myocardial fiber shortening and ultimately the stroke volume of the heart. In addition to calcium, norepinephrine, the adrenergic transmitter intrinsic to the wall of the myocardium, acts on myocardial β-receptors which also augment contractility through ATP generation.

In recent years, significant advances have been made in the evaluation of myocardial contractility in man as well as in the laboratory. The maximum velocity of shortening of the unloaded muscle, or V_{Max}, has proved to be an effective and exacting measurement of the contractile state of the myocardium—but has the disadvantage of being primarily a laboratory determination. The cardiac catheterization laboratory has provided the opportunity of measuring ventricular pressure changes over unit time (dP/dT/T), and the rate of pressure-rise can be used as an estimate of myocardial contractility. There is no single study in the acute care setting which adequately assesses myocardial contractility. However, measurements of the presystolic ejection period (PEP) and

---

* The law of Laplace defines the change in wall tension of a chamber or vessel. The tension varies directly with the distending pressure and exponent of the radius, and is the inverse of wall thickness:

$$\text{wall tension} = \text{distending pressure} + \frac{\text{radius}^N}{\text{wall thickness}}$$

In the heart, then, myocardial wall tension varies roughly with end-diastolic pressure and the square of the radius.

echocardiographic determinations are noninvasive clinical adjuncts which seem to be useful in assessing ventricular function and performance. The presystolic ejection period represents the time required to generate the pressure necessary to open the aortic valve; this relates to dP/dT. The ratio of presystolic ejection and left ventricular ejection time (LVET) reflect the time required until the aortic valve opens (PEP) and the time that stroke volume is ejected (LVET). This ratio has proven clinically useful as a measure of contractility. Increased contractility will increase dP/dT, shorten PEP, lengthen LVET, and thus lower the ratio. Echocardiography can be useful in situations of depressed contractility by evaluating myocardial wall geometry during pressure development and ejection.

PERIPHERAL CIRCULATION

The resistance (arterial) and capacitance (venous) beds are the prime extrinsic determinants of cardiac output within the limits of a given state of myocardial contractility. In other words, the amount of venous blood returned to the heart (more than any other factor) will of necessity determine the amount which can be pumped. This occurs independently of diastolic ventricular pressure. In addition, the resistance to ventricular ejection (afterload) determines, in large part, the amount of work a left ventricle must perform. The healthy myocardium can alter its performance as dictated by the systemic circulation through broad ranges of both preload and afterload. The myocardium deprived of oxygen (ischemic disease), or one subjected even to modest increases in peripheral resistance, or states in which venous return is excessive (systemic AV fistula), has narrow performance limits which circumscribe its ability to pump. Changes in the peripheral circulation, more than any other single factor, will alter the pumping capacity of both the normal and diseased myocardium.

The peripheral vascular bed is basically controlled by intrinsic regulation. Sympathetic discharge provides only 15 to 20 percent of the vascular tone at rest. However, humoral vasoconstriction mechanisms are extremely important in redistribution of cardiac output during activity. In congestive heart failure, both in man and animals, there is a marked increase in releasable norepinephrine available.[2] There is, therefore, a marked increase in peripheral vascular resistance at rest and during exercise in patients with chronic congestive heart failure. This increase can be further increased by circulating catecholamines. Since development of myocardial wall tension (afterload-induced) is a prime determinant of myocardial oxygen consumption, these mechanisms result in additional stress for the compromised heart.

The whole theory of normal cardiac output regulation is based upon the hypothesis that the tissues control the amount of blood flow that they need. This intrinsic control of blood vessels ultimately results from the activity of the single unit smooth muscle in the precapillary resistance vessels.[2] Yet, it is not clear what controls the intrinsic relaxation of the precapillary resistances, although histamine, acetylcholine, adenine, and other vasoactive substances have been suggested. Vasodilatation may be induced by oxygen deficit in the vessel wall produced by skeletal muscle activity. This effect, alone or in combination with an increase in local hydrogen ion concentration (fall in pH), produces relaxation of vascular smooth muscle.

Neural or sympathetic regulation may produce instantaneous changes in the peripheral circulation. Blood flow is usually reduced to areas of low metabolic needs in order to maintain blood flow to necessary areas like the heart and brain which have high oxygen requirements and absent or weak α-adrenergic innervation. The reduced capability for vasoconstriction in these areas (even in the presence of high levels of circulating endogenous catecholamines) insures continued blood flow during stress or compromised cardiovascular function.

Both central and peripheral regulatory mechanisms markedly affect the homeostatic function of the circulation. Changes in afterload, whether created by application of an aortic cross clamp, as in aneurysm surgery, or increased arterial muscle tone, as in hypertension, create abnormal peripheral vascular resistances. The left ventricle must then compensate for the increase in afterload. In the chronic situation (hypertensive cardiovascular disease), this compensation is attained by cardiac muscle hypertrophy with recruitment of contractile units. But when hypertrophy is excessive, oxygen delivery is compromised leading to left ventricular dilatation and further increase in oxygen requirements. If this increase cannot be met, decompensation and cardiac failure ensues. As cardiac output falls, a further increase in peripheral vascular resistance occurs because of the increased release of systemic norepinephrine, causing a further burden on an already compromised heart. Application of an aortic cross clamp, with its marked increase in afterload, causes a similar picture of chamber dilatation and failure—but in a more rapid sequence in patients with compromised oxygen delivery undergoing aneurysm surgery.[3] In the chronic situations such as hypertension, peripheral resistance vessels become noncompliant, or "stiff," and the cycle of cardiac failure is thereby aggravated. A return of resistance toward normal following diuresis suggests an increased salt and water retention within vascular walls as an additional event which further perpetuates the cycle of cardiac failure.

This body of knowledge, however theoretical and incomplete, must be applied to cardiac functions in the acute care setting, if an appropriate therapeutic intervention is to be chosen.

DETERMINATION OF CARDIOVASCULAR DYSFUNCTION

The introduction of the flow-directed pulmonary artery catheter in the early 1970s by Swan and Ganz has allowed accurate assessment of the cardiovascular and respiratory systems previously unavailable to the clinician. In addition, pressure, flow, and blood oxygen content determinations allow for rapid calculation of most cardiovascular and respiratory parameters in the critically ill patient.

Listed below are common abbreviations and formulas utilized in common intensive care unit calculations.

CARDIORESPIRATORY PARAMETERS: ABBREVIATIONS

CARDIAC		RESPIRATORY	
Cardiac output	CO	Hemoglobin concentration	Hb
Systolic blood pressure	SP		
Diastolic blood pressure	DP	Inspired oxygen tension	FIo_2
Mean arterial pressure	MAP	Arterial carbon dioxide tension	$Paco_2$
Heart rate	HR		
Mean pulmonary artery pressure	MPA	Arterial oxygen tension	Pao_2
		Arterial oxygen saturation	Art Sat
Pulmonary artery occlusion or wedge pressure	PAO	Mixed venous oxygen saturation	Ven Sat
Central venous pressure	CVP	Mixed venous oxygen tension	Pvo_2
Body surface area	BSA		
Stroke work conversion factor	0.0136	Dissolved oxygen coefficient	0.0031
Stroke volume	SV	Hemoglobin oxygen binding	1.39
Cardiac index	CI		
Stroke index	SI	Alveolar oxygen tension	PAo_2
Right ventricular stroke work	RVSW	Pulmonary capillary oxygen content	C_C
Left ventricular stroke work	LVSW	Mixed venous oxygen content	C_V
Systemic vascular resistance	SVR	Arterial oxygen content	C_A
Pulmonary vascular resistance	PVR	Arterial venous oxygen content difference	$C_A—C_V$
Myocardial oxygen consumption correlate	MVO_2C	Oxygen delivery	O_2 del
"Pump failure" correlate	PF	Oxygen consumption	O_2 cons
		Oxygen utilization	% util
		Intrapulmonary shunt	Qsp/Qt
		Shunt index	Sh I
		Shunt flow	SF
		Pulmonary capillary flow	PCF

CARDIORESPIRATORY PARAMETERS: FORMULAS

$$MAP = DP + \tfrac{1}{3}(SP - DP) \quad (normal = 80\text{-}90 \text{ torr})$$

$$SV = CO/HR \quad (normal = 50\text{-}60 \text{ ml})$$

$$CI = CO/BSA \quad (normal = 3.5\text{-}4.0 \text{ ICU population})$$

$$SI = SV/BSA \quad (normal = 35\text{-}40 \text{ ICU population})$$

$$RVSW = SV \times (MPA - CVP) \times 0.0136 \quad (normal = 10\text{-}15 \text{ gm/sq m})$$

$$Ratio = RVSW/CVP$$

$$LVSW = SV \times (MAP - PAO) \times 0.0136 \quad (normal = 60\text{-}80 \text{ gm/sq m})$$

$$Ratio = LVSW/PAO$$

$$SVR = \frac{(MAP - CVP) \times 80}{CO} \quad (normal = 1200 \text{ dynes cm}^{-5})$$

$$PVR = \frac{(MAP - PAO) \times 80}{CO} \quad (normal = 200 \text{ dynes cm}^{-5})$$

$$MVO_2C = \frac{SP \times HR}{100} \quad (higher \text{ values} = greater \text{ consumption})$$

$$PF = \frac{DP \times Ven\ Sat \times 100}{PAO} \quad (survival \text{ associated with} > 250)$$

$$PAO_2 = (760 - 47) \times FIO_2 - \frac{Paco_2}{0.8}$$

$$C_c = (PAO_2 \times 0.0031) + (Hb \times 1.39 \times 1)$$
$$(assumes\ 100\%\ Hb\ sat;\ normal = 18.3 \text{ ml/100 ml})$$

$$C_v = (Pvo_2 \times 0.0031) + (Hb \times 1.39 \times Ven\ Sat)$$
$$(normal = 13 \text{ ml/100 ml})$$

$$C_A = (Pao_2 \times 0.0031) + (Hb \times 1.39 \times Art\ Sat)$$
$$(normal = 19 \text{ ml/100 ml})$$

$$O_2\ del = C_A \times CO \times 10 \quad (normal = 1000 \text{ ml/min})$$

$$C_A - C_V = C_A - C_V \quad (normal = 3.5\text{-}4.5 \text{ ml/100 ml})$$

$$O_2\ cons = (C_A - C_V) \times CO \times 10 \quad (normal = 250 \text{ ml/min})$$

$$\%\ util = \frac{C_A - C_V}{C_A} \quad (normal = 0.2\text{-}0.25)$$

$$Qsp/Qt = \frac{C_c - C_A}{C_c - C_V} \quad (normal < 0.10)$$

$$Sh\ I = \frac{Qsp/Qt}{CO} \quad (no \text{ range established})$$

$$SF = Qsp/Qt \times CO \quad (normal < 0.5 \text{ liters/min})$$

$$PCF = CO - SF \quad (normal = 4.5\text{-}6.5 \text{ liters/min})$$

SYMPATHOMIMETIC AMINES

Many sympathomimetic amines have been prepared since the first efforts in the early 1900s. Most were prepared because their ability to vasoconstrict reflected an early focus on simple blood pressure measurement in the selection of agents to augment cardiac function, rather than myocardial energetics. The drugs in clinical usage all have similar cardiac and systemic vascular effects. The major differences are in magnitude of α- or β-receptor stimulation.

α-Effects	β_1-Effects	β_2-Effects
Vasoconstriction: skin mucosa, abdominal viscera, sweat glands	Positive chronotropic effect	Bronchial muscle relaxation
	Positive inotropic effect	Skeletal muscle vasodilatation
Pilomotor muscle	Increased automaticity	
Pupil dilation		
Decrease intestinal motility	Coronary artery dilatation	

CARDIAC ACTION

The biochemical basis for the effects of the catecholamines on the heart are now known to be the result of the conversion of ATP to adenosine 3/5 monophosphate (cyclic 3/5 AMP) by adenylcyclase, mediated by β-adrenergic receptors. Cyclic AMP was initially discovered in the course of investigation of the effects of adrenergic agents on carbohydrate metabolism. The relationship to 3/5 cyclic AMP is not unique to catecholamines since the activity of many trophic hormones can be related to a capacity to increase adenylcyclase activity in their respective organs. Glucagon and thyroid hormone can also activate myocardial adenylcyclase activity. This effect is presumed to account for the increased contractility seen in hyperthyroid patients and also that produced by glucagon (see p. 227).

The myocardial action of catecholamines appears to be the same for the entire group—positive inotropic and chronotropic effects. They differ only in the dose required to produce a given effect.

PERIPHERAL VASCULAR ACTION

The peripheral vascular bed contains α-receptors which cause vasoconstriction and β-receptors which cause vasodilatation, particularly in skeletal muscle beds. More recently, dopaminergic receptors have been described which cause vasodilatation in renal and mesenteric beds. The prediction of precise peripheral vascular responses to a given sympathomimetic amine can be difficult due to the interaction of several factors:

1. Intravascular volume status.
2. Vasodilatation in one bed may occur with vasoconstriction in another.
3. Vasodilatation which occurs at low doses of some catecholamines may be overriden as dose is increased.
4. Vasodilatation may be produced in some beds as a result of excessive oxygen utilization, not direct action.
5. Hydrogen ion concentration in tissues alter both dilator and constrictor responses.[4]

These interactions must be kept in mind during discussion of the naturally occurring catecholamines.

NOREPINEPHRINE (LEVOPHED)

History   Pressor effects of suprarenal extracts were demonstrated by Oliver and Schöfer in 1895.[5] This produced the basis for study of large numbers of naturally occurring and synthetic sympathomimetic drugs. In 1910 Barger and Dale demonstrated a series of amines that had the ability to mimic the actions of epinephrine, hence the term sympathomimetic amines.[5a] One of the compounds they studied was norepinephrine. Because epinephrine was extracted from the adrenal gland, epinephrine was termed *adrenalin* by early workers, as it is today in Europe. Norepinephrine, for the same reason, is often referred to as noradrenalin.

Cardiac Effects   The ability of norepinephrine to stimulate β-receptors in the myocardium, and thus increase both heart rate and strength of contractions, is unquestioned. It is also the predominant substance released in vivo by the sympathetic nerve endings in the myocardium to cause augmented cardiac function. During the intravenous administration of 1 to 5 μg/min, the predominant effects are those of an increase in mean aortic pressure with little change in heart rate or cardiac output. However, this causes a 15 percent increase in tension index, indicative of a marked increase in myocardial oxygen consumption.

Systemic Effects   The predominating α-adrenergic stimulation overshadows the β-adrenergic effects on the myocardium. Vasoconstriction occurs in essentially all vascular beds except for coronary arteries and cerebral vessels. This includes both arterial and venous circuits. These effects can be particularly damaging in the kidney, since they can produce ischemic renal failure.

Current Usage   Because of its predominant vasoconstrictor response, there is little to recommend its use except in certain patients with acute myocardial infarction, and then only to achieve a specific end. The uniform response to norepinephrine infusions is an elevation of mean blood pressure which thus may augment coronary perfusion. However, there is little change in cardiac rate and cardiac output usually falls. The predictable decline in output is a response to intense systemic vasoconstriction and contraindicates the use of norepinephrine except in the rare acute care setting in which the increased coronary perfusion pressure results in an overall beneficial effect. If only blood pressure is being recorded, there is a distinct hazard that there is a "presumed" beneficial effect which cannot be documented by flow, cardiac output or myocardial oxygen consumption measurements.[6,6a]

Preparation: Levarterenol Bitartrate 1 mg/5 ml One milligram is placed in 250 ml diluent and a microdrop infusion set administration is utilized.

NOREPINEPHRINE	
Action	Predominant α-agonist in vivo; some β-adrenergic activity seen at clinical doses
Indications	Limited usefulness except for myocardial infarction or inadequate coronary perfusion
Contraindications	Causes marked increase in ventricular afterload
How supplied	1 mg/5 ml levarterenol bitartrate in 250 ml D5W
Dosage	1–4 μg/min

EPINEPHRINE

History The history of epinephrine parallels that of norepinephrine.

Cardiac Effects Epinephrine is a powerful cardiac stimulant. It acts on β-receptors of the myocardium and cells of the pacemaker and conducting tissue. Heart rate increases because of the positive chronotropic effect. Epinephrine shortens systole more than diastole, so that duration of diastole per minute is increased. This increase in heart rate is associated with an increasing conduction velocity in the bundle of His, Purkinje fibers, and ventricles. The membrane potential is increased in Purkinje fibers in particular. In conditions favoring excessive depolarization, such as an ischemic heart, endogenous catecholamine liberation produced by elevated carbon dioxide, or in the presence of anesthetics which further sensitize the myocardium (e.g., halothane), ventricular arrhythmias may be produced. This arrhythmogenic effect can be blocked by β-blocking drugs. It is not clear why some α-blocking drugs, such as phenoxybenzamine, may also attenuate these arrhythmias as well. However, some evidence suggests that α-receptors do exist in certain areas of the heart, particularly in the atria, since isolated atrial strips respond to epinephrine with increased contraction, even in the presence of β-blockade.[7]

Systemic Vascular Effects   Skeletal muscle vessels are dilated by low dose (0.5 to 1 μg/min) stimulation of β-receptors. This explains the initial fall in blood pressure seen with low dose epinephrine infusions. This response is accentuated in patients with hypovolemia. Larger doses stimulate α-receptors as well as β-receptors, leading to an overall increase in peripheral vascular resistance and a rise in blood pressure. Epinephrine constricts precapillary sphincters and markedly reduces cutaneous blood flow following infusions in humans. In addition, this constriction occurs in the bowel mucosa and renal vasculature as well. The venous bed is constricted, initially producing a slight increase in venous return and distribution in the heart volume with subsequent augmentation of cardiac output. Pulmonary vascular pressures are increased, but probably as the consequence of left atrial pressure elevation and increased pulmonary blood volume. There is a direct pulmonary vasoconstrictor effect as well. The effect of epinephrine upon cerebral blood flow is similar to the other sympathomimetics, and is directly related to systemic flow: no direct constrictor response can be demonstrated in humans.[8]

Respiratory Effects   Epinephrine stimulates respiration and, when β-activity predominates (in low doses), it is a potent bronchodilator. This has been the basis for its extensive low dose, subcutaneous usage in patients with asthma, or hyperreactive bronchi, secondary to histamine, cholinesterase, pilocarpine, bradykinin, slow reacting substance or prostaglandin F2αC. This is also the basis for its use in anaphylactic reactions, in addition to systemic support of blood pressure and cardiac function.

Current Concepts   Epinephrine has a major role in the cardiovascular support of acutely ill patients. The augmentation of myocardial contractility without the overwhelming α-activity of norepinephrine makes it a suitable agent in a variety of clinical situations.[9] Like all drugs with β₁-effects, the increase in myocardial oxygen consumption seen in normal hearts may be modified in the failing heart by effecting a reduction of end-diastolic volume as contractility increases. This reduces wall tension and hence reduces oxygen consumption. Separation of the positive inotropic effect from the marked chronotropic effect which characterizes the effect of Isoproterenol (see below) thus can have an overall salutary effect upon oxygen consumption in the failing heart. The concomitant α-stimulation at doses of 1 to 2 μg/min may produce undesirable elevation of afterload which diminishes cardiac output and/or leads to an elevation of myocardial oxygen consumption. This can be antagonized by concomitant administration of α-blocking drugs (phenoxybenzamine) or direct smooth muscle relaxants such as sodium nitroprusside (pp. 233–43).

Only careful assessment of cardiac output and left atrial or pulmonary capillary wedge pressures can determine the overall performance of the diseased heart in stress during epinephrine infusion. Like all sympathomimetic amines, the mere elevation of systemic blood pressure is not an indication of the performance and energy cost to the myocardium. The arrhythmogenicity of epinephrine must also be considered in patients who are ischemic, or who also are in electrolyte imbalance.

Preparation   Adrenalin or epinephrine, 1 mg (1:1000) in 250 ml is administered through a microdrip infusion. It should be administered directly into the central circulation, not into a peripheral vein—unless there is some reason that central infusion cannot be accomplished.

EPINEPHRINE	
Action	α- and β-Agonist
Indications	Useful in: Profound hypotension of diverse etiologies to maintain organ perfusion Support of myocardial contractility and heart rate following cardiopulmonary bypass
Contraindications	Increase in myocardial irritability, careful attention must be paid to the magnitude of change in peripheral vascular resistance
How supplied	1 mg epinephrine (adrenalin) in 250 ml D5W
Dosage	Predominant β-effects: 0.5–1.5 μg/min; α and β effects: > 1.5 μg/min

ISOPROTERENOL

History   Isoproterenol was first studied by Konzett in 1940. It is a naturally occurring catecholamine and is almost entirely a β-adrenergic stimulant.

Cardiac Effects   Stimulation of β-receptors in the myocardium produce cardiac effects similar to those of epinephrine infusions. In the normal heart there is an increase in heart rate and cardiac contraction. The increase in rate is due both to the direct stimulation of the β-receptors in the SA node and to the sympathetic reflexes activated by its systemic marked muscle bed vasodilatation. This tachycardia is often the limiting factor in its use and is aggravated by a relative or absolute hypovolemia. Myocardial demands for oxygen perhaps increase less in the dilated than in the ischemic heart, but the systemic vasodilatation produces a decrease in perfusion pressure which leads to a severe reduction in myocardial oxygen delivery. For these reasons, its use in patients with myocardial ischemia has been, and should be, limited. Isoproterenol has been shown to increase myocardial lactate production in patients in cardiogenic shock.[10] Isoproterenol in ischemic disease "wastes" more oxygen than it delivers and has very limited usefulness in patients with compromised oxygen delivery. On the other hand, patients with normal coronary vasculature—congential heart surgery with primary pump failure, or patients requiring positive inotropic support after trauma—may benefit from its use. The chronotropic effects are useful as a temporizing measure in the treatment of heart block as well.

Isoproterenol has been shown to produce focal necrosis of myocardial cells, probably as a result of the marked oxygen supply/demand imbalance that it produces.[11] This response is less likely at lower dosages (1 to 2 mg/min).

Systemic Vasculature The deleterious effects of isoproterenol infusion on the heart may also be aggravated by the redistribution of systemic blood volume and a reduction of systemic blood pressure which reduces myocardial oxygen delivery. Sandler found that renal flow increased only slightly in patients with congestive heart failure despite a large increase in cardiac output.[12] The kidney thus receives a lesser increment of flow than other vascular beds (such as muscle with active vascular dilatation). Thus, isoproterenol produces a relative "steal" from vital organs such as the heart and kidney and delivers the increased flow to the less important vascular beds which have greater β_2 activity. There is little reason, therefore, to recommend its use in patients with any myocardial oxygen supply/demand imbalance. It probably has its greatest usefulness in endotoxic shock and in selected postcardiac surgical patients requiring inotropic support in nonischemic disease.

Preparation Supplied 1 mg in 5 ml isoproterenol. This should be diluted in 250 ml of diluent and administered directly into the central circulation.

ISOPROTERENOL	
Actions	β-adrenergic agonist
Indications	Inotropic support, especially when myocardial oxygen supply is not compromised
	Acceleration of heart rate in heart block as temporary measure
Contraindications	Development of tachyarrhythmias and ventricular irritability
	Creation of increased myocardial demand without increased supply
	Muscle bed vasodilatation may unmask relative hypovolemia and produce a fall in blood pressure
How supplied	1 mg in 5 ml; add 1 mg to 250 ml D5W and administer preferably into central circulation
Dosage	0.5–3 μg/min (7–45 microdrops) initial dose; clinical response is best guide.

DOPAMINE

History Dopamine is the immediate precursor of norepinephrine and epinephrine in the endogenous pathway of their synthesis. It is found in particularly high concentrations in sympathetic nerves and adrenal glands. In addition, it is present in areas where norepinephrine does not occur, such as the brain. Dopaminergic nerves and receptors have specialized actions in the brain as well as in the splanchnic and renal vasculature.

Cardiac Activity Like the other catecholamines, dopamine increases myocardial contractility and heart rate by direct action on the β-adrenergic receptors. It may also liberate some increased endogenous catecholamine stores. Both the direct and indirect actions of dopamine can be antagonized by β-blocking drugs.[13] The recent enthusiasm for dopamine has stemmed from its demonstrated positive inotropic effect without a marked chronotropic response[6] thereby producing less overall myocardial oxygen supply/demand imbalance. Recent studies[9] are contradictory in their reported beneficial effects on the heart. Several explanations for this may exist. Dopamine on a microgram for microgram basis is less potent than the other catecholamines. In addition, its dose-related α- and β-stimulation effects are different from epinephrine, whose action it most closely mimics. A dosage of 1 to 5 μg/kg/min causes stimulation of primary dopaminergic receptors—primarily in the kidney and mesenteric circuits—with little α- or β-stimulation.[14] As dosage increases from 5 to 10 μg/kg/min, β-adrenergic effects become more prominent; with increasing infusions above 15 μg/kg/min, α-adrenergic effects become dominant. At that point they begin to antagonize dopaminergic receptors and hence the beneficial effects on renal and splanchnic blood flow. This also produces increased afterload mediated by increasing systemic vasoconstriction. It appears that if only modest β-activity is required to stimulate the myocardium, a dose of 10 to 15 μg/kg/min will produce effective clinical improvement without activating adverse α-adrenergic effects. Its chronotropic effects are also minimal since the overall β-stimulation is not as great as with other catecholamines. In addition, systemic vascular resistance declines (if, indeed, any change occurs), with little change in perfusion pressure. All of this leads to improved myocardial supply/demand relationships.[9] However, when infusion rates exceed 15 μg/kg/min, the effects of dopamine on the myocardium are not dissimilar from epinephrine in inotropic and chronotropic response. Although cardiac performance is improved, it will only occur at an ever increasing oxygen cost. This increase in cost occurs because chronotropic, intropic, and systemic vascular effects become indistinguishable from modest (3 to 6 μg/min) epinephrine infusions. This may be particularly harmful to the ischemic myocardium.[15] The relative freedom from arrhythmogenic potential of low-dose dopamine also disappears at "epinephrinomimetic" dosages.

Systemic Effects The unique and clinically useful properties of dopamine which distinguish it from the other catecholamines are related to its ability at low doses (1 to 5 μg/kg/min) to stimulate the dopaminergic receptors. These receptors cause vasodilatation of renal and mesenteric vascular beds in particular,[13] and perhaps cerebral circulation as well.[16] The effects on mesenteric and renal vascular beds are not antagonized by propranolol, atropine, or antihistamines; however, some are antagonized by haloperidol and various phenothiazines. Droperidol, on the other hand, had no antagonistic effect upon dopamine, and mediated increases in renal blood flow.[17] The increase in renal blood flow in normal subjects is usually accompanied by incremental increases in glomerular filtration rate and sodium excretion. A redistribution of renal blood flow has been postulated to account for the sodium diuresis.[18] The ability to increase renal and mesenteric flow is unique to dopamine and provides a potential for preservation of renal function in a variety of shock states. However, as infusion rates begin to exceed 3 to 5 μg/kg/min, α-receptor stimulation increases and may override this beneficial effect on renal blood flow.

Dopamine increases renal blood flow in patients with cirrhosis,[14] and Bennett[19] has shown angiographic evidence of improved cortical to medullary flow ratios with subpressor doses in patients with hepatorenal syndrome. However, he could not show evidence of increased survival. This remains a promising area to study.

Clinical Usefulness The specific peripheral effects of dopamine make this catecholamine particularly useful when low dose infusions can restore cardiovascular stability and also result in an augmented renal function. When significant myocardial depression or ischemia is present, dopamine would not appear to offer any significant advantage over epinephrine, i.e., if infusion rates greater than 15 μg/kg/min are required to attain the desired clinical response. As with epinephrine, antagonism of the undesirable vasconstrictor effects (utilizing drugs such as sodium nitroprusside) creates a particularly useful combination.

Preparation Dopamine (Intropin), 200 mg in 250 ml of appropriate diluent, is administered through a central venous route. It should be noted that dopamine infusions are usually calculated by a μg/kg/min range rather than the μg/min range common with the other catecholamines. This reflects the relative weakness in terms of potency, i.e., whereas a 70-kg patient might require epinephrine 2 to 5 μg/min, 10 to 15 μg/kg/min of dopamine (700 to 1000 μg/min) would be required to achieve a similar effect.

DOPAMINE	
Actions	Stimulates α-receptors, β-receptors, and dopaminergic receptors
Indications	Support of circulation in a variety of low output states

	In low doses (see below) as a primary agent to augment renal blood flow and promote diuresis
Contraindications	Production of oxygen supply/demand imbalance
	Over 20 μg/kg/min activity predominates and will antagonize one dopaminergic effect and increase ventricular afterload
How supplied	Dopamine (Intropin) 200 mg in 5 ml; add to 250 ml of diluent
Dosage	Predominant dopaminergic effects 1–5 μg/kg/min
	α- and β-effects at 5–20 μg/kg/min
	Above 20 μg/kg/min, α-effects predominate

DOBUTAMINE

History Dobutamine is a recently synthesized cardiospecific inotropic agent useful in a variety of states characterized by cardiac failure. Preliminary studies indicate that equivalent inotropic stimulation was obtained at a dobutamine-to-isoproterenol ratio of 43:1.[20] Loeb, however, studied ratios of 500:1 in a clinical series.[21] There was little difference noted between dobutamine and isoproterenol in any parameters in patients with nonischemic congestive heart failure. Dobutamine, however, caused less tachycardia than isoproterenol at the dose ratios studied. A comparison of dobutamine and dopamine at dosages producing similar increases in cardiac output showed that dobutamine reduced left ventricular filling pressure on the average of 9 torr while dopamine increased left ventricular filling pressure 3 to 4 torr with similar changes in heart rate.[22] Dobutamine can thus be considered a more potent inotropic agent, i.e., the increased output was accomplished at a lower filling pressure, and therefore this point must be on a "higher" Starling curve (Fig. 4-1). Dobutamine does not seem to share dopamine's special effects on renal or mesenteric vasculature. This potential disadvantage of the drug might be overcome by concomitant administration of dopamine (1 to 2 μg/kg/min) when minimal inotropic support is required along with augmentation of renal blood flow.

Dosage The range of dosage for dobutamine is from 1 to 30 μg/kg/min.

OTHER SYMPATHOMIMETICS

Other commercially available sympathomimetics are categorized in terms of their effects in Table 4-1. Their overall actions do not specifically differ from the previously described catecholamines except in dose and duration of action.

TABLE 4-1

Other Sympathomimetics and Their Effects

Drug	Proprietary Name	Receptor Stimulation		Mechanism of Action (D = direct, I = indirect)
		α	β	
Epinephrine	Adrenaline	+++	++ predominates in low dose	D
Isoproterenol	Isuprel	−	++++	D
Norepinephrine	Levophed	++++	+*	D
Dopamine	Intropin	+++	++†	D
Ephedrine	—	+++	++	I and D
Metaraminol	Aramine	+++	++	I and D
Methoxamine	Vasoxyl	++++	−	D
Mephentermine	Wyamine	+++	++	I
Phenylephrine	Neosynephrine	++++	−	D (some I)

* β-Effects seen in vivo when no α-receptors are present as occurs within the myocardium.
† Also stimulates dopaminogenic receptors.

CARDIAC GLYCOSIDES (DIGITALIS)

History The beneficial effects of digitalis (used herein synonymously with the entire class of cardiac glycosides) in the therapy of patients with heart disease, has been known since Withering's classic *Account of the Foxglove.* Withering and others, however, did not attribute the beneficial effects to any primary cardiac activity even in cases of dropsy. They attributed its benefit to its diuretic action on the kidney. Withering did note, however, that foxglove "had power over the motion of the heart." It has only been within the last sixty years that digitalis has been used specifically for its cardiac effects, although in 1799 Ferrian described the action of digitalis as primarily on the heart and saw its diuretic activity as a secondary action. In the nineteenth century, digitalis preparations were prescribed for a wide spectrum of ailments—often in toxic doses.

Cardiac Effects Cardiac glycosides act at the cellular level to inhibit sodium and potassium transport across the cell membrane by inhibition of the transport enzyme, potassium-sodium-activated ATPase. Inhibition of this transport system causes the substantial efflux of potassium from the myocardium which occurs with digitilization. This alone, however, does not explain the inotropic activity of digitalis. The glycosides have not been shown to have an important direct effect on contractile proteins, intermediate metabolism, or substrate availability. Furthermore, contractile effects are not secondary to catecholamine release.[23,24] Recent studies have attempted to link the inotropic effects of digitalis to the presence of increased calcium ions. Several hypotheses have been proposed to explain the mechanism of sodium-potassium ATPase glycoside binding with an increase in intracellular Ca^{++} concentration. Gervis[25] has shown that glycoside interaction with sodium-potassium ATPase leads to an increased pool of cell membrane-bound calcium. This still leaves unanswered the question of how the calcium enters the cell to increase contractile protein function, but contributes to the understanding of where this postulated increased calcium may originate.[26,27] An excellent review of possible cellular mechanisms of action of digitalis has been published by Smith and Haber.[28]

Until the 1960s, the cardiac action of digitalis was thought to be limited to the failing myocardium. Braunwald demonstrated that digitalis augmented the contractile state of the myocardium even in normal humans, but that reflex adjustments in the other determinants of cardiac output prevented the ready appreciation of this inotropic effect.[29]

Demonstration of the positive inotropic effect in the normal heart helps explain the disparity of earlier investigations relating to myocardial oxygen consumption and digitalis. Covell[30] demonstrated that the administration of digitalis to the normal heart increased both contractility and wall tension, two prime determinants of myocardial oxygen consumption (MVO_2). In the failing heart, however, decreased oxygen consumption can be explained by a decrease in left ventricular end-diastolic pressure (the result of the augmented contractility) which produces a decrease in end-diastolic volume and consequently a decline in wall tension on the basis of the Laplace relationship. The clinical result seen is a summation of these changes. MVO_2 may be increased in the normal heart, but it is reduced in a failing one. Clinically, the pain of angina is diminished by digitalis when some element of cardiac enlargement and failure exists (an overall decrease in MVO_2); whereas in others, angina can be exacerbated if little or no cardiac decompensation (dilatation) is present (overall increase in MVO_2).

In addition to augmenting myocardial contractility, the cardiac glycosides preferentially decrease conduction and prolong the functional refractory period of the AV node. These effects are observed in the therapeutic range of digitalis and are manifested in the electrocardiogram by a prolonged P-R interval. The decreased conduction and prolonged refractory period allow regulation of ventricular response in chaotic atrial rhythms, such as atrial fibrillation. In such instances, MVO_2 will be decreased proportionately to the decrease in heart rate.

Systemic Circulation In normal subjects, digitalis tends to increase the tone of peripheral resistance vessels.[31] While this increase in afterload is potentially detrimental to patients in shock or with an already compromised MVO_2, studies in man during cardiopulmonary bypass[29] suggest this effect is transient.

The venous bed shows a biphasic effect similar to the effect on MVO_2. Mason [32] showed evidence of venous constriction in normal subjects caused by the cardiac glycosides; however, in patients with congestive heart failure, venodilatation occurred. It has been postulated that this paradoxical response is due to the lowering of the markedly elevated circulating levels of catecholamines present in congestive failure as cardiac function is improved by digitalis therapy.

Other Action The predominant noncirculatory action is an augmentation of vagal activity, commonly manifested by bradycardia in both experimental animals and humans. Clinically, we utilize this principle by withholding a digitalis dose when the pulse rate is already slow, suggestive evidence of increasing blood levels of digitalis. In addition to the augmentation of vagal activity, a reduction of the chronotropic effects produced by epinephrine and sympathetic stimulation can also occur with high doses of digitalis.[33]

Current Concept of Use

Heart Failure Cardiac glycosides are of potential value in most patients with symptoms and signs of congestive heart failure due to ischemic, valvular, hypertensive, and congenital heart diseases. Patients with cardiomyopathies and cor pulmonale may also show some improvement with digitalis. Improvement in depressed contractility will increase cardiac output, promote diuresis, and reduce filling pressures in the ventricles. However, signs and symptoms of idiopathic hypertrophic subaortic stenosis (IHSS) are often exacerbated with digitalis since the increased strength of contraction can actually increase the muscular obstruction. Similarly, in patients with infundibular pulmonic stenosis which occurs in the tetralogy of Fallot, augmentation of contractility may further reduce the already diminished pulmonary blood flow by increasing the obstruction of the pulmonary outflow tract.

The usefulness of digitalis after acute myocardial infarction is uncertain. One-half of the patients after myocardial infarction develop congestive heart failure of a mild nature, and 12 percent develop severe heart failure and pulmonary edema.[34] However, patients with mild congestive heart failure after myocardial infarction do not improve significantly after digitalis; therefore, digitalis has not been recommended for congestive failure following an infarction.[35] The failure to improve cardiac function may be secondary to the previously described peripheral vascular effects. Elevation of serum CPK has been demonstrated in patients who have received digitalis after uncomplicated myocardial infarction, suggesting further cellular damage.[36]

When heart failure is due to tachyarrhythmias, digitalis may be of some benefit. However, the use of β-adrenergic blocking drugs has a more theoretically beneficial rationale because overall oxygen consumption should be more predictably reduced.

Cardiac Rhythm Disturbances Digitalis is of potential use in four types of supraventricular tachyarrhythmias. They are:

1. Paroxysmal supraventricular tachycardia, whether atrial or junctional in origin (direct effect on AV node).
2. Atrial fibrillation with rapid ventricular response (direct effect on AV node).
3. Atrial flutter (direct cardioversion should probably be attempted initially since a large loading dose of digitalis renders cardioversion more hazardous because of a greater tendency to produce ventricular fibrillation).
4. Wolfe-Parkinson-White syndrome and associated tachyarrhythmias (these may be terminated or prevented by digitalis).

Prophylactic digitalization of patients with diminished cardiac reserve has been debated as a measure to optimize cardiovascular performance prior to major surgical procedures. Meyer[37] reviewed the indications for preoperative digitalization and proposed that the following be considered:

1. Previous history of heart failure.
2. Increased heart size on a standard PA chest X-ray.
3. Coronary flow disturbance.
4. Age greater than 60.
5. Patients over 50 undergoing pulmonary surgery.
6. Whenever massive blood loss is anticipated.
7. Presence of atrial fibrillation.
8. Patients to undergo cardiovascular surgery.
9. Patients with rheumatic valvular lesions.

All of these patient groups have shown improved cardiovascular function during anesthesia and surgery since the negative inotropic effects of anesthesia and surgical stress can be effectively antagonized by the administration of digitalis. Other investigators have confirmed these indications.[38-40]

The use of digitalis in patients without overt congestive heart failure undergoing the stress of critical illness, has a similar rationale. The increased systemic demands for cardiovascular function in acute illness can be met by the use of digitalis during such stress. Recent studies also suggest that digitalis compounds offer a protective effect upon the maintenance of contractility in sepsis, which so often accompanies critical illness.[41] Digitalization can be accomplished at and through the time of acute stress—that portion of the hospital admission necessitating maximum cardiac function; it may then be discontinued before hospital, or even I.C.U., discharge.

Increased oxygen consumption in the nonfailing, nondilated heart and the possibility of inducing digitalis toxicity must always be kept in mind. If adequate extracellular potassium and magnesium levels are maintained, the risk of toxicity is so low that it does not outweigh the potential benefit to be gained by digitalization during times of acute stress.

Dosage and Administration Contrary to former teachings, full digitalization to near toxicity in the I.C.U. setting is neither necessary nor desirable to enhance myocardial contractility. Digitalization is not an "all or none" state. Improved contractility is dose related; that is, any dose will strengthen myocardial contractility until toxic arrhythmias occur.[42] Within ten minutes following an intravenous injection of 0.5 to 1.0 mg of digoxin, a marked improvement in contractility can be noted, though peak action may not be seen for 6 hours. Once the desired effect has been obtained, it is not necessary to continue administering the drug just because a "digitalizing dose" has not yet been reached. The goal, therefore, is to correct heart failure with the minimal effective dose.

The amount of digitalis administered, or "optimal digitalization," should be judged by the clinical improvement desired in a particular patient, and the quantitation of improvement should be accurately measured with serial cardiac output measurements and other parameters. In patients with flutter or fibrillation, the ventricular rate response provides a valuable endpoint for optimum dosage. Since carotid sinus massage can evoke rhythm disorders, such as second degree AV block, accelerated AV junctional rhythm, ventricular premature beats, or bigeminy as toxic levels are approached, it too can prove to be a useful clinical test. If carotid sinus massage evokes an arrhythmia, potential digitalis toxicity can be presumed and further doses withheld before any actual clinical manifestations occur.

Toxicity Unfortunately, digitalis can produce, as toxic manifestations, many of the very rhythmic disturbances it may be employed to treat. Toxic manifestations of digitalis include the appearance of conduction disturbances in both the atrial and ventricular muscles. Digitalis may produce virtually all cardiac arrhythmias, including frequent premature beats and atrial tachycardia with AV block, nodal tachycardia, and other degrees of AV block (commonly the Wenckebach phenomenon). Digitalis will enhance the automaticity of the His-Purkinje system because of the enhancement of phase 4 depolarization.[43] Moe has also demonstrated that digitalis action does not affect conduction and ventricular fibers uniformly. The enhanced automaticity produced thus predisposes the heart to ventricular arrhythmias based on a re-entry mechanism that may progress to ventricular tachycardia and fibrillation.[44]

With these complications in mind, all schedules for digitalis administration should be selected in view of potential toxicity. The creatinine clearance can be used as a rough guideline to maintain adequate digitalis therapy without inducing toxicity. About 35 percent of the total body digitalis content is lost daily in patients with normal renal function, but this diminishes to 14 percent or less in patients who are in renal failure. The 14 percent can be accounted for by secondary hepatic metabolism.[45] Jelliffe has constructed a nomogram which takes into account age, body mass, and renal function in terms of the normal maintenance and digitalizing doses (Fig. 4-2).

Several endogenous factors are known to influence sensitivity to the cardiac glycosides. These include serum potassium, magnesium, and calcium concentrations. In addition, tissue oxygenation, acid-base balance, age (perhaps), renal function, thyroid function, autonomic nervous system tone, interaction with other drugs, and the type and severity of the underlying heart disease all play a role in determining an individual's sensitivity to the relative toxic effects of digitalis.

Interactions

Potassium Digitalis results in a loss of intracellular potassium by NaK ATPase inhibition. In addition, a low extracellular concentration will produce digitalis toxicity with nontoxic "digoxin" plasma levels. This is seen frequently in patients in the acute care setting receiving diuretics or unreplaced nasogastric drainage. Vigorous potassium replacement is indicated when digitalis toxicity is manifested by conduction disturbances (AV block); caution should be used if concomitant administration of potassium is necessary, since elevated potassium concentrations also tend to impair AV conduction.

Magnesium It is well appreciated that magnesium deficiency also predisposes to digitalis intoxication. This should always be considered a potential cause for arrhythmias in patients receiving digitalis. Situations in the intensive care unit which predispose to magnesium loss include gastrointestinal losses, long-term parenteral nutrition, and diuretic therapy. Hypomagnesemia has been reported to result in increased myocardial binding of digitalis.[46]

Myocardial potassium losses (see above) induced by digitalis that are partially responsible for the resultant arrhythmias, are inhibited by magnesium administration in experimental animals.[46] Magnesium sulfate can be administered 1 gm (8 mEq) I.V. over 15 minutes without any untoward effects.

Calcium Calcium potentiates the effects of digitalis. When calcium is given to digitalized patients, or when digitalis is given in the presence of hypercalcemia, extreme caution should be used, since an increased arrhythmogenic potential may be created.

Fig. 4-2. Approximation of digitalizing and maintenance doses according to age, body mass, and renal function. The estimated dose should be validated in the critically ill patient by measured digoxin levels. (From Jelliffe: Am J Med 57:63, 1974.)

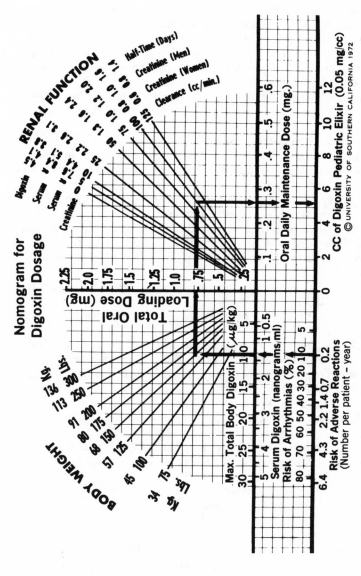

Nomogram for Digoxin Dosage

Available as plastic wallet-sized card for $1.50 each plus postage from Nomograms, Business Office, USC School of Medicine, 2025 Zonal Avenue, Los Angeles, CA 90033.

© UNIVERSITY OF SOUTHERN CALIFORNIA 1972

Other Factors Hypoxia and acid-base disturbances may decrease tolerance to the cardiac glycosides, perhaps secondary to changes in serum or, perhaps, intracellular electrolyte levels. Thyroid disease also alters sensitivity to digitalis. In hypothyroidism, toxicity is often evident at serum levels lower than usually associated with toxicity, whereas hyperthyroid patients are relatively resistant to digitalis.[47] Age also plays a role in digitalis tolerance. Younger patients tolerate high serum levels, whereas toxicity may develop at low serum levels in the older age group; unfortunately, earlier appearance of toxic manifestations also occur in older patients. These effects, which may be secondary to deteriorating renal function in older patients, must be remembered since these are the very patients who require enhancement of myocardial contractility.

Serum Digitalis Concentration Since the advent of accurate methods of assaying plasma digitalis levels, efforts have been made to determine the blood levels which correlate with toxicity. Although several methods have been devised, radioimmunoassay is the most commonly used. The plasma level is only a reflection of the tissue bound levels, and in studies by Gullner,[48] the ratio of myocardial to plasma digitalis was on the order of 24:1. This was a constant and reproducible finding in patients receiving maintenance digitalis administration. Therefore, the following conclusions regarding the use of serum levels appear to be justified:

1. They are useful in ascertaining whether patients have recently received digitalis.
2. There is some correlation between maintenance dose and plasma levels.
3. Plasma levels may help to determine whether aberrant rhythms are or are not related to digitalis toxicity. Beller[49] has shown that patients with known digitalis toxicity had mean serum levels of 2.3 plus or minus 1.6 μg/ml, while nontoxic patients averaged 1.0 plus or minus 0.5 μg/ml. However, there was considerable variation and overlap.
4. There is a gross correlation between inotropic effect and serum levels as determined by systolic time intervals.[48]
5. Ventricular rates of patients with atrial fibrillation do not correlate with plasma levels, even though ventricular rates provide an excellent clinical guide to digitalis tolerance.[50]
6. Serum levels have been shown not to correlate with different brands of digoxin given in the same dose.[50]

Thus, the technique exists, but the desired clinical correlates have not been defined sufficiently to be a day-to-day therapeutic guide or indicator of arrhythmogenic potential/activity. Elucidation of the important correlates will most probably be forthcoming, but the interpretation of digitalis levels must still be viewed as a "gray" area. High levels do suggest impending toxicity, or confirm toxicity potentially caused by digitalis.

DIGITALIS

Actions	Augments myocardial contractility by increasing cellular Ca^{++}
Indications	Any condition requiring augmentation of myocardial contractility or control of cardiac rate
Contraindications	Development of digitalis toxicity
How supplied	Digoxin (Lanoxin) parenteral use 0.25 mg/ml
Dosage	Initially 0.25–0.75 mg I.V. followed by additional 0.5 to 0.75 mg in divided doses until desired effect is obtained; usual range, 1.0–1.75 mg administered in 8–12 hours

CALCIUM

Calcium is the fifth most abundant element in the body and is necessary for the body to perform many essential functions. It is essential for nerve and muscle function where it plays a major role in tissue excitability. Calcium is also necessary for blood coagulation and is essential for cardiac function (p. 203).

Recently, the importance of ionized calcium levels has been demonstrated in critically ill patients.[51] Drop and Laver studied patients in low flow states who developed low ionized calcium levels and who were minimally responsive to calcium infusions. Of greatest importance is the lack of correlation between ionized and total calcium levels; especially important is the fact that ionized calcium is often significantly lower than would be predicted from the total calcium.

Cardiac Effects Without question, calcium has a positive inotropic effect demonstrated in the isolated heart,[52] intact experimental animals,[53] and humans.[54] Stanley,[55] in a unique study with calves, compared the effect of Ca^{++} (5 and 10 mg/kg) in animals before and after implantation of an artificial heart. This has differentiated the effects of calcium in intact animals between its cardiac and various extracardiac effects. In the pretransplant calves, there was a transient, but definite, increase in cardiac output. Following transplantation, cardiac output increased, but less than in the intact animal. In both groups there was a fall in systemic vascular resistance. Flow is therefore augmented by both a positive inotropic effect as well as a fall in systemic resistance with a concomitant increase in flow. Seifen[52] also found that an observed increased heart rate correlated with an increase in ionized calcium. As with all inotropic drugs, there was a concomitant increase in myocardial oxygen consumption.

Systemic Circulation Although early data on the effects of calcium on isolated vascular beds was contradictory, this probably represents an inability to separate cardiac from peripheral vascular effects. The use of the artificial heart in an intact animal[55] has clarified the action of calcium on the systemic vascular bed showing a fall in systemic vascular resistance.

Current Concepts   Recent studies have shown a reduced ionized calcium level in a variety of critically ill states, including respiratory failure[51] and massive blood transfusions.[56] In addition, Ca^{++} also reverses the cardiovascular depression caused by general anesthetics.[57] Howland, however, did not demonstrate any change in measured cardiovascular parameters, even when ionized calcium levels were markedly decreased.[58]

Our clinical impression is that the administration of calcium chloride in situations associated with low ionized calcium or myocardial depression will often produce effects longer than the transient changes seen in normocalcemic patients. Calcium is also indicated in patients who have ganglionic blockade for induced controlled hypotension when reversal of the hypotension is desired. In this regard, Drop[59] demonstrated a significant increase in cardiac output without a change in systemic vascular resistance, which was already decreased by ganglionic blockade.

Calcium also is useful in hemorrhagic and septic shock, perhaps related to the decreases in interstitial calcium noted when micropuncture techniques are used in experimental shock preparations. While the pathophysiologic mechanisms that result in "ionized hypocalcemia" are still unknown, the facts (and therapeutic implications) are clear. Ionized calcium deficits are common and respond to ionized calcium infusions.

Administration   Caution *must* be used when administering the drug. Slow infusions (100 mg $CaCl_2$/min) are used; usual dosage is 1 to 2 gm. Care and reduced dosage are especially important in patients who have received digitalis or who have demonstrated hypokalemia. The electrocardiogram must be continuously monitored and observed. Any premature ventricular activity must abort further drug infusion. Although hypokalemia enhances the arrhythmogenic potential of calcium, concomitant administration of potassium may make calcium administration safe if it is deemed necessary in an acute situation. Calcium can be administered as either a chloride or gluconate, but available Ca^{++} in calcium chloride is 0.72 moles compared to 0.36 moles in the gluconate. Therefore, calcium chloride is preferred (if the above guidelines are observed) since it has a greater and more rapid effect.

CALCIUM	
Action	Direct positive inotropic effect; reduction of systemic vascular resistance
Indications	Low ionized calcium levels frequently associated with a variety of critical illnesses

Contraindications	Should be administered with caution in digitalized and/or hypocalcemic patients; EKG monitoring must always be performed and observed
How supplied	Calcium gluconate or calcium chloride 1 gm in 10 ml
Dosage	1 ml slowly each minute until a desired response is achieved—usually not more than 1-2 gm

GLUCAGON

History Heralded as a potentially useful inotropic agent, glucagon was introduced into clinical practice in 1968.[60] Glucagon is a naturally occurring amino acid compound liberated in small amounts from the pancreas. Its primary action is to stimulate glycogenolysis and gluconeogenesis endogenously since it is directly delivered to the liver. Its chief systemic action as an inotropic agent rests in its ability to increase AMP by stimulation of adenyl cyclase—simulating the action of catecholamines. Its effects are not blocked by β-receptor blocking drugs, do not produce irritability, and in fact, can be considered as antiarrhythmogenic. Glick[61] and Luoff[62] have reviewed the use of glucagon and discussed its role in heart failure. Several points can be emphasized from these reports.

First, one of the principal drawbacks of glucagon administration is that it produces severe nausea and vomiting. However, the administration of an antiemetic overcomes these effects so that the drug may be continued. Second, although some patients in severe heart failure respond to glucagon, it is difficult at this time to define with any degree of certainty those who will benefit from its administration. Third, it has been used to antagonize excessive myocardial failure in patients who have received β-blocking drugs. Fourth, in some patients who have developed functional bundle branch blocks following myocardial infarction, administration of glucagon may induce normal conduction.

In short, the drug may have only a limited place in the therapy of heart failure, especially in terms of time-course effectiveness, but should also not be considered totally useless.

Dosage The inotropic effects are obtained by infusions of 3 to 10 mg of glucagon per hour. When gastrointestinal side effects or improvement of cardiac failure occur, the infusion should be reduced.

α- AND β-ADRENERGIC ANTAGONISTS

The growing understanding of the relationship of the heart's consumption of oxygen (MVO_2) and the importance of microcirculatory flow in low output states has led to the study of compounds antagonistic to sympathomimetic amines. Each will be discussed separately. This represents an almost complete turnaround in the philosophy applied to the pharmacologic therapy of heart failure. At the present time, one might almost mathematically postulate that "the pendulum has swung to the other extreme"; however, *all* the theoretic principles espoused will and must eventually be synthesized into an overall scheme. We can only present the available and most useful clinical candidates today.

α-ADRENERGIC BLOCKING AGENTS

α-Adrenergic blocking drugs competitively antagonize the action of sympathetic drugs at the α-adrenergic receptor. While many compounds show some blocking activity (phenothiazines, general anesthetics, etc.), only dibenzyline (Phenoxybenzamine), tolazoline (Prisciline), and phentolamine (Regitine) are primary α-blocking agents with useful clinical activity.

Cardiovascular Effects   All α-blocking drugs reduce peripheral vascular resistance with a progressive increase in cardiac output. In addition, the use of phentolamine in patients with pheocromocytoma allows the physiologic reexpansion of intravascular volume (plasma volume) after the endogeneous catecholamines have been antagonized. Coronary and cerebral vascular beds are not influenced by α-adrenergic blockade. Experimental evidence in dogs[63] suggests that, in cardiogenic shock, the elevated pulmonary vascular resistance (PVR) can be antagonized by α-adrenergic blocking agents. Unfortunately, this may be a species-related phenomenon. Our experience with phentolamine and tolazoline in adults with an elevated pulmonary vascular resistance (ARDS, postcardiopulmonary bypass, septicemia) has only been sporadically encouraging in this regard, and reports in infants with increased pulmonary vascular resistance[64] have been inconsistent. At this time, we can only say that when a reduction of pulmonary vascular resistance is desired and is not readily accomplished with other pharmacologic compounds, the use of α-blocking drugs may be tried with occasionally gratifying results.

Clinical Usage   Pretreatment in patients with pheochromocytoma with 30 to 60 mg of phenoxybenzamine each day 2 to 3 weeks preoperatively will effectively restore plasma volume. In addition, α-adrenergic blocking drugs have been employed in these cases to treat cardiogenic shock and left ventricular failure by reducing systemic vascular resistance and improving microcirculatory flow.[65,66] Because cardiac output is increased, phentolamine has been ascribed inotropic properties. Rabinowitz[67] demonstrated that phentolamine *lacks* a direct positive inotropic response, but attenuates the peripheral effects of norepinephrine, which produces a reflex increase in cardiac output as systemic resistance declines. The use of α-blocking drugs (like other peripheral dilators), must be accompanied by careful attention to intravascular volume. If intravascular volume is inadequate, the resulting fall in systemic resistance can lead to profound and long-lasting hypotension which can result in inadequate coronary and cerebral perfusion. This was particularly evident in the Regitine test formerly used to diagnose pheochromocytoma. Plasma volume expanders and vasoconstrictors should be readily available to counteract any untoward effects. Above all, however, careful assessment of the intravascular volume status prior to the administration of α-blocking drugs is essential. The simple clinical observation is that these drugs, after many years of study, are not primary therapeutic agents. However, in patients with refractory heart failure or low output states persistent reduction of peripheral resistance may improve cardiovascular function markedly.

Dosage   It is very difficult to give a "cookbook" dose schedule for the α-blocking drugs. The wide range of patient variability and volume states makes very careful titration mandatory. The rule, "Start small, you can always give more," is especially pertinent.

As a general guideline, however, when intravascular volume status is judged reasonable, by CVP and/or PCW pressure measurements, phentolamine 2.5 ± 2.0 mg can be infused intravenously over 5 to 30 minutes. In our experience, slightly larger doses, and hence more concomitant volume administration, are often necessary when a reduction of pulmonary artery pressure is the desired effect. Only by direct measurement of cardiac output, mean pressures, and calculation of systemic and pulmonary vascular resistance can objective evidence of benefit be determined. Similar guidelines for tolazoline should be followed.

α-BLOCKING DRUGS	
Action	Competitive α-adrenergic antagonists
Indication	Plasma volume expansion in preoperative pheochromocytoma; treatment of low output states; may have a role in the reduction of pulmonary vascular resistance
Contraindications	Hypovolemia
How supplied	Regitine (phentolamine), 5 mg ampules with diluent; Priscoline (tolazoline), multidose vials (250 mg in 10 ml or 25 mg/ml); Dibenzyline (phenoxybenzamine) available P.O. only
Dosage	See text (above)

β-ADRENERGIC BLOCKING AGENTS

Although Ahlquist proposed α and β to identify the different actions of sympathomimetic amines in 1948,[68] it was not until 1957 that Slater and Pauel developed dichloroisoproterenol (DCI) with specific β-blocking properties. In 1967 Lands subdivided the β-adrenergic receptors into β_1- and β_2-receptors. β_1-receptors are found in the heart and small intestines and β_2-receptors are found in the arterioles and bronchi. Propranolol is the only intravenous β-blocking drug available at this time in the United States. The β_1- and β_2-antagonistic effects of this drug are about equal.[69] Practalol, available in Europe, has a greater cardiac specificity. This can be an important difference, since it may reduce the respiratory (bronchospastic) effects of β-blockade.

Cardiovascular Effects β-Adrenergic stimulation, in general, causes an increase in oxygen consumption in the heart. Direct action of the β-antagonists on the coronary circulation is limited,[70] and any increase in cross-sectional area in normal coronary arteries is due to the metabolic products (such as adenosine) that accumulate with relative tissue-oxygen debt. When coronary artery disease exists, and increased flow to meet metabolic needs is not possible, myocardial ischemia results. β-blocking drugs have been utilized to reduce the β-effects of inotropic and chronotropic agents which make excessive metabolic demands relative to any change in oxygen delivery. Therefore, propranolol has been found very useful in the treatment of angina; it may even reduce the need for nitroglycerin as well.[71]

Propranolol is also effective in treating many widely divergent tachyarrhythmias. It will reduce sinus, superventricular, and ventricular rates by a decrease in spontaneous depolarization of ectopic pacemakers. It will also slow conduction in the atria and across the atrioventricular node. Propranolol is particularly effective in antagonizing arrhythmias of digitalis intoxication and has minimal effects on digitalis-induced augmentation of cardic contractility.

Propranolol has been employed to treat hypertrophic cardiomyopathies since, in physiologic terms, it should have an opposite effect to the obstruction to ventricular outflow which can be increased by isoproterenol. This can be used in both left ventricular outflow tract obstruction (IHSS) and tetralogy of Fallot where infundibular right ventricular muscular obstruction also occurs.[73] Propranolol has been shown to decrease the renal release of renin[74] by a non-β-blocking action, and is therefore a useful adjunct in the treatment of hypertension. In addition, propranolol is useful in pre- and intraoperative control of β-adrenergic effects of pheochromocytoma, especially when combined with α-adrenergic blockade.

Although the exact mechanism is not yet clear, β-blocking drugs have been shown to be remarkably effective in treating the cardiovascular,[75] peripheral,[76] and hypercalcemic effects of thyrotoxicosis and thyroid storm.

Clinical Usage   It is tempting to attribute all of propranolol's clinical effects to β-blocking activity; but as its usage has increased, non-β-blocking effects, such as its action in hypertension and thyrotoxicosis, have been clearly shown to be quite significant.[77] However, its chief advantages and disadvantages remain primarily associated with its effects upon the β-adrenergic system. Intermittent claudication has been recorded after chronic administration in patients with peripheral vascular disease.[78] The most life-threatening complication reported has been the production of acute heart failure or heart block, seen especially in acutely ill patients whose systemic vascular resistance is already increased. Patients with excessive afterload treated with propranolol can rapidly suffer cardiac dilatation.[79] Although this initially contraindicated its use in acute myocardial infarction, recent evidence[80] suggests that infarct size can actually be reduced. This would make sense in MVO_2 supply-and-demand relationships. This, then, is another area in which concepts have been postulated by clinical utility but have yet to be proven. Again, the data base necessary to interpret all the changes requires a global view of the many interrelated variables.

In patients with underlying bronchospastic disease, propranolol should be used with great care and cogent preparation. Because β-adrenergic tone is blocked, patients with a tendency to bronchospasm may be affected by the administration of propranolol. Hypoglycemia has been mentioned as a side effect of propranolol therapy, but this is probably an exaggerated concern, except in insulin-dependent diabetic patients.[81]

Preoperative Considerations When or if to discontinue β-adrenergic blockage therapy in the perioperative period is still somewhat controversial. Viljoen[82] suggested that cardiac surgery was dangerous in patients on propranolol. However, acute withdrawal of propranolol has been associated with a higher incidence of rebound angina and infarction.[83] Since usage of the drug has increased and operative management has attained clinical expertise, fewer patients are now being withdrawn from the medication. Our present philosophy is to continue propranolol administration pre- and intraoperatively regardless of the disease or dose involved if objective benefits have been obtained. Of course, this necessitates careful monitoring. If patients were given the drug to relieve angina, we reinstitute the drug in the postoperative period as soon as possible, either through the intravenous or oral route. It now appears that the risks of discontinuing the drug are far greater than letting its effect continue if careful monitoring is maintained. Preoperatively, the magnitude of existing β-blockade can be assessed easily by testing to see whether an increase in pulse rate is produced by simple exercise such as stair climbing. If the expected response is diminished or prevented, effective β-blockade truly exists. This will serve to alert the anesthesiologist and intensivist to the necessity for monitoring, and to be ready to intervene with appropriate measures to counteract established β-blockade.

The use of propranolol in the acutely ill has increased markedly in recent years. Tachycardias and most tachyarrhythmias have detrimental effects on MVO_2 and cardiac function within acceptable limits.

The concern of producing cardiac dilatation is real, but is outweighed by the demonstrable clinical benefit usually obtained if the dosage of the drug is carefully titrated.

Dosage and Administration   Propranolol is administrated intravenously in increments of 0.25 to 0.5 mg at intervals of 2 to 5 minutes until the desired response is achieved. When tachyarrhythmias are being treated, the response is usually seen at relatively low doses. It is rather unusual to require more than 2 to 3 mg to treat the majority of arrhythmias or the myocardial irritability seen in the acutely ill patient.

There is a wide variability in dose response of patients to propranolol, and this has made interpretation of the duration of action and frequency of administration controversial. Pharmacokinetic factors responsible for this variation include plasma drug binding, differences of bioavailability, the presence of active metabolites, and the route of administration.[81] Duration of effect is also controversial, because plasma levels may not reflect the active tissue concentrations. While Viljoen[82] suggested that a two-week period was necessary to eliminate the effects, Romagnoli[84] showed response to isoproterenol 24 hours after withdrawal of propranolol.

Propranolol should *always* be administered cautiously. Elevated systemic vascular resistance should be treated prior to any but modest dosages of propranolol. Excessive bradycardia can be reversed successfully by atropine. The competitive antagonist, isoproterenol, may require slightly higher doses than usually employed, but can also be effective. There are three drugs which have different biochemical activity and may be useful in antagonizing unwanted inotropic depression: digitalis, calcium chloride, and glucagon.

Contraindications to the use of β-adrenergic blockade include the presence of heart failure and cardiac dilatation, second- or third-degree heart block, and bronchospastic disease. When practolol or similar compounds become available in this county, bronchoconstriction should be eliminated as a contraindication since they are cardioselective in β-activity.

β-BLOCKING DRUGS (PROPRANOLOL)	
Action	Competitive β-adrenergic antagonist
Indications	Restore MVO_2 supply/demand relationships by (a) negative chronotropic and (b) negative inotropic effect
	Treatment of tachyarrhythmias of all types
	Perioperative treatment of thyrotoxic patients
	Adjunctive therapy in hypertension
Contraindications	Congestive heart failure, unless induced by MVO_2 imbalance
	Bronchospastic disease
	Potentially harmful in peripheral vascular disease

| How supplied | Propranolol 1 mg/1 ml |
| Dosage | 0.25–0.5 mg I.V. up to 3 mg in 20 min; may be repeated if filling pressures are carefully measured |

PERIPHERAL VASODILATORS

Many potential agents are available to decrease vascular resistance. Some (the α-blocking drugs) have already been discussed. Because of the clinical usefulness of sodium nitroprusside, it will be emphasized. Ganglionic blocking drugs and other direct acting smooth muscle relaxing drugs will be presented only in order to give a complete picture.

SODIUM NITROPRUSSIDE

History Sodium nitroprusside was introduced into medical practice by Playfair[85] in 1849, as a color indicator in a test designed to detect acetone aldehydes and alkali sulfides. Claude Bernard reported its ability to lower blood pressure in the 1850s. Hermann[86] and Davidsohn[87] postulated that all of the actions of nitroprusside could be ascribed to the liberation of cyanogen. In 1929, Johnson[88] first suggested that the low therapeutic doses of nitroprusside needed to treat hypertensive crises could be therapeutically separated from its toxicity caused by liberation of cyanide. However, it was not until 1955 that Page et al.[89] applied Johnson's knowledge of the hypotensive effects of sodium nitroprusside in the clinical setting, specifically for the treatment of hypertensive emergencies. Beginning in the 1950s and early 1960s clinical reports began to appear indicating that sodium nitroprusside was effective in a variety of clinical circumstances, including malignant hypertension, induction of hypotensive anesthesia, and treatment of phentolamine-resistant pheochromocytoma.[90] General clinical use of sodium nitroprusside was limited, however, because of the unavailability of a commercial, sterile preparation until, in 1974, Roche Laboratories marketed sodium nitroprusside (Nipride). Since then, many reports of its clinical use have appeared. Much of the current enthusiasm for its use is the result of increased understanding of the regulation of the peripheral circulation and of myocardial function. In addition to its cardiovascular effects, sodium nitroprusside can alter the functions of other organ systems by its inherent action on all blood vessels.

Cardiovascular Effects Sodium nitroprusside is a nonspecific vascular smooth muscle relaxant which affects both arteriolar resistance and venous capacitance beds. The reduced myocardial oxygen consumption and improved myocardial function resulting from a decrease in systemic vascular resistance have fostered clinical use of drugs which, like sodium nitroprusside, have this primary effect. The concomitant reduction in preload by increasing venous bed capacity is usually of secondary importance. Miller,[91] in a study of the effects of sodium nitroprusside in patients with chronic ischemic heart disease, demonstrated dramatic improvement in ventricular function due to reduction in peripheral resistance. Optimum cardiac function was achieved with repletion of intravascular volume (preload) to achieve the filling pressures equal to those that existed before treatment. The marked improvement in cardiac index was not accompanied by any significant change in heart rate or any direct effect on the myocardium. The only significant change was a marked reduction in systemic vascular resistance. Palmer and Lasseter,[92] in a recent review, concluded that nitroprusside is a direct vascular smooth muscle dilator, and that the improvement in cardiovascular function it induced is not a result of any action on the autonomic nervous system, the central nervous system, or cardiac muscle, even at doses 100 times greater than those needed for vascular smooth muscle dilatation. Sodium nitroprusside also antagonizes potassium- and/or epinephrine-induced contractions of vascular smooth muscle.[92] In addition, nitroprusside has been shown to be a direct dilator of vessels within the substance of the myocardium, which results in increased coronary blood flow and a marked decrease in coronary vascular resistance.[93]

Renal Effects Bastron and Koloyanides[94] measured para-aminohippuric acid (PAH), inulin clearance, and sodium excretion in the isolated kidney before and after the administration of sodium nitroprusside. They observed increases in both renal blood flow and sodium excretion. However, in the intact animal, when perfusion pressure falls, a predictable reduction in PAH and inulin clearance occurs. There is also a compensatory release of renin in response to the decline in blood pressure.

Central Nervous System Ivankovich[95] found that sodium nitroprusside dilates the cerebral circulation similarly to other vascular beds. This can result in increased intracranial pressure resulting from increased cardiac output and/or cerebral blood flow. In our experience, the increase in intracranial pressure is variable, and in the clinical setting it is difficult to be sure which of the two mechanisms is more important at any given time. These effects on cerebral blood flow, however, can have serious implications in patients whose intracranial pressure is already increased when an infusion of sodium nitroprusside is chosen to treat the underlying hypertension. Intracranial pressure monitoring is mandatory in this situation. In our experience during neurosurgical procedures with the cranium open, when hypotension has been induced with sodium nitroprusside, no deleterious swelling of the brain has occurred. This is especially true when other maneuvers to reduce cerebral mass are employed. During hypotensive anesthesia, Griffiths[96] demonstrated a decrease in cerebral vascular resistance but no significant decrease in cerebral blood flow or cerebral metabolic oxygen consumption, despite approximately 42 percent reduction in blood pressure. This would indicate that oxygen requirements are met by the increased flow. Sodium nitroprusside does impair normal cerebral autoregulation, however, and abrupt reversal of hypotension can cause large increases in cerebral blood flow with potentially harmful effects.

Pulmonary Circulation Wildsmith[97] et al. demonstrated a marked decrease in Pao_2 in patients during sodium nitroprusside-induced hypotension which they attributed to an increase in ventilation/perfusion $(\dot{V}/\dot{Q})$ scatter comparable to a similar change that occurs with aging. The $(\dot{V}/\dot{Q})$ scatter probably results from direct pulmonary artery dilatation. High FIO_2 and careful monitoring of arterial blood gases are mandatory when induced hypotension with nitroprusside is being employed. Cawley and Chaney[98] found an increase in intrapulmonary shunt $(\dot{Q}s/\dot{Q}t)$ in dogs with regional atelectasis during the administration of sodium nitroprusside. Our preliminary work in patients following cardiac surgery and nitroprusside administration also suggests a decline in arterial oxygenation with an increasing shunt $(\dot{Q}s/\dot{Q}t)$ in those patients who have increased ventilation/perfusion abnormalities. Gallagher and Etling[99] found that shunt did not change in patients with elevated systemic resistance whose primary disease process was acute respiratory failure; this is consistent with our findings in the adult respiratory distress syndrome.

We have used the dilating effects of sodium nitroprusside on the pulmonary vasculature to reduce the high pulmonary vascular resistance associated with the adult respiratory distress syndrome (Fig. 4-3). High pulmonary vascular resistance has been postulated to be a significant etiologic factor in acute respiratory failure in sepsis and other acute respiratory failure states.[100] The gradient of pulmonary arterial diastolic pressure to pulmonary capillary wedge pressure is normally close to zero, since there is little difference between these values. In respiratory failure, pulmonary vascular resistance may markedly increase with the development of a substantial pulmonary arterial diastolic to pulmonary-capillary wedge-pressure gradient. Frequently, this can be abolished with infusions of nitroprusside in high doses (see Fig. 4-3). Whether such therapy can significantly reduce the morbidity or mortality of adult respiratory distress syndrome remains unsettled.

Clinical Usage

Hypertensive Crisis The original, and still important, indication for the use of sodium nitroprusside is in hypertensive emergencies. Koch-Weser,[101] who reviewed a variety of drugs used in the treatment of severe hypertension, found sodium nitroprusside to be the most potent and predictably effective agent for the treatment of the hypertensive

Pt. L. H., 12-6-76
ARDS
HYPERCOAGUABLE

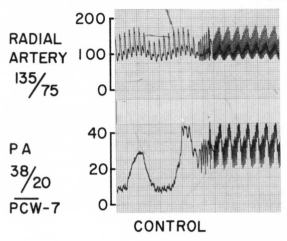

RADIAL
ARTERY
$^{135}/_{75}$

P A
$^{38}/_{20}$
$\overline{PCW}$-7

CONTROL

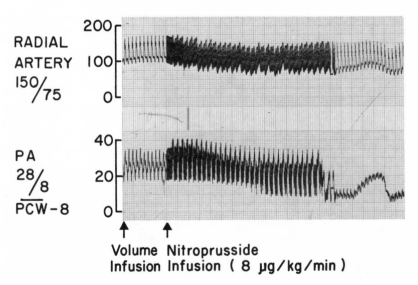

RADIAL
ARTERY
$^{150}/_{75}$

P A
$^{28}/_{8}$
$\overline{PCW}$-8

Volume Nitroprusside
Infusion Infusion (8 μg/kg/min)

Fig. 4-3. Nitroprusside infusion in this patient had a marked effect upon pulmonary artery pressure with little change in systemic pressure. PA pressure decreased from 40/20 to 8/3 rapidly; when the infusion was terminated pulmonary artery pressure again increased.

emergency. As in other clinical situations, its use must be carefully monitored inasmuch as cerebral autoregulation is impaired and wide variation in cerebral blood flow may occur. This is particularly critical if lower limits of acceptable blood pressure cannot be well defined. Ahearn and Crim[102] treated seven patients with malignant hypertension for an average of six days with nitroprusside administered by constant infusion pump, while continuously monitoring arterial pressure. Other oral antihypertensive drug therapy was instituted in the course of this infusion and a gradual reduction of the continuous rate of nitroprusside administration was accomplished. Resolution of symptoms occurred in all cases in response to nitroprusside and supplemental oral therapy. It is our practice in the intensive care unit to institute longer acting compounds, such as hydralazine (p. 247–48), when it appears that long-term control will be necessary and desirable.

Cardiogenic Shock The therapeutic effects of sodium nitroprusside in acute myocardial infarction and heart failure have been widely studied. Shell,[103] Chatterjee,[104] Guiha,[105] Mukherjee,[106] and others have reported beneficial effects on the compromised myocardium. Improvement in ventricular function and diminution of pulmonary arterial and left atrial pressure were uniformly observed. Cardiac output increased as long as left ventricular filling pressure was maintained; peripheral circulatory flow improved at a reduced level of myocardial oxygen consumption.

The effects of intramyocardial arteriolar vasodilatation in the early stages of ischemic injury are the subject of recent discussion. Chianiello, et al.[107] compared the effects of infusions of sodium nitroprusside and nitroglycerine in ischemic heart disease during acute myocardial infarction. The primary effect of nitroglycerine is on the venous capacitance vessels, with a less pronounced effect on the arteriolar resistance vessels. Nitroprusside, because of its effect on arteriolar resistance, might be detrimental in some circumstances when an acute ischemic area is present. Pharmacologic dilatation of normal vessels within the substance of the myocardium was postulated to cause a relative "intramyocardial steal." Comparison of the two drugs in acute ischemic injury revealed no difference in cardiac output or heart rate. With surface electrocardiographic mapping, however, the summated effect on the ST segments showed that nitroprusside increased the size of the ischemic area, while nitroglycerin decreased it. While it is difficult to negate the many clinical reports of patients with acute ischemic episodes who have benefited from infusion of nitroprusside, the different effects of nitroglycerin and nitroprusside warrant some forethought in making a selection. Further study of patients, particularly during evolution of an acute infarction, may resolve these issues to define clinical guidelines.

Open Heart Surgery Nitroprusside has proven to be a valuable adjunct in overcoming the decreased cardiac output that sometimes occurs during and after cardiac surgery. Benzing et al.[108] found systemic vascular resistance decreased by 53 percent, and mean arterial pressure fell 10 percent. In a selected group of patients with low cardiac indices and high peripheral resistance immediately following corrective surgery, a dramatic improvement in cardiac index (to 77 percent) was seen when nitroprusside was instituted. The combination of nitroprusside and potent inotropic drugs (such as epinephrine or dopamine) to maximize cardiac function and minimize systemic resistance, and improve microcirculatory flow provides maximum pharmacologic support at an acceptable oxygen cost. A nonspecific vasodilator, such as nitroprusside, has distinct advantages over isoproterenol, which produces limited vasodilatation while its other sympathomimetic effects may adversely affect oxygen demand.

Mitral Valve Regurgitation Grossman et al.[109] noted marked improvement in ventricular function and an increased ejection fraction following the administration of nitroprusside to patients with mitral insufficiency. The lowered aortic impedance permits preferential aortic ejection which results in a lesser volume pumped back through the mitral valve. The effects of a constant infusion of nitroprusside in a patient with severe acute mitral regurgitation are illustrated in Figure 4-4. Minimal changes in arterial blood pressure are accompanied by a dramatic decline in the pulmonary-capillary wedge (left atrial) pressure tracings. Supplemental fluid volume should be given as filling pressures decline to low normal levels.

Congenital Heart Disease Synhorst et al.[110] studied vasodilator therapy in animals with experimentally produced ventricular septal defects. Systemic vasodilatation markedly reduced the pulmonary-to-systemic blood flow ratio and improved systemic output. It is attractive to postulate that manipulation of the ratio between systemic and pulmonary vascular resistance, which is the prime determinant of the magnitude of the left-to-right shunt in acyanotic congenital heart disease, can increase systemic flow and alleviate the heart failure associated with large left-to-right shunts. This would allow better preoperative preparation. Our preliminary data from nitroprusside infusion[111] in two infants just preceding pulmonary banding demonstrated a reduction in cardiac filling pressures without a reduction in systemic blood pressure, suggesting increased systemic flow. It is also attractive to consider the chronic administration of vasodilators such as hydralazine or phentolamine, in addition to digitalis and diuretics to manage these patients until they reach an appropriate age for definitive correction.

Fig. 4-4. Effect of nitroprusside infusion upon the PAD–PCW gradient. Note that the gradient, originally 14 torr, decreased to a near normal value of 6 torr after nitroprusside. This gradient indirectly represents pulmonary vascular resistance.

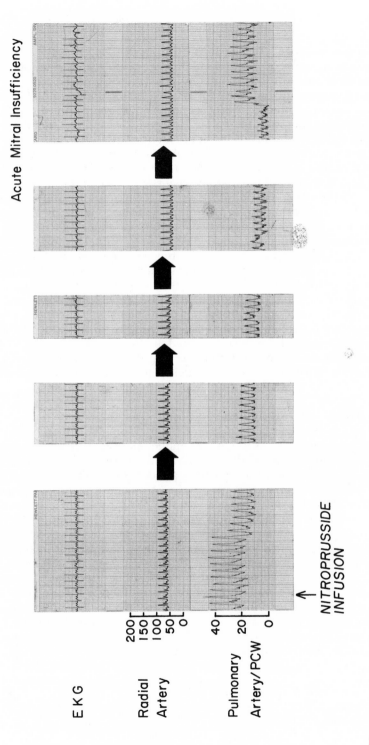

Acute Mitral Insufficiency

EKG

Radial Artery

200
150
100
50
0

Pulmonary Artery/PCW

40
20
0

NITROPRUSSIDE INFUSION

Miscellaneous Uses Taradash and Jacobsen[112] successfuly used nitroprusside to improve microcirculatory flow and cardiac output in the therapy of idiopathic lactic acidosis. Ergot poisoning[113] has also been treated successfully with nitroprusside infusion. Palmer and Lasseter[114] and others suggested the use of sodium nitroprusside as medical therapy of dissecting thoracic aneurysms. However, recent data from their laboratory indicate that an increase in extent of dissection can result from sodium nitroprusside infusion. The marked improvement in ventricular function that occurs with reduction of systemic resistance accelerates the first derivative of the maximum aortic pressure (aortic dP/dT max), which can further extend the dissection. This complication can be attenuated by depressing the myocardium with large doses of propranolol. It would appear, however, that the ganglionic blocking drug trimethaphan, which produces a relative decrease in dP/dT, remains the drug of choice in the initial therapy of acute aortic dissection. Without question, the spectrum of clinical indications for sodium nitroprusside will be subject to change as more extensive experience accumulates. This is particular true since the hemodynamic events that occur are more complex than the simple production of hypotension. As in thoracic aortic aneurysms or ischemic heart disease, these consequences may not always be beneficial. On the other hand, in disease states in which microcirculatory flow is compromised[115] or platelet aggregation occurs[116] such as disseminated intravascular coagulation, nitroprusside may prove particularly beneficial.

Metabolism and Toxicity The enthusiasm for the clinical effectiveness of sodium nitroprusside has been tempered somewhat by recent reports of at least three deaths during the induction of hypotensive anesthesia. Greiss et al.[117] discussed these deaths and reported lethal cyanide levels in blood and urine in at least one patient. The metabolic scheme for the biodegradation of sodium nitroprusside is illustrated in Figure 4-5. Smith and Kruszyna[118] have shown that the interaction of erythrocytes and sodium nitroprusside involves a nonenzymatic reaction liberating cyanide. At least one molecule of this cyanide is inactivated by the formation of methemoglobin. The remaining four molecules in association with rhodanase and endogenous thiosulfate form the less toxic compound thiocyanate. A small portion of this thiocyanate may be oxidized by the thiocyanate oxidase in the tissues to liberate free cyanide. Since cyanide can be released from nitroprusside and has been found in lethal concentration in at least one reported death, it is probably the prime etiologic factor in fatal reactions. The amount of available cyanide, and hence the total amount of nitroprusside administered, is crucial. The

Fig. 4-5. Schematic representations of the metabolism and excretion of nitroprusside. Note the reactions which lead to toxicity of both cyanide and thiocyanate and the effect of hydroxycobalamine (vitamin B_{12A}).

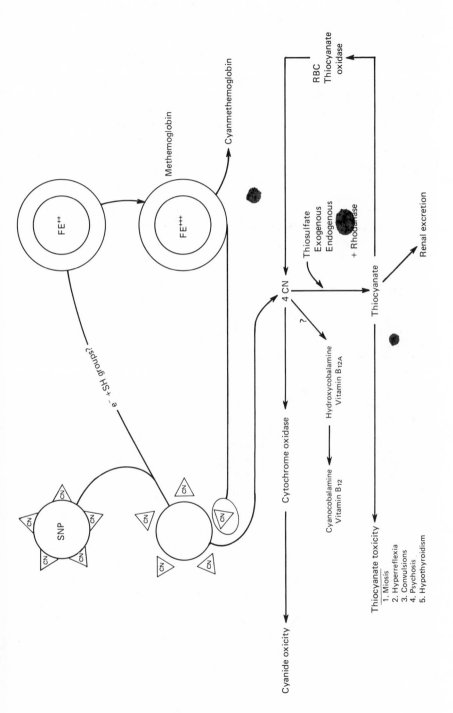

241

rate of administration of nitroprusside is also important. Davies[119] characterized at least three distinctly different responses to nitroprusside: (1) total dose is less than 3 mg/kg; (2) constant and apparently normal dose response requiring total doses greater than 3 mg/kg; (3) tachyphylaxis and nearly total resistance to infusion of the drug. In at least the second and third groups, metabolic studies would indicate the presence of tissue acidosis and a picture like that of cyanide toxicity.

The resistance that some patients show to sodium nitroprusside infusion can be explained in several ways. Patients who require high doses of sodium nitroprusside may have inappropriately low levels of thiocyanate. A deficiency in endogenous thiosulfate or an abnormality of tissue rhodanase necessary for the conversion of cyanide to thiocyanate, could explain the low thiocyanate levels. The possibility of inhibition of rhodanase by other drugs has not been ruled out. Tachyphylaxis would suggest that the biodegradation system is initially intact, but progressively becomes less effective. Reduced amounts of endogenous thiosulfate or progressive inhibition of rhodanase may be the cause. The administration of thiosulfate might be useful in patients who become tachyphylactic after an apparent normal initial response, since low endogenous levels of thiosulfate could be the metabolically limiting step. The cyanide-thiosulfate interaction may be congenitally absent, as in Leber's optic atrophy, or "environmentally" induced as in tobacco amblyopia, accounting for the finding of elevated cyanide and decreased thiocyanate levels in these patients.

Other adverse effects of nitroprusside which may be important clinically would include the formation of methemoglobin,[120] hypothyroidism following several days of continuous therapy,[121] and the effect recently observed by Saxon and Kahlove[116] of a direct platelet inhibition secondary to a possible effect on thrombosthenin, a platelet smooth muscle-like protein necessary for the second platelet release response. Recent evidence points to a synergism between nitroprusside and a new antihypertensive drug, clonidine,[122] producing rather profound hypotension. As the uses for nitroprusside increase, other clinical problems will undoubtedly be reported.

Treatment of Toxicity Inasmuch as the direct lethal effects of nitroprusside infusion appear to be related to cyanide levels, the potential for toxicity should always be considered when using the drug. Any patient showing resistance or tachyphylaxis should have the drug discontinued promptly. In addition, progressive acidosis in patients receiving the drug should be assumed to be cyanide toxicity until proven otherwise. The infusion should be stopped and treatment for cyanide poisoning should be considered. Currently, cyanide toxicity is managed by (1) inhalation of amyl nitrate every 2 minutes; (2) intravenous infusion of sodium nitrate in a dose of 5 mg/kg in 20 ml of water over 3 to 4 minutes; (3) intravenous infusion of sodium thiosulfate, 150 mg/kg in 50 ml of water over 15 minutes. This form of therapy is designed to form methemoglobin which has a higher affinity for cyanide than does the cytochrome system. It yields cyanmethemoglobin; following this, administration of thiosulfate allows conversion of cyanmethemoglobin to thiocyanate and methemoglobin. Thiocyanate is then excreted by the kidneys. Patients with impaired renal function may not excrete thiocyanate normally and must be carefully watched for thiocyanate or cyanide intoxication. The hazard of this form of therapy is the production of methemoglobin in such excess that oxygen-carrying capacity is reduced even though the cytochrome system is functional. At least one fatal case secondary to this therapy has been reported. Recently, Posner and associates[123,124] reported the promising use of hydroxycobalamine (vitamin B_{12A}), which in the presence of cyanide forms cyanocobalamine, or vitamin B_{12}. Cottrell[125] has also reported successful reduction of cyanide levels in patients with the use of hydroxycobalamine. At present this indication is not approved by the Food and Drug Administration, but it appears likely that approval will be gained shortly. There is presently no indication that cyanocobalamine is toxic, even in excessive doses, when administered to subhuman primates. This should be a promising drug for either prophylactic or therapeutic use.

Clinical Usage Individual patient response is dependent upon the intravascular volume and overall cardiovascular status of the patient. A dose of 50 mg sodium nitroprusside dissolved in 250 ml (0.02 percent solution) or 500 ml (0.01 percent) is administered 0.1 to 0.5 mg/min.

SODIUM NITROPRUSSIDE	
Action	Direct vascular smooth muscle relaxant
Indications	Cardiogenic shock
	Post-open-heart surgery
	Control of peripheral vascular resistance in low flow states
	Hypertensive crisis
	Mitral regurgitation
	Reduction of pulmonary vascular resistance
	Induced hypotension
Contraindications	Hypovolemia
	Potential redistribution of intramyocardial blood flow in acute ischemia
Special problems	Development of toxicity
How supplied	Sodium nitroprusside (Nipride) 50 mg in powder form (solution must be protected from light)

GANGLIONIC BLOCKERS

There are many drugs with activity as autonomic ganglionic blocking agents. Although hexamethonium was the prototype, only trimethaphan is of clinical importance in the acute care setting today. This compound is not only employed to reduce blood pressure in acutely ill patients, but also to induce hypotension during surgical procedures for the purpose of limiting blood loss.

Cardiovascular Effects   Trimethaphan affects blood pressure primarily by its action on venous capacitance and arteriolar resistance vessels mediated by blocking of sympathetic motor reflexes.[126] Both arterial blood pressure and cardiac output usually decrease.[127] The ganglionic blocking effect seems to exert a negative inotropic effect similar to β-blockade[128] on the heart and has been postulated to be responsible for the reduction in cardiac output during trimethaphan influsion. Cardiac index also declines in cardiac surgical patients when trimethaphan infusion[129] has been employed.

In critically ill patients with head injuries, intracranial pressure can be reduced by trimethaphan whereas it is often exacerbated by sodium nitprusside.[130] This difference presumably occurs because cardiac index diminishes and there is no cerebral vascular dilatation as induced by sodium nitroprusside. When elevated intracranial pressure (ICP) and systemic hypertension coexist, trimethaphan is the drug of choice—so long as careful attention is paid to cerebral perfusion pressure (CPP). This is defined as mean arterial pressure minus intracranial pressure. (CPP = BP − ICP).

When treating coexisting systemic hypertension and intracranial hypertension, careful attention must be paid to maintenance of cerebral perfusion pressure. These pressure recordings must be made with a transducer at the level of the brain. CPP less than 75 torr is associated with alteration of EEG, evoked potential, and cerebral blood flow compatible with deterioration of cerebral function.[131]

Clinical Usage   Trimethaphan is, in part, metabolized by pseudocholinesterase which accounts for its short duration of action. Consistent blood pressure control may be difficult however because of tachyphylaxis. In addition, tachycardia, potentially detrimental to patients with heart disease, may also require therapy with propranolol. Again, Palmer has recommended trimethaphan rather than sodium nitroprusside for medical therapy of acute aortic dissection because ventricular contractility is depressed while it is often enhanced by sodium nitroprusside.

Dosage   Trimethaphan is prepared by adding 500 mg of trimethaphan to 500 ml of 5 percent dextrose in water and titrated until the desired pressure is achieved. As with all dilating agents, intravascular volume must be monitored and maintained. The decline in cardiac index may be detrimental in many critically ill patients. Central venous administration is preferred for trimethaphan, as well as for all other vasoactive substances.

GANGLIONIC BLOCKING DRUGS (TRIMETHAPHAN)	
Action	Predominant sympathetic ganglionic blocker
Indication	Blood pressure reduction, especially when augmentation of cardiac contractility is not necessary
Contraindications	Hypovolemia
	States where tachycardia are potentially harmful
Special problems	Early tachyphylaxis
	Potential neuromuscular paralysis with excessive dosage
How supplied	Trimethaphan (Arfonad) 500 mg ampule diluted in 500 ml D5W

NITROGLYCERINE

Historically, nitroglycerine has been the mainstay of therapy for angina.[132] It has, until recently, been considered to be contraindicated in patients with overt myocardial infarctions. However, a rebirth of interest in, and enthusiasm for, nitroglycerine has occurred, creating a new spectrum of potential uses.

Cardiovascular Effects Nitroglycerine was traditionally thought to be a coronary vasodilator. It has become increasingly apparent that coronary vessels with atheromatous plaques are not likely to dilate in response to pharmacologic agents. (There is documented evidence of relief of coronary spasm, however, in Prinzemetal's angina.) In addition, vessels distal to an obstructed coronary are maximally dilated because ischemia is already present. It is now apparent that the beneficial effects of nitroglycerine are primarily caused by a reduction of myocardial wall tension[133] as a result of an increase in the venous capacitance bed which lowers myocardial filling pressures. This may occur without changes in peripheral arteriolar resistance and with little or no change in cardiac index. The universal nature of vasodilatation by sodium nitroprusside is now considered to be potentially detrimental to an ischemic myocardium, particularly when compared to nitroglycerine. The dilatation by nitroprusside of coronary resistance vessels leading to nonischemic areas, results in an intramyocardial "steal" by directing flow away from the critical areas and may also increase the area of ischemia.

When evolving myocardial infarction is the cause of "pump failure" in the acute care setting, the use of nitroglycerine is an attractive alternative to nitroprusside, particularly in view of its low toxic potential. When LVEDP is elevated because an ischemic myocardium functions poorly, cardiac output may increase as more favorable ventricular function ensues. However, nitroglycerine predominantly reduces preload and these effects may not provide the desired increase in microcirculatory flow so frequently desirable in the critically ill patient. In that case, sodium nitroprusside should be of greater value. This should not detract from its potential benefit if myocardial ischemia is complicating any critical illness. Thus, the nitroglycerine and nitroprusside seem to have greater specificity for treating certain illnesses, a perspective that has evolved with increasing clinical experience.

Dosage and Administration The major limitation to more general usage of nitroglycerine in the acute care setting is the lack of an FDA approved intravenous solution. Most hospital pharmacies, however, can prepare nitroglycerine infusions by dissolving nitroglycerine tablets (0.4 mg each) in D5W, removing the talc-containing supernatant by centrifugation, and passing the remainder through a 0.22 millipor filter and diluting with D5W to achieve the final concentration of 30 μg/ml. This is then injected directly I.V. (30 to 60 μg) or prepared as an infusion with a final concentration of 30 to 60 μg/ml. Nitroglycerine can also be used as in the past; the tablets themselves may be placed in the sublingual area. Nitroglycerine must also be shielded from light. The prepared concentrate should be used within 30 days of preparation.[134] Nitroglycerine is also available for transcutaneous absorption as Nitrol paste. This provides a more continuous level than sublingual tablets for the patient who no longer needs a continuous infusion. Dosage is titrated in a unique way—the tube is squeezed and a measured length of paste is applied to the skin. This may be lengthened or shortened according to the effect desired.

	NITROGLYCERINE
Action	Smooth muscle relaxant with predominant venous capacitance activity
	Will antagonize coronary artery spasm, i.e., Prinzmetal's angina
Indications	Reduction of LVEDP by reducing preload
	Alleviation of myocardial ischemia induced by coronary spasm or subendocardial ischemia seen with an elevation of LVEDP
	Reduction of blood pressure
Contraindications	Hypovolemia
	Less effective than nitroprusside in augmenting cardiac output in absence of ischemia
Special problems	Lack of commercially available intravenous preparation
Preparation	Nitroglycerine tablets 0.4 mg sublingual or dissolved
	Application of cutaneous paste
	I.V. infusion 30–120 μg/min

HYDRALAZINE

Frequently, a long acting vasodilator is more desirable than one requiring constant intravenous infusion. The beneficial effects of nitroprusside result primarily from its reduction of arteriolar resistance and not its action on the venous capacitance vessels. Since hydralazine has actions very similar to nitroprusside on the arteriolar resistance bed, it can be a very attractive substitute when long-term reduction in afterload is desirable. Hydralazine is also employed to optimize cardiac function in preoperative cardiac surgery patients with mitral or aortic regurgitation by reducing peripheral resistance and augmenting ventricular ejection. Hydralazine can be used to provide a stable "baseline level" of vasodilatation to which nitroprusside can be added in smaller doses to provide "fine-tuning" in seeking optimal function.[135]

Cardiovascular Effects The action of hydralazine is greater on arterioles than on venules. Recently Pierpont[136] has shown that combination hydralazine-nitroglycerine therapy is equivalent to nitroprusside for a longer period of time. Hydralazine, in our experience, has provided a satisfactory method of continuing the vasodilating effect without the necessity of continuous infusion or the risk of toxicity inherent in long-term nitroprusside therapy.

Dosage and Complications Initial conversion from nitroprusside to hydralazine is accomplished with 5 to 10 mg increments of hydralazine given intravenously every 10 to 20 minutes until the desired effect is achieved. This has occasionally necessitated administering over 200 mg in a 12-hour period. Long-term oral administration has been associated with induction of an acute rheumatoid state or a syndrome indistinguishable from disseminated lupus erythermatosis. However, we have not encountered this problem even at high dose levels in the relatively short-term (up to three weeks) therapy necessary in most acute care situations.

HYDRALAZINE	
Action	Vascular smooth muscle relaxant (primarily arterioles)
Indication	Antihypertensive
	Reduction of systemic vascular resistance in congestive heart failure
	Replacement for or concomitant with sodium nitroprusside for blood pressure and/or cardiac output manipulation
Contraindications	Hypovolemia
	May produce undesirable tachycardia which can be treated with propranolol and/or volume administration

Special problems	Rare development of a rheumatoid state or sys-
	temic lupus erythermatosis with high doses
Dosage and	Hydralazine (Apresoline) 10–20 mg I.V. every 20
Administration	min initially, then 20–50 mg I.V. every 6 hr

MISCELLANEOUS DRUGS

Alpha methyl dopa and diazoxide can also be used to reduce systemic vascular resistance. Alpha methyl dopa is neither as potent nor as rapid in onset as hydrazaline and often requires 24–48 hours to achieve its effect. Occasionally, patients with mild preexisting but untreated hypertension can be treated with this drug when potency and rapid onset are undesirable because "overshooting," and the production of hypotension, would be potentially dangerous. A dosage of 250 to 500 mg may be administered every 4 to 6 hours, or a total of 1 to 3 gm daily. The sedation that often accompanies alpha methyl dopa therapy may be either advantageous or not, depending upon the particular patient in the I.C.U. setting. For instance, a restless patient, straining at invasive monitoring lines, will be easier to manage, but it may impede the weaning of an elderly, somnolent patient from the respirator.

Diazoxide often will reduce blood pressure significantly within a short period of time and maintain the reduction for 4 to 6 hours. It is most effective when combined with a "loop" diuretic which decreases intravascular volume and increases sodium excretion. This combination may overcome the retention of sodium in the vascular walls caused by diazoxide and is occasionally useful in the treatment of transient (and supposedly self-limited) hypertension in the I.C.U. For instance, acute exacerbation of renal hypertension after corrective surgery usually disappears in 12 to 24 hours, if surgery has been successful. A single dose of diazoxide may be sufficient therapy. If cardiovascular compromise and/or critical intravascular volume changes are suspected, this approach might be too empirical; invasive monitoring might then define abnormalities more exactly. Continuous infusion therapy may also be preferred when short-term changes seem likely.

THERAPY OF INADEQUATE CARDIOVASCULAR FUNCTION

The therapy of inadequate cardiovascular function must begin with the identification of any specific etiologic factors present. The most critical factor is the recognition of the low output state. Blood pressure, urine output, or central venous pressure may not suggest a critically low cardiac output. This can be induced by excessive demand—septicemia or pancreatitis; hypertension, with marked increases in systemic resistance; trauma or related stressful states—or it can be the direct result of primary pump failure. Most often, in the critical setting a combination of factors interact to produce a situation in which cardiac output is inadequate for systemic demands. For example, the patient with long-standing hypertension who requires major surgery creates an excessive demand on a heart with limited reserve. Moreover, the reference "normal cardiac index" obtained from healthy patients at rest in a cardiac catheterization laboratory is rarely adequate to meet the systemic demands of stress, the postoperative state, infection, or, most critically, the multisystemic insult compounded by inadequate host defense in the I.C.U. patient. In these situations, augmentation of overall cardiovascular function seems mandatory.

A simple solution is rarely possible, except in cases of acute blood loss in the healthy patient where restoration of circulating blood volume solves the problem. But, as demonstrated in Vietnam, even in a healthy heart, significant overall multifaceted impairment of the cardiovascular system can occur. Because acute disease is often superimposed upon an existing chronic impairment, careful assessment of cardiac function is the only reasonable solution.

Monitoring, data accumulation, and analysis are essential. Rational choices and evaluation of therapy can only be made when objective assessment of the determinants of cardiac function are known. These include specific measurements of cardiac output, systemic resistance, oxygen consumption, and right and left ventricular work.

A sudden crisis in the I.C.U. must generate a simultaneous diagnostic and therapeutic approach. A rapid clinical evaluation must assess the presence of an adequate airway and blood pressure compatible with organ perfusion (MAP > 70 torr or a systolic pressure of 100 torr). If the pressure is inadequate, a central venous route is immediately established and epinephrine or dopamine, infused at the lowest level necessary to obtain an adequate perfusion pressure, is begun. This should only be considered a transient measure to "buy some time." Once perfusion pressure is restored (or if it is initially adequate), a flow-directed pulmonary artery catheter is inserted. Cardiac output and filling pressures are then measured. After performing the calculations presented earlier,* specific areas of hemodynamic dysfunction can be identified and corrected. Each patient will, of course, demonstrate a unique picture so that principles alone must serve as building blocks to construct a "therapeutic edifice."

However, it can be stated that the ultimate goal of cardiovascular support is to optimize cardiac function with a minimal oxygen cost to the heart. The best method of achieving this goal is to concentrate on the most energy consuming tasks that the heart must perform, i.e., pressure-work, creating wall tension and excessive heart rate. Continuous evaluation of hemodynamic parameters is required to achieve this end.

---

* Calculator programs are available upon request from the volume editor.

If, for example, the cardiac index is 3 liters/min, $C_A - C_V$ content difference is 6 ml/dl, systemic vascular resistance (SVR) is calculated to be 3000 dynes cm^{-5}, and pulmonary capillary wedge pressure (PAO) is 20 torr, then a reduction of SVR to 1500 dynes cm^{-5} would probably increase the cardiac index, reduce the $C_A - C_V$ difference, and decrease the pulmonary capillary wedge pressure. All of this could be accomplished with peripheral vasodilatation and would be accompanied by a reduction in oxygen cost as well. An inotropic drug (dopamine or epinephrine) would probably increase MVO_2 with little change or further increase in SVR. If O_2 delivery to the myocardium were normal, this increased demand could perhaps be met; however, this would not be an optimal choice of therapy for either the myocardium or the systemic vasculature. If vasodilatation diminished pulmonary-capillary wedge pressure, then the judicious administration of fluids to increase filling pressures can optimize stroke volume by the Frank-Starling mechanism at a low O_2 cost.

It is often necessary, however, to augment contractility with positive inotropic agents. This is usually most effective when systemic resistance is concomitantly reduced and when intravascular volume is already adequate, but it is often necessary to begin inotropic support before a reduction of SVR can be tolerated.

Ideally, one would strive to obtain the following hemodynamic parameters:

1. A cardiac index that will maintain the $C_A - C_V$ difference about 3 to 4 vol percent. (In critically ill patients, this is usually in the 3 to 4 liters/min/sq m range.)
2. An SVR between 1000 to 1500 dynes cm^{-5}
3. A PAO of 12 to 18 torr. This minimizes pulmonary venous pressure and allows subendocardial blood flow in the myocardium. If the LVEDP (PAO) rises above 25 torr, subendocardial flow may be compromised and the risk of pulmonary edema increases.

Another consideration involves patients with elevated pulmonary vascular resistance; in this instance it would seem desirable to lower resistance in the lung in order to reduce right ventricular work as well.

By understanding pharmacologic principles, it is then possible to maximize the desired effects of a drug while minimizing its undesirable effects. Evaluation of the specific etiology and development of a therapeutic plan can now be undertaken.

ETIOLOGY OF ACUTE HEART FAILURE

Simply stated, an inadequate cardiac output occurs when: (1) demands exceed the heart's ability to pump, (2) inadequate oxygen is delivered to the myocardium for the amount of work the heart is performing, or

(3) inadequate volume is returned to the left ventricle. Patients can be divided into those with normal or compromised myocardial oxygen delivery; each group will be presented with a variety of systemic insults, inasmuch as both sets of factors alter the approach to therapy.

Examples of inordinate demands placed upon the ventricle would include chronic hypertension with progressive hypertrophy and inability of the myocardium to eject against the increased resistance. Aortic stenosis and the cardiomyopathies fall into this general classification. Cardiogenic shock and the inadequate cardiac output associated with ischemia of the myocardium are examples of inadequate oxygen supply to the myocardium and hence primary "pump failure." Inadequate volume return to the left ventricle is obvious in acute vascular injuries, but may be less well appreciated as a complicating effect of pulmonary edema, inadequate ventricular return evidenced by overloading the pulmonary capillary bed, protracted fever, or in the early postoperative state, "third space" losses and decreases in functional extracellular volume resulting in decreased intravascular volume.

THE ROLE OF INTRAVASCULAR VOLUME

The monitoring and maintenance of the adequacy of intravascular volume in the critically ill patient cannot be overemphasized. Manipulation of the cardiac work performed by adjusting volume according to a Starling ventricular function curve is the "cheapest" in terms of oxygen cost. This is especially true when adequate volume is associated with normal or reduced systemic vascular tone. Adequate volume is especially essential in disease states where filling pressures must be maintained higher than normal. If inotropic support or vasodilators cause end-diastolic volume to fall to normal or subnormal levels, there will be a subsequent and undesirable fall in cardiac index. This is especially likely with the use of sodium nitroprusside[137] because of its effect on venous capacitance. Restoration of filling pressures (diastolic volume) can then lead to a marked increase in stroke volume at a relatively modest energy cost to the myocardium. Careful attention to central venous pressure or, preferably, pulmonary-capillary wedge pressure (left atrial pressure) is mandatory in preventing the use of excessive pharmacologic support (high energy cost) instead of increasing intravascular volume (low energy cost). Patients with ischemia, old infarcts, or ventricular hypertrophy, commonly have poor ventricular compliance (high filling pressures at less than normal ventricular volumes). In order to achieve adequate end-diastolic volumes, much higher filling pressures must be employed to generate maximum cardiac performance. However, the relationship between the filling pressure, stroke volume, and stroke work must be carefully titrated because of the inherent risk of creating pulmonary edema. This occurs when left atrial pressure is elevated and overdistention of the heart ultimately decreases its work output (Law of Laplace).

THERAPY OF PATIENTS WITH ADEQUATE OXYGEN DELIVERY

Agents which increase myocardial contractility and, to some degree, systemic resistance, continue to have a role in clinical practice despite the potential for producing a marked increase in myocardial oxygen consumption. Patients with normal coronary arteries, whose intravascular volume is adequate or being restored, and whose cardiac output persists at a low level, will show dramatic improvement with infusions of catecholamines, the use of digitalis preparations, or any of the other inotropic agents previously discussed. The increased oxygen demand *can* be met by oxygen delivery.

This is particularly true in the postcardiac surgical patient after valvular and congenital heart surgery;[138] in the patient who has suffered massive trauma; or in the patient in septic shock.[139] In addition, the patient with an overdose of a cardiovascular depressant (e.g., a barbiturate) and the one with central nervous system trauma will show return of cardiac performance and a measurable increase in cardiac output with inotropic support. The use of catecholamine infusions in patients with massive trauma will maintain maximum cardiac function and critical organ perfusion pressures until further volume loss can be contained and intravascular volume restored. However, agents which simply elevate systemic vascular resistance, and hence treat blood pressure alone, have a very limited role in the therapy of any form of cardiac decompensation short of overt cardiac standstill and cardiopulmonary resuscitation. Regulation of catecholamine infusions by the resulting blood pressure should be considered as an unacceptable intensive care unit practice. Rather, a dose (in μg per minute) is chosen and tested for its overall effects upon cardiac output, resistance, and filling pressure. If the results do not meet the predetermined expectations, re-evaluation of all hemodynamic parameters must be undertaken. Therapy can then be further modified. The titration, or the measurement of blood pressure, on the other hand, gives little evidence as to the overall state of cardiovascular function.

Occasionally, drugs which decrease the myocardial work are beneficial even in patients with normal myocardial oxygen delivery. For instance, sodium nitroprusside can be used in patients with mitral insufficiency (see p. 238). In patients with severe cardiomyopathies, or in tamponade, augmentation of contractility would seem to be desirable, but in practice is often ineffective. However, reduction of the total work the heart must perform often effects an overall improvement in function.[140]

THERAPY OF PATIENTS WITH
INADEQUATE OXYGEN DELIVERY

Cardiogenic shock is a name applied to the functioning of a heart faced with inadequate oxygen delivery. Therapeutic modalities have undergone numerous changes in recent years as concepts of oxygen delivery and utilization have evolved. Positive inotropic and vasopressor support alone are of less theoretic and clinical usefulness since the therapeutic perspective now focuses upon reducing myocardial oxygen consumption rather than producing more oxygen debt.[141] The only other method that is applicable is to increase oxygen delivery by coronary artery bypass grafting, or, for a short-term effect, by intra-aortic balloon counter pulsation. These continue to undergo investigation in the acute setting. Forrester[141] has shown that non-oxygen-consuming therapeutic modalities have reduced morbidity and mortality. Those agents that reduce afterload (sodium nitroprusside, hydralazine) or wall tension (nitroglycerine), or those that reduce inotropic or chronotropic activities, i.e., MVO_2 (propranolol), have proven their usefulness in acute cardiac ischemia (Table 4-2).

Practically speaking, there is often a concomitant need to augment contractility and reduce end-diastolic volume while reducing the resistance work the heart must perform. Since a single suitable drug is not yet available, the combination of a positive inotropic agent (epinephrine or dopamine) and a vasodilator (sodium nitroprusside or nitroglycerine), with careful attention to maintaining optimal volume and filling pressures, has proven to be particularly advantageous in patients who are ischemic and have increased systemic demands for maximal cardiac output. Chronotropic effects must be minimized in this approach, and only the minimal amount of catecholamine[141] necessary to augment contractility should be used. Dobutamine, a new synthetic catecholamine,

TABLE 4-2

Drugs Used in the Treatment of Heart Failure and Their Effects on Hemodynamics and Myocardial Oxygen Consumption

Drug	Hemodynamics		MVO_2*	
	CO†	PCW‡	Effect	Mechanism
Digitalis	↔	↔	↑	↑ Contractility (see p. 203–4)
Norepinephrine	↔	↔	↑	↑ HR,§ Contractility (low dose) ↑ SP‖ (high dose)
Isoproterenol	SL ↑	SL ↓	↑↑	↑ HR, Contractility
Diuretics (Furosemide)	←	↓	↓	↓ Heart size
Vasodilatation (Nitroprusside)	↑	↓	↓	↓ SP, Heart size
β-Blockade (Propranolol)	SL ↓	↔ or ↑	↓	↓ HR, Contractility, SP

Modified from Forrester JS, Swan HJC: Crit Care Med 2:290, 1974
* MVO_2 = Myocardial oxygen consumption
† CO = cardiac output
‡ PCW = Pulmonary capillary wedge pressure
§ HR = Heart rate
‖ SP = Systemic pressure

combines inotropic with minimal chronotropic effect and simultaneously reduces systemic resistance.[142] This is a most desirable combination and may prove to make dobutamine an important drug. While at first glance isoproterenol might appear to have similar advantages, its marked chronotropic effect and lack of predictable effect upon afterload make isoproterenol particularly devastating in ischemic disease.[143]

Without question, perfusion pressure must be maintained, particularly in the areas of fixed resistance in the coronary bed where flow is totally pressure-dependent. However, if overall myocardial oxygen demand is reduced, lower perfusion pressures can be tolerated even with improved function, since the need for oxygen is concomitantly reduced. Summaries of drugs, their effects on MVO_2, and their hemodynamic effects are given in Table 4-2.

CONCLUSION

It is axiomatic that a specific etiology for the cause of inadequate cardiac output be determined. However, acute therapy must often be accomplished, almost without regard to etiology. The desired principles are no different, but must be applied at first somewhat empirically. If primary ventricular failure is suspected, then inotropic support within the limits of myocardial oxygen delivery should be started. If ischemia, relative or absolute, appears likely, then efforts should be initially directed to reducing myocardial work and hence matching its oxygen consumption with available oxygen delivery. Constant hemodynamic surveillance is absolutely essential, including measurement of filling pressures, cardiac output, and calculations of stroke work, stroke volume, and resistances. It must be remembered that the right and the left side of the heart function separately and that left ventricular decompensation can occur while right sided pressures are consistently within the normal range.[144] Blood pressure, the common clinical parameter, can only be put into its proper perspective as a reflection of the adequacy of systemic flow when all other parameters are also known from direct measurement.

Finally, the cheapest work the heart can perform, i.e., utilization of the Starling mechanism, is "volume enhanced" work. Thus, regardless of the etiology of cardiac failure, vasoactive and cardiotonic drugs should never be substituted for intravascular volume simply to achieve a "normal" blood pressure.

REFERENCES

1. Sonnenblick EH, Ross J, Braunwald E: Oxygen consumption of the heart: newer concepts of its multifactorial determination. Am J Cardiol 22:328, 1968

2. Zelis R, Mason D: Compensatory mechanisms in congestive heart failure—the role of peripheral resistance vessels. N Engl J Med 282:962, 1970

3. Attia RR, Murphy JD, Snider M et al: Myocardial ischemia due to infrarenal aortic cross clamping during surgery in patients with severe coronary artery disease. Circ Res 53:961, 1976

4. Bendixen H, Laver MB, Flacke W: Influence of respiratory acidosis on circulatory effects of epinephrine in dogs. Circ Res 13:64, 1963

5. Oliver G, Schöfer EA: The physiologic effects of extracts from the suprarenal capsules. J Physiol (Lond) 18:230, 1895

5A. Barger G, Dale HH: Chemical structure and sympathomimetic action of amines. J. Physiol (Lond) 41:19, 1910

6. Diamond G, Forrester J, Danzig J et al: Acute myocardial infarction in man: comparative hemodynamic effects of N. E. and glucogen. Am J Cardiol 26:612, 1971

6A. Kones RJ: The catecholamines: reappraisal of their use of acute myocardial infarction and the low cardiac output syndromes. Crit Care Med 1:203, 1973

7. Benfey BG, Varma DR: Interactions of sympathomimetic drugs, propranalol and phentalamine on atrial refractory period and contractility. Br J Pharmacol 30:603, 1967

8. King BD, Sokoloff L, Wechler RL: The effects of 1-epinephrine and L-norepinephrine upon cerebral circulation and metabolism in man. J Clin Invest 31:273, 1952

9. Steen PA, Tinker JH, Pluth JR et al: Efficacy of dopamine, dobutamine, and epinephrine during emergency from cardiopulmonary bypass in man. Circulation 57:378, 1978

10. Mueller HS, Ayres SM, Gregory S et al: Effects of isoproterenol, L norepinephrine and intra-aortic balloon counter pulsation on hemodynamic and myocardial metabolism in shock following acute myocardial infarction. Circulation 45:335, 1972

11. Scroff J, Wexler BC: Isoproterenol induced myocardial infarction in rats. Circ Res 27:1101, 1970

12. Sandler H, Dodge HT, Murdough HV: Effect of isoproterenol on cardiac output, and renal function in congestive heart failure. Am Heart J 62:643, 1961

13. Goldberg L: Dopamine—clinical uses of an endogenous catecholamine. N Engl J Med 291:707, 1974

14. Goldberg LI: Cardiovascular and renal actions of dopamine: potential clinical applications. Pharmacol Rev 24:1, 1972

15. Meuller HS, Evon R, Ayres SM: Effect of dopamine on hemodynamic and myocardial metabolism in shock following acute myocardial infarction in man. Circulation 57:361, 1978

16. VonEssen D: Effects of dopamine, noradrenaline and hydroxytryptamine on cerebral blood flow in the dog. J Pharm Pharmacol 24:668, 1972

17. Birch AA, Boyce WA: Effects of droperidol-dopamine interaction on renal blood flow in man. Anesthesiology 47:70, 1977

18. Hardaker T, Wechsler AS: Redistribution of renal intracortical blood flow during dopamine infusions in dogs. Circ Res 33:437, 1973

19. Bennett WM, Keefe E, Melnyk C et al: Response to dopamine HC1 in the Hepatorenal syndrome. Arch Intern Med 135:964, 1975

20. Robie NW, Nutter DO, Moody C: In vivo analysis of adrenergic receptor activity of dobutamine. Circ Res 34:663, 1974

21. Loeb HS, Khan IM, Saudye A et al: Acute hemodynamic effects of dobutamine and isoproterenol in patients with low output cardiac failure. Circ Shock 3:55, 1976

22. Loeb HS, Bredakis J, Gunnar RM: Superiority of dobutamine over dopamine for augmentation of low cardiac output in patients with chronic low output cardiac failure. Circulation 55:315, 1977

23. Fawz G: Effects of reserpine and pronethalal on the therapeutic and toxic actions of digitalis in the dog heart lung preparation. Br J Pharmacol 29:302, 1967

24. Koch-Weser J: Beta receptor blockade and myocardial effects of cardiac glycosides. Circ Res 28:109, 1971

25. Gervis A, Lane LK et al: A possible molecular mechanism of the action of digitalis. Circ Res 40:8, 1977

26. Reuter H, Seitz NJ: The dependence of calcium efflux from cardiac muscle on temperature and external ion compensation. J Physiol (Lond) 195:451, 1968

27. Langer GA: The intrinsic control of myocardial contraction; ionic factors. N Engl J Med 285:1067, 1971

28. Smith TW, Haber E: Digitalis. N Engl J Med 289:945, 1973

29. Braunwald, Bloodwell RD, Goldberg LI et al: "Studies on Digitalis" IV. Observations in man on the effects of digitalis preparations on the contractility in the non-failing heart and on total vascular resistance. J Clin Invest 40:52, 1961

30. Covell JW, Braunwald E, Ross J: Studies on digitalis: effects of oxygen consumption. J Clin Invest 45:1535, 1966

31. Ross J, Waldhausen JA, Braunwald E et al: "Studies on Digitalis" I. Effects on peripheral vascular resistance. J Clin Invest 39:930, 1961

32. Mason DT, Braunwald E: "Studies on Digitalis" X. Effects of ouabain on forearm vascular resistance and venous tone on normal subjects and patients in heart failure. J Clin Invest 43:532, 1964

33. Nadeau RA, James TN: Antagonistic effects on the sinus node of acetylstrophanthidin and adrenergic stimulation. Circ Res 13:388, 1963

34. Schick D, Schever J: Current concepts of therapy with digitalis glycosides: Part II. Am Heart J 87:391, 1974

35. Karliner JS, Braunwald E: Present status of digitalis treatment of acute myocardial infarction. Circulation 45:891, 1972

36. Varonkov Y, Shell WE, Smirnov V et al: Augmentation of serum CPK activity by digitalis in patients with acute myocardial infarction. Circ Res 55:719, 1977

37. Meyer J: Concerning the question of pre, intra and post operative digitalis administration. Survthesiol Anes, 16:9, 1972

38. Johnson LW, Dickstein RA, Fruehan T et al: Prophylactic digitalization for coronary artery bypass surgery. Circ Res 53:819, 1976

39. Deutsh S, Dalen JE: Indications for prophylactic digitalization. Anesthesiology 30:648, 1969

40. Shields TW, Ujiki CT: Digitalization for prevention of arrhythmias following pulmonary surgery. Surg Gynecol Obstet 126:743, 1968

41. Coalson JJ, Woodruff HK, Greenfield LJ: Effects of digoxin on myocardial ultrastructures in endotoxin shock. Surg Gynecol Obstet 135:908, 1972

42. Klein M, Negard NS, Corwin B et al: Correlation of the electrical and mechanical changes in the dog heart during progressive digitalization. Circ Res 29:635, 1971

43. Mason DT, Braunwald E: Digitalis, new facts about an old drug. Am J Cardiol 22:151, 1968
44. Moe GK, Mendy R: The action of several cardiac glycosides on conduction velocity and ventricular excitability in the dog heart. Circulation 4:729, 1951
45. Jelliffe RW: Reduction of digitalis toxicity by computer-assisted glycoside regimens. Ann Intern Med 77:891, 1972
46. Neff MS, Mendelsohn S, Kim KE et al: Magnesium sulfate in digitalis toxicity. Am J Cardiol 29:379, 1972
47. Shick D, Scheuer J: Current concepts of therapy with digitalis glycosides II. Am Heart J 87:391, 1974
48. Gullner HG, Stinson EB: Correlation of serum concentration with heart concentration of digoxin in human subjects. Circulation 50:653, 1974
49. Beller S: Digitalis intoxication: a prospective clinical study with serum level correlations. N Engl J Med 284:989, 1971
50. Smith TW, Habert E: Digoxin intoxication: The relationship of clinical presentation to serum digoxin concentration. J Clin Invest 49:2377, 1970
51. Drop LJ, Laver MB: Low plasma ionized calcium and response to calcium therapy in critically ill man. Anesthesiology 43:300, 1975
52. Seifen E, Flacke W, Alpen MH: Effects of calcium on isolated mammalian heart. Am J Physiol 207:716, 1964
53. Pitt B, Sugishita Y, Gregg DE: Coronary hemodynamic effects of calcium on the unanesthetized dogs. Am J Physiol 216:1456, 1969
54. Denlinger JK, Kaplan JA, Leckey J et al: Cardiovascular responses to calcium administered intravenously to man during halothane anesthesia. Anesthesiology 42:390, 1975
55. Stanley TH, Isern-Armarol J, Lie WS: Peripheral vascular versus direct cardiac effects of calcium. Anesthesiology 45:46, 1976
56. Olinger GN, Hellenott C, Mulder DG: Acute clinical hypocalcemic myocardial depression during rapid blood transfusion and post-operative hemodyalsis. J Thorac Cardiovasc Surg 72:503, 1976
57. Price HC: Myocardial depression by nitrous oxide and reversal by calcium. Anesthesiology 44:211, 1976
58. Howland WS, Schweizer O, Carlon GE: Cardiovascular effects of low levels of ionized calcium during massive transfusion. Surg Gynecol Obstet 145:581, 1977
59. Drop LJ, von Pohl J, Cullen DJ: Hemodynamic response to intravenous calcium chloride following operation and during hypotensive anesthesia. ASA Abst, p. 107, 1973
60. Lucchesi BR: Cardiac actions of glucogon. Circ Res 22:777, 1968
61. Glick G: Glucagon: a perspective. Circulation 45:513, 1972
62. Lvoff R, Wilcken D et al: Glucagon in heart failure and in cardiogenic shock. Experience in 50 patients. Circ Res 45:534, 1972
63. Romero LH, Matsay GJ, Beckman CG et al: Effects of alpha stimulation and alpha blockade on pulmonary vascular segment resistance in canine cardiogenic shock. J Surg Res 16:185, 1974
64. Guetzman BW, Sunshine P, Johnson JD et al: Hypoxia and pulmonary vasospasm response to tolazoline. J Pediatr 89:617, 1976
65. Gould L, Reddy CVR: Use of phentolamine in acute myocardial infarction. Am Heart J 88:144, 1974
66. Majid PA, Shomou B, Tyler SH: Phentolamine for vasodilation treatment of severe heart failure. Lancet 2:978, 1971
67. Rabinowitz B, Parmly WW: Interaction of phentolamine and noradrenaline

on myocardial contractility and adenycyclase activity. Cardiovasc Res 8:243, 1974

68. Ahlquist RP: A study of adrenergic receptors. Am J Physiol 153:586, 1948
69. Goldstein RE: A comparison of beta blocking drugs. Circulation 47:443, 1973
70. Anderson R, Holmberg S, Svednyr R et al: Adrenergic alpha and beta receptors in coronary vessels in man: an in vitro study. Acta Med Scand 191:241, 1972
71. Prichard BNC: Beta adrenergic receptor blocking drugs in angina pectoris. Drugs 7:55, 1974
72. Koch-Weser J: Nonbeta blocking actions of propranolol. N Engl J Med 293:998, 1975
73. Furberg CD: Beta adrenergic receptor blocking drug in hypertropic cardiomyopathy, autonomically medicated cardiovascular function disorders and Fallot's tetralogy. Drugs 7:106, 1974
74. Pattingen WA, Mitchell HC: Renin release, saralasin and the vasodilation beta blocking drug interaction in man. N Engl J Med 292:1214, 1975
75. Mackin JF, Canary JJ, Pittman CS: Thyroid storm and its management—current concepts. N Engl J Med 291:1396, 1974
76. Grossman W, Robin NI, Johnson LW: Effects of beta blockade on the peripheral manifestations of thyrotoxicosis. Ann Intern Med 74:875, 1971
77. Rude RK, Oldham SB, Singer FR: Treatment of thyrotoxic hypercalcemia with propranolol medical intelligence. N Engl J Med 294:431, 1976
78. Rodger JC: Intermittant claudication; complication beta blockade. Br Med J 1:1125, 1976
79. Nies AS, Shand DG: Clinical pharmacology of propranolol. Circulation 52:6, 1975
80. Kloner RA, Fishbein MC, Cotran RS: Effects of propranolol on microvascular injury in acute myocardial ischemia. Circulation 55:872, 1977
81. Shand DG: Propranolol drug therapy. N Engl J Med 293:280, 1975
82. Viljoen JF, Estafamous G, Kellner GA: Propranolol and cardiac surgery. J Thorac Cardiovasc Surg 64:826, 1972
83. Miller RR, Olson HC, Amsterdam EA: Propranolol withdrawal rebound phenomenon. N Engl J Med 293:416, 1975
84. Romagnoli A, Keats A: Relationships between pre-operative propranolol blood levels and response to isoproterenol. ASA Abst, p. 159, 1973
85. Playfair L: On the Nitroprussides—A New Class of Salts. London: RJE Tayler, 1849
86. Hermann L: Ueber die Wirkung des, Nitroprussidnatriums. Arch Ges Physiol 39:419, 1886
87. Davidsohn K: Versuche uber die Wirkung des, Nitroprussidnatriums. Dissertation, Albertus Universitat, Konigsberg, Prussia, 1887
88. Johnson CC: Actions and toxicity of sodium nitroprusside. Arch Int Pharmacodyn Ther 35:480, 1926
89. Page IH, Corcoran AC, Dustan HP et al: Cardiovascular actions of SNP in animals and hypertensive patients. Circ Res 11:188, 1955
90. Nourok DS, Glassock RJ, Solomon DH: Hypothyroidism following prolonged sodium nitroprusside therapy. Am J Med Sci 248:129, 1964
91. Miller RR, Vismara LA: Clinical use of sodium nitroprusside in chronischemic heart disease: effects on peripheral vascular resistance and venous tone and ventricular volume, pump and mechanical performance. Circulation 57:328, 1975

92. Palmer RF, Lassetter KC: Sodium nitroprusside. N Engl J Med 929:294, 1975
93. Rose GG, Henderson RH: Systemic and coronary hemodynamic effects of SNP. Am Heart J 87:83, 1974
94. Bastron RD, Kaloynanides GJ: Effect of SNP on function in isolated and intact dog kidney. J Pharmacol Exp Ther 181:244, 1972
95. Ivankovich AD, Miletich DJ, Albrecht RF et al: SNP and CBF in anesthetized and unanesthetized goat. Anesthesiology 44:21, 1976
96. Griffiths DPG, Cummins BH, Greenbaum R: Cerebral blood flow and metabolism during hypotension induced with SNP. Br J Anaesth 46:671, 1974
97. Wildsmith JAW, Drummond GB, MacRae, WR: Blood-gas changes during induced hypotension with SNP. Br J Anaesth 47:1205, 1975
98. Calley PS, Cheney FW: Sodium nitroprusside increases $\dot{Q}s/\dot{Q}t$ in dogs with regional atelectasis. Anesthesiology 47:338, 1977
99. Gallagher TJ, Etling T: Failure to alter intrapulmonary shunt with sodium nitroprusside (sic). Crit Care Med 6:118, 1978
100. Sibbald WJ, Paterson NAM, Holliday RL et al: Pulmonary hypertension in sepsis. Chest 730:583, 1978
101. Koch-Weser J: Hypertensive emergencies. N Engl J Med 290:211, 1974
102. Ahearn DJ, Crim CE: Treatment of malignant hypertension with SNP. Arch Intern Med 123:187, 1974
103. Shell WE, Sabel BE: Protection of jeopardized ischemic myocardium by reduction of afterload. N Engl J Med 291:481, 1974
104. Chatterjee K, Parmly WW, Gary W: Hemodynamic and metabolic response to vasodilation therapy in acute myocardial infarction. Circulation 48:1183, 1973
105. Guiha NH, Cahn JN, Mikulic E et al: Treatment of refractory heart failure with infusions of nitroprusside. N Engl J Med 291:587, 1974
106. Mukherjee D, Feldman MS, Helfont RH: Nitroprusside therapy. JAMA 235:2406, 1976
107. Chianiello M, Gold HK, Leinbach RC et al: Comparison between the effects of SNP and TNG on ischemic injury during acute myocardial infarction. Circulation 54:766, 1976
108. Benzing G, Helmsworth JA, Schrieber JT: Nitroprusside after open heart surgery. Circulation 54:467, 1976
109. Grossman W, Hanshaw CW, Munro AB: Lowered aortic impedance as therapy for severe mitral regurgitation. JAMA 230:1011, 1974
110. Synhorst DP, Lauer RM, Doty DB: Hemodynamic effects of vasodilation agents in dogs with experimental USD. Circulation 54:472, 1976
111. Glass DD: unpublished data
112. Taradash MR, Jacobsen LB: Vasodilation therapy of idiopathic lactic acidosis. N Engl J Med 293:468, 1975
113. Carliner NH, Denune DP, Finch CS: SNP treatment of ergotomine-induced peripheral ischemia. JAMA 227:308, 1974
114. Palmer RF, Lasseter KC: Nitroprusside and aortic dissecting aneurysm (correspondence). N Engl J Med 294:1403, 1976
115. Glass DD: Intra-operative coagulation defects: etiology, diagnosis and treatment. ASA Annual Refresher Course Lectures 224:1976
116. Saxon A, Kahlove HE: Platelet inhibition by sodium nitroprusside—a smooth muscle inhibitor. Blood 47:957, 1976
117. Greiss L, Tremblay NAG, Davies DW: Toxicity of sodium nitroprusside. Can Anaesth Soc J 23:48, 1976

118. Smith RD, Kruszyna H: Nitroprusside produces cyanide poisoning via a reaction with hemoglobin. J Pharmacol Exp Ther 191:557, 1974
119. Davies DW, Greiss, L, Kadar D et al: SNP in children: observations on metabolism during normal and abnormal responses. Can Anaesth Soc J 22:553, 1975
120. Bower PJ, Peterson JN: Methemoglobinemia after SNP therapy. N Engl J Med 293:865, 1975
121. Nourak DS, Gwinup G, Hamuic GJ: Phenotalamine resistant pheomocytoma treated with sodium nitroprusside. JAMA 183:541, 1963
122. Cohen IM, Mattel MM, Francis GS et al. Danger in sodium nitroprusside therapy. Ann Intern Med 85:205, 1976
123. Posner MA, Toby RE, McElroy H: Hydroxyocobalanin therapy of cyanide intoxication in guinea pigs. Anesthesiology 44:157, 1976
124. Posner MA, Rodky FL, Toby RE: Nitroprusside induced cyanide poisoning. Anesthesiology 44:330, 1976
125. Cottrell JE, Casthely P, Brodie JD et al: Prevention of nitroprusside induced cyanide toxicity with hydroxycobalamine. N Engl J Med 298:809, 1978
126. Koch-Weser J: Hypertensive emergencies. N Engl J Med 290:211, 1974
127. Scott DB, Stephen GW, Marshall RC et al: Circulatory effects of controlled arterial hypertension with trimethaphan during nitrous oxidehalothane anesthesia. Br J Anaesth 44:523, 1972
128. Stephen GW, David IT, Scott DB: Hemodynamic effects of beta receptor blocking drugs during nitrous oxide halothane anesthesia. Br J Anaesth 43:320, 1971
129. Stinson EB, Halloway MD, Deatsy G et al: Comparative hemodynamic responses to chlorpromazine, nitroprusside, nitroglycerin and trimethaphan immediately after open heart operation. Circulation (Suppl I) 51:26, 1975
130. Stoyka WW, Shutz H: Cerebral response to sodium nitroprusside and trimethaphan controlled hypotension. Can Anaesth Soc J 22:275, 1975
131. Astrup J et al: Cortical evoked potential and extracellular K^+ and H^+ at critical levels of brain ischemia. Stroke 8:51, 1977
132. Murrell W: Nitroglycerin as a remedy for angina. Lancet 18:, 1879
133. Greenberg H, Duyer EM, Jameson AG et al: Effects of nitroglycerin as the major determinants of myocardial oxygen consumption. Am J Cardiol 36:420, 1975
134. Armstrong PW, Walker DC, Burton JR: Vasodilation therapy in acute myocardial infarction. Circulation 52:1118, 1975
135. Sladen RN, Rosenthal MH: Selective afterload reduction with parenteral hydralazine. ASA Abstracts, p. 145, 1978
136. Pierpont GL, Cohn JN, Franciosa JA: Combined oral hydralazine-nitrate therapy in left ventricular failure. Chest 73:8, 1978
137. Miller RR, Vismara LA: Clinical use of sodium nitroprusside in chronic ischemic heart disease: effects on peripheral vascular resistance and venous tone and in ventricular volume and mechanical performance. Circulation 51:328, 1975
138. Kauchoukous NT, Karp RB: Management of post-operative cardiac surgical patients. Am Heart J 92:513, 1976
139. Hinshaw LB: Role of the heart in pathogenesis of endotoxin shock. J Surg Res 17:134, 1974
140. Fowler NO, Dabel M, Holmes JC: Hemodynamic effects of nitroprusside and hydralazine in experimental cardiac tamponade. Circulation 57:563, 1978

141. Forrester JS, Swan HJC: Acute myocardial infarction. A physiologic basis of therapy. Crit Care Med 2:283, 1974
142. Sakamoto T, Yamada T: Hemodynamic effects of dobutamine in patients following open heart surgery. Circulation 55:525, 1977
143. Ramanathan KB, Bodenheimer MM, Banka VS: Contracting effects of dopamine and isoproterenol in experimental myocardial infarction. Am J Cardiol 39:431, 1977
144. Civetta JM, Gabel JC, Laver MB: Disparate ventricular function in surgical patients. Surg Forum 22:109, 1971

FIVE

Renal Function in the Critically Ill Patient

Clyde H. Beck, Jr.

Each minute, one-fifth of the cardiac output, or approximately 1 liter of blood, is pumped through the 300 gm of normal kidney tissue. Of the 500 ml of plasma delivered to the kidneys each minute, 100 ml (±20 ml) of protein-free filtrate is created as it crosses the glomerular basement membranes. Under normal circumstances, 99 percent of this filtered volume is reabsorbed and 1 ml of urine produced each minute (Table 5-1). Normal kidneys may, however, produce 15 to 20 ml of urine per minute if an individual is water loaded. This is possible only if there is enough solute available to produce such a high volume of very dilute urine. Table 5-2 indicates the range of normal values for the urine from healthy individuals. Note that the urine can be diluted to approximately one-sixth the plasma osmolality of 285 mOsm/liter. It can be concentrated to four times this value. The urine may be rendered essentially salt free or have a sodium concentration of double the serum value.

Glomerular filtration is measured best by creatinine clearance and best followed serially with serum creatinine determinations.[1,2] The creatinine clearance is greatly influenced by effective renal blood flow. For a certain percentage of decrease in effective renal blood flow, the creatinine clearance will be decreased to a significant, but somewhat lesser degree. Any pathophysiologic process that decreases the effective renal blood flow to the 2 million glomeruli in the normal human kidneys will have this effect of lowering the creatinine clearance; thus, a decrease in left ventricular function, hypovolemia, and microemboli to the kidneys can lead to decreased renal perfusion.

Table 5-3 lists the more common causes of decreased renal blood flow. When any of these conditions lead to a rise in BUN or serum creatinine, we will refer to that state as prerenal azotemia. At times, the identification of a prerenal state may enable the physician to identify a previously unrecognized pathophysiologic process. Clinical tests for diagnosing a prerenal state are discussed in a later section of this chapter.[3]

In the proximal tubule of the kidney, 65 to 75 percent of the filtered sodium chloride and water are reabsorbed in an isotonic fashion (Table 5-4 and Figure 5-1). In addition, glucose, bicarbonate, phosphorus, uric acid, and amino acids are similarly reabsorbed. They quantitatively par-

TABLE 5-1
Normal Renal Blood and Urine Flow Values

Parameter	Approximate Flow
Cardiac output	5 liter/min
Renal blood flow	1 liter/min
Renal plasma flow	0.5 liter/min
Glomerular filtration rate	0.1 liter/min
Urinary output	.001 liter/min

TABLE 5-2

Normal Range of Urine Composition and Volume

mOsm	50–1200 mOsm/liter
U Na	1–260 mEq/liter
U K	10–250 mEq/liter*
H⁺	300–400 mEq/day†
Volume	0.5–30 liter/day

* High value possible with progressive K loading over 5–6 days; not possible acutely
† High value possible with progressive H⁺ loading over 5–6 days; not possible acutely

TABLE 5-3

Causes of Renal Hypoperfusion and Prerenal Azotemia

Hypovolemia
  External fluid loss
    Hemorrhage
    Losses from skin, gastrointestinal tract, or kidneys
  Internal fluid loss
    Sequestration as seen after surgery
    Trauma
Cardiovascular failure
  Decreased cardiac output
    Primary decrease in myocardial function
    Arrhythmia
    Tamponade
  Vascular pooling
    Sepsis
    Acidosis
    Anaphylaxis

TABLE 5-4

Sites of NaCl and H_2O Reabsorption in Nephron
(Percent of Glomerular Filtrate Reabsorbed)

	NaCl	H_2O
Proximal tubule	65	67
Loop of Henle	25	5
Distal tubule	slight	8
Collecting duct	9	19
Total	99	99

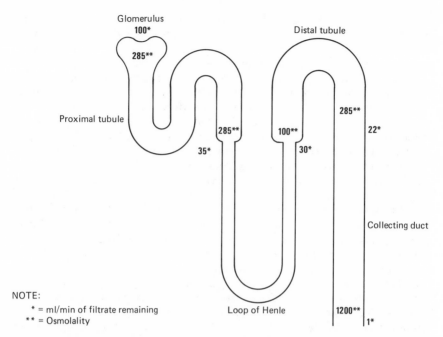

Fig. 5-1. Glomerular infiltrate absorption in a normal patient with antidiuretic hormone and aldosterone affecting the nephron. The numbers in the tubule give osmolality, those outside, remaining filtrate (ml/min).

allel sodium in the completeness of the reabsorptive process. Drug toxicities, including those induced by specific antibiotics, may interfere with the reabsorption of these substances and produce low plasma levels or high urine levels of each, individually or in numerous combinations.[4]

In the loop of Henle, an additional 5 percent of the filtered water is reabsorbed with even a greater fraction of the filtered sodium being actively returned to the peritubular blood by a chloride pump in the ascending limb of the loop. Thus, the fluid leaving the loop and entering the distal tubule is hypotonic with regard to the plasma. The loop of Henle establishes a concentrated renal medulla. This process is necessary for both concentration and dilution of the urine.

In the distal tubule and collecting duct, further sodium may be extracted from the tubular fluid, leaving the urine almost sodium free in sodium-avid states such as congestive heart failure, nephrotic syndrome, and severe hypovolemia. Aldosterone, if present, plays an important role in the reabsorption of the last few mEq of sodium in the distal tubule and collecting duct. Similarly, if antidiuretic hormone is present in response to a rise in serum osmolality of 5 to 10 mOsm/liter, or due to severe volume depletion, the urine will be maximally concentrated. If the glomerular filtration rate is high, a large fraction of filtered sodium will escape to the distal tubules and subsequently be excreted. Aldosterone will usually not be present in such states, since the effective intravascular volume is adequate and there is no stimulus for aldosterone production and release. In states where the patient's serum osmolality is 5 to 10 mOsm/liter below the normal value of 285 mOsm/liter, antidiuretic hormone will not be present in the blood. If the renal circulation is adequate, the urine will remain dilute after leaving the loop of Henle and become more dilute as further solute is reabsorbed in the distal tubule and collecting duct. In many hypotonic and hyponatremic critically ill patients, antidiuretic hormone will not be turned off appropriately, and the patient may not excrete a water load normally. This problem is discussed in the section on hyponatremia (pp. 286–90).

The nearly complete reabsorption of filtered bicarbonate in the proximal tubule conserves this important body buffer. In the distal tubule, the urine is maximally acidified to a pH of 5.0. Less than a mEq of hydrogen ion is excreted by virtue of this change in pH. The 50 to 100 mEq of hydrogen ion that must be removed by the kidney each day are excreted by titrating acids, such as Na_2HPO_4. More importantly, conversion of tubular fluid ammonia (NH_3) to the nonreabsorbable ammonium ion (NH_4^+) also occurs as hydrogen ion is secreted into the distal tubule. Significant metabolic acidosis can occur if either the proximal tubule leaks bicarbonate or the distal tubule is unable to maximally lower the urinary pH to 5.0. Numerous systemic diseases affecting the kidney and many drug toxicities may cause this type of normal anion gap acidosis.[6]* Additional causes of normal anion gap as well as increased anion gap acidosis are discussed later (pp. 296–97). These may be seen in a critical care unit.

Urine flow from the nephron may be obstructed anywhere from the minor calyces of the kidney to the end of the urethra. Moderate obstruction to urine flow can cause nonoliguric azotemia of as much clinical significance as that caused by prerenal states or renal parenchymal damage.

There are a number of diagnostic tests that can assist the clinician in determining whether a patient has prerenal, postrenal or renal parenchymal azotemia. Table 5-5 lists these tests and their expected values. The normal BUN to serum creatinine ratio is 20:1. If this ratio is increased (as it would be, for example, in a patient with a BUN of 90 mg% and a creatinine of 2 mg%), one should suspect hypoperfusion of the kidneys. In such a prerenal state, a urine osmolality of greater than 450 mOsm/liter and urinary sodium of less than 15 mEq/liter suggest excellent tubular function and healthy kidneys.

Remember, however, that critically ill patients commonly have preexisting renal disease, are prone to renal failure, and can receive potentially

---

* The anion gap is a value determined by subtracting the sum of the serum chloride and bicarbonate from the serum sodium concentration. This value is normally between 6 and 16 mEq/liter of determined ions.

TABLE 5-5

Tests to Differentiate between Prerenal, Renal,
and Postrenal Azotemia

	Prerenal	Renal	Postrenal
Urine output	0.6–1. liter	0.3 liter to normal	0 to normal
BUN/creatinine	> 20/1	20/1	20/1
Sediment	Hyalin casts	Hyalin and granular casts, many epith, white and red cells	Frequently normal
U Osm	> 450 mOsm/ liter	300 ± 100 mOsm/ liter	300 ± 100 mOsm/ liter
U Na	< 15 mEq/ liter	30–60 mEq/liter	Low, then 30–60 mEq/liter*
$F_E Na$	< 1%	> 3%	> 3%
U/P Creatinine	> 40/1	< 20/1	< 20/1

* For 24 hours after acute obstruction, the U Na may be less than 15 mEq/liter

toxic therapeutic substances. Thus, renal functional impairment from multiple etiologies is the rule.

Calculations of the fractional excretion of sodium may help in diagnosing a prerenal state if the urine volume is low.[3] This value may be determined using the following formula:

$$F_E NA = \frac{\text{urine sodium/plasma sodium}}{\text{urine creatinine/plasma creatinine}} \times 100$$

where the urine and plasma, sodium and creatinine concentrations are measured in the same units (mEq/liter and mg% respectively). This test is the best measure of renal tubular health. In prerenal states, a fractional excretion of sodium that is less than 1 percent is suggestive of normal tubular function.

The urinary sediment may be quite abnormal with hyalin and granular casts even in the case of renal hypoperfusion. Thus, an abnormal sediment need not indicate renal parenchymal damage. However, a patient with obstruction to urinary flow and associated azotemia may have a normal urine output, a relatively unremarkable urinary sediment, and isosmotic (isotonic) urine with abundant sodium in it. Table 5-6 lists the more common causes of obstructive uropathy. These should be considered in every case of azotemia since specific therapy may be available if the correct diagnosis is made.

Damage to the renal parenchyma itself may create some findings in the diagnostic tests in Table 5-5 that are similar to those found in pre- and postrenal azotemia.[8] Such patients may have no urine output

TABLE 5-6
Common Etiologies of Urinary Tract Obstruction

Nephrolithiasis
Tumors—in and adjacent to any part of the collecting system
Ureteral ligation—especially important if there is only one functioning
   kidney
Ruptured bladder
Prostatism and urethral stricture
Crystal sludge by uric acid or sulfa

or a normal urine output.[9,10] Most commonly they are oliguric with a 24-hour volume between 300 and 600 ml. The urine contains abundant sodium, is isosmotic, and has an abnormal sediment frequently containing pigment stained casts. The BUN/creatinine ratio of 20:1 is maintained and the fractional excretion of sodium is usually greater than 3 percent.

The importance of adequate cardiovascular monitoring is emphasized in numerous sections of this text. By maintaining good cardiac filling pressures, normal cardiac output, and normal blood pressure, the critical care physician is indirectly doing the best he can to maximize effective renal blood flow. There is no direct clinical measure of effective renal blood flow. However, a normal 24-hour urine volume of greater than 600 ml and a stable serum creatinine in the normal range suggest adequate renal perfusion. Maintenance of good blood pressure in the extremities, good peripheral tissue perfusion, and no apparent decrease in cardiac output on physical exam do not assure adequate renal blood flow. Any decrease in the urine output of a critically ill patient must be quickly evaluated by a review of the patient's recent history, medications, weight, fluid intake and output, and physical exam. If an adequate explanation for a decrease in urine flow or rise in BUN and creatinine is not forthcoming, further quantitative evaluation of the patient's cardiovascular status must be obtained. Currently, this requires the placement of a Swan-Ganz thermodilation catheter. A brief episode of only 5 minutes of hypotension to two-thirds of the patient's normal blood pressure, or a mean blood pressure of approximately 60 mm Hg, may be sufficient to cause an episode of acute renal failure. This is a grim occurrence in the I.C.U. since it is followed by an average of 14 days of inadequate renal function. Even with intense dialysis and good nutrition during this azotemic period, the mortality rate is greater than 50 percent.[11,12] The diagnosis of ischemic ARF is made when the patient (1) has had a clinical event likely to cause renal injury, (2) does not have other likely causes for parenchymal damage to the kidney (see Tables 5-7 and 5-8), and (3) meets the criteria for parenchymal damage listed in Table 5-5.

At the same time that circulatory disturbances are being investi-

TABLE 5-7
Common Nephrotoxins

Antibiotics
  Amphotericin B
  Cephalosporins—especially cephaloridine
  Polymyxin
  Aminoglycosides—gentamicin, kanamycin, and neomycin in particular
  Penicillins—including methicillin, ampicillin
Anesthetics
  Methoxyflurane
Iodinated radiographic contrast media
Organic solvents—chlorinated hydrocarbons
Heavy metals
  Mercury
  Cadmium
  Lead
Endogenous toxins
  Hemoglobin or its associated red blood cell breakdown products
  Myoglobin
Abnormal concentrations of physiologic substances
  Hypercalcemia
  Hyperuricemia
  Hypokalemia

---

gated, obstruction to urine flow must be excluded as a cause of oliguria. Even if there is no intra-abdominal reason to suspect ureteral obstruction and no drug or medical condition that may have plugged the tubules with an abnormal protein or drug crystal, an abdominal ultrasound study should be performed to exclude urinary tract obstruction; a reversible

TABLE 5-8
Nontoxic Causes of Renal Parenchymal Damage

Ischemia
  Shock, sepsis, anaphylaxis, severe acidosis
Pregnancy related
  Uterine hemorrhage, eclampsia, postpartum renal failure
Glomerulitis
  Poststreptococcal, visceral abscess, related collagen vascular disease
Vasculitis
  Periarteritis, hypersensitivity angiitis
Malignant hypertension
Acute diffuse severe pyelonephritis with or without papillary necrosis
Intravascular clotting states
Intratubular precipitation
  Myeloma protein, uric acid, sulfonamide

---

lesion must be reversed if the patient is to survive. Ascertaining the proper placement or patency of a urinary bladder catheter is a "cost effective" diagnostic test and by restoring urinary output may even be therapeutic!

ENDOGENOUS TOXINS

A routine urinalysis at the time of declining renal function or oliguria may be extremely helpful. Myoglobinuria frequently accompanies ischemic or infectious damage to muscle. The urine may be yellow-brown when this pigment is present. The presence of hemoglobin or myoglobin in the urine is easily detected by the orthotolidine reaction for occult blood found on most combination laboratory dip sticks used for urine testing. Further laboratory tests of the urine, such as immuno-electrophoresis and starch gel electrophoresis, can identify which pigment is present. Since myoglobin has a molecular weight of only 17,000, it is easily cleared by the kidneys. Thus, a history of dark urine *before* hospitalization from a patient with muscle damage and azotemia should suggest a myoglobin insult to the kidneys. If the BUN rises more than 20 mg% per day, associated with a serum creatinine rise greater than 2 mg% per day and a creatinine phosphokinase of greater than 20,000, myoglobinuric renal failure should be suspected.[13] Serum uric acid and potassium values also rise faster than the usual expected rate in acute renal failure.

Hemoglobinuria from hemolysis may also cause a red-brown urine and acute renal failure. The hematocrit may fall rapidly and the serum potassium may rise to such high levels that it cannot be controlled. The toxic substance in this case appears to be the stroma of the red cell rather than the hemoglobin itself.

While diagnostic measures searching for muscle or red blood cell breakdown are proceeding, an attempt should be made to increase the patient's urine volume to greater than 2 liters a day with a saline and mannitol diuresis. If hemoglobin is the suspected pigment, alkaliniza-tion of the urine to a pH greater than 7.0 with sodium bicarbonate may aid the renal clearance of this pigment and associated toxic intracellular substances. Carbonic anhydrase inhibitors, such as acetazolamide, work too slowly for this purpose. Even if these pigmenturias have been present for a number of hours, augmenting intravascular volume and inducing diuresis will frequently prevent damage to the kidneys. Clearly, volume overloading the patient while obtaining such a diuresis may lead to decreased left ventricular function and renal hypoperfusion which may worsen the situation. Kidneys that are hypoperfused for any reason may be more susceptible to insult by these pigments. Bilirubin, on the other hand, while it alters urinary sediment by creating pigmented hyalin and granular casts, does not cause significant impairment of renal function.

DRUG AND CHEMICAL TOXICITY

Table 5-7 includes a list of drugs and chemicals that can lead to renal parenchymal damage by various mechanisms.[4,10] Clearly, drugs such as penicillin that can cause an anaphylactic reaction and shock should be avoided in the patient with even a question of penicillin allergy. Drugs such as amphotericin can cause decreased renal blood flow and modest azotemia. The penicillin group of antibiotics may directly decrease renal function by causing a hypersensitivity reaction with concomitant glomerulitis. This syndrome may be suspected in patients who have moderate azotemia, mild hypertension, and microscopic hematuria with red cell casts. This constellation of findings is also associated with a whole host of infections that may cause a glomerulitis in the critically ill patient. Bacterial infections with streptococcus, coagulase-negative and -positive staphylococci, pneumococci, and *Hemophilus influenzae* may cause such a glomerulitis. Infected heart valves, in particular, may lead to a more severe form of this glomerular process with markedly elevated BUN and creatinine.[14] Drug-related and infection-related acute renal failure may be immunologic in origin. Thus, the clinical and laboratory abnormalities, including the suppression of serum complement levels, may be the same. It may be difficult to decide, therefore, whether to continue a life-saving antibiotic or discontinue it because of probable renal damage from the drug. Frequently, the date of onset of the renal abnormality and the institution of a new drug will coincide and convince the clinician to discontinue the medication. Substitution of a drug from another generic category may provide a workable compromise if bacteriologic studies indicate it is possible.

Proximal tubular leak syndromes may occur with drugs such as out-of-date tetracycline. A normal anion gap acidosis, hypouricemia, hypophosphatemia, glucosuria, and amino aciduria constitute the Fanconi syndrome and suggest a drug-related insult to the proximal tubule.

Interstitial nephritis caused by drugs may simply present as nonoliguric azotemia with an unremarkable urinalysis. However, the presence of a skin rash suggestive of a drug reaction, fever, eosinophilia, and eosinophils in the urine (by Wright's stain), makes the case stronger for an interstitial drug insult. Treatment with a corticosteroid such as prednisone 60 mg per day may abort such a process and prevent a protracted course of acute renal failure with its attendant complications.

In the distal tubule, amphotericin may cause anatomic damage to the nephron and renal tubular acidosis as well. An abundance of carbenicillin, ticarcillin, and other penicillins with negative chemical charge in the lumen of the distal tubule may lead to obligate losses of potassium and hydrogen ion. By this mechanism, these antibiotics may lead to severe hypokalemia and metabolic alkalosis.

Antibiotics, such as carbenicillin, contain between 3 and 5 mEq of sodium per gram. Thus, patients receiving these drugs must be observed for weight gain, edema, and electrolyte imbalance.

Antibiotics such as dimethylchlortetracycline, as well as other drugs mentioned in the section under hyponatremia, may lead to an insensitivity of the collecting duct to endogenous antidiuretic hormone. A clinical state of nephrogenic diabetes insipidus may ensue.

METABOLIC FACTORS

Metabolic abnormalities such as hypercalcemia and hypokalemia may cause azotemia. Hypercalcemia may cause acute renal failure by inducing an osmotic diuresis, paralyzing the concentrating mechanism of the kidney and altering the hemodynamics of the systemic and glomerular circulations.[15,16] Patients with increased serum calcium values initially become hypertensive only to develop cardiovascular collapse if they become volume depleted. With the resultant decrease in renal perfusion, they may become even more hypercalcemic.

Treatment must include volume repletion, diuresis with mannitol and/or furosemide, avoidance of the calcium-retaining thiazide diuretics, and rapid assessment of the cause of hypercalcemia. Disease-specific immediate treatment of hypercalcemia must also be considered. In cases where hypercalcemia is tumor related, glucocorticoids may be used for their antitumor effect. Up to several hundred mg of cortisone or its equivalent may be needed daily. Mithramycin may also be given for tumor-related hypercalcemia. The usual dose is 25 μg/kg body weight over a 4- to 24-hour period. This may lower the serum calcium for up to 48 hours. If the patient has impaired renal function or cannot tolerate a saline diuresis, hemodialysis may rapidly return an elevated calcium value to normal.

Hypokalemia not only decreases the concentrating ability of the kidneys, but also causes mild azotemia by an unknown mechanism.[17] However, a BUN of greater than 60 mg% or a serum creatinine of greater than 4 mg% usually implies an additional cause of renal function impairment. Potassium replacement corrects both the azotemia and concentrating defect although it may take days for the azotemia to completely resolve.

Intrarenal obstruction by the precipitation of crystals must be quickly corrected. If the serum uric acid rapidly rises to levels of 15 mg% or greater, acute renal failure may develop from sludging of sodium urate crystals in the tubules.[13] Since normal urine may contain urate crystals, such crystalluria alone cannot be used to make or exclude the diagnosis of hyperuricemic renal failure.

A serum uric acid determination should therefore be included in the workup of developing acute renal failure.[18] Historical information including previous gouty attacks or antimetabolite therapy of a tumor is obviously helpful.

Alkaline diuresis may prevent damage to the kidneys of a severely hyperuricemic patient. Allopurinol therapy in an initial dose of 100 mg per day advancing to at least 300 mg per day will decrease the excretion of uric acid in the urine by diminishing its production. If the patient is already azotemic, acute hemodialysis usually leads to good recovery of renal function.

Sulfa crystals may be seen in the urine of patients receiving more than 6 gm per day of even the most soluble sulfa drugs. Tubular plugging may occur just as it does with sodium urate.

Drug toxicities, the antibiotics in particular, have been mentioned earlier in this chapter.[19] Drugs, such as penicillin and the aminoglycoside family of antibiotics, may cause renal failure even if given in proper dosage for patient's weight and creatinine clearance. Identification of drug nephrotoxicity and discontinuance of the offending drug may prevent further renal functional impairment.

MANEUVERS THAT MAY PREVENT OR MODERATE ACUTE RENAL FAILURE

Once an obvious circulatory abnormality, obstruction to urine flow, and toxic nephropathy have been excluded as the cause of oliguria or rising BUN and creatinine, a trial of an intravenous diuretic is indicated.[9] Furosemide (120 to 240 mg I.V.) may be given at the same time that 25 gm of the osmotic diuretic mannitol is administered. If a diuresis of 75 to 100 ml per hour occurs for several hours after this therapy, these drugs should be continued every 4 to 6 hours. It has not been established that such diuretic treatment with increased urine flow prevents acute renal failure or significantly modifies its course.

However, patients who are initially oliguric after a renal insult, may have a better prognosis if made nonoliguric by this treatment. They then have the same prognosis as patients who were nonoliguric from the onset of renal dysfunction. If the urine output is less than 50 ml per hour after this treatment, the continued use of this regimen serves no useful purpose, but may lead to furosemide-induced ototoxicity. Additional mannitol may mobilize intracellular water causing circulatory overload, especially in a patient with borderline left ventricular function.

In a patient with oliguric or nonoliguric acute renal failure, the serum creatinine may rise 1 to 1.5 mg% per day. If the serum creatinine is 2 mg% the first day after renal insult, the creatinine clearance is usually less than 10 ml/min. Thus, the oliguric patient with rising serum creatinine must have drug doses immediately adjusted since he has severely damaged kidneys. Drugs that are nephrotoxic must be avoided. Many drugs, while not nephrotoxic, contain substances that accumulate in dangerous amounts when given in standard therapeutic doses to patients with renal failure. Table 5-9 lists many of the drugs that must be used cautiously in this regard.

TABLE 5-9

Drugs Leading to the Accumulation of Toxic Substances
in Renal Failure

Magnesium containing
  Antacids, laxatives, antihypertensive therapeutic regimens
Potassium containing
  Salt substitutes, massive potassium penicillin therapy
Sodium containing
  Antacids, Na–K exchange resins, sodium penicillin, carbenicillin (4.7
  mEq Na/gm), ampicillin
Calcium containing
  Antacids as $CaCO_3$
Phosphorus containing
  Enemas, antacids
Antianabolic effect
  Tetracycline
Catabolic effect
  Corticosteroids
Uric acid, increased serum level
  Diuretics, oncologic chemotherapeutic agents
Alkalosis inducing
  Sodium bicarbonate, calcium carbonate, large doses of penicillin or
  carbenicillin
Acidosis inducing
  Ammonium chloride, ascorbic acid, isoniazide, mandelamine, fura-
  dantin

ACUTE DIALYSIS

Table 5-10 lists the indications for acute dialysis. These criteria apply
to any critically ill patient with azotemia of any etiology not immediately
reversible by nondialytic means.[20,21] Hemodialysis is usually preferable
since the treatment is shorter, more efficient, and easier for the patient.

TABLE 5-10

Indications for Dialysis in the Intensive Care Unit

Obtundation, combativeness, or decreased cooperation—all thought to be due to
  the level of azotemia
Uremia related seizures
Fluid overload or hyponatremia (serum Na < 120 mEq/liter)
Hyperkalemia uncontrolled by medical measures
Bleeding in the presence of nonuremia-related causes of abnormal clotting if
  the BUN is greater than 75 mg%
Prophylactic treatment to balance volume needed for nutrition or drug therapy
BUN > 100 mg% in an oliguric patient

Fewer infections and respiratory complications result with this treatment. For patients with an unstable cardiovascular system, concomitant arrhythmias or BUN of over 200mg%, peritoneal dialysis may be the treatment of choice. A stiff catheter may be placed percutaneously at the bedside and dialysis instituted immediately with hypertonic dialysate-containing dextrose.

POTASSIUM

Ninety-nine percent of the potassium contained in the human body is in the intracellular water. Serum potassium determinations are only one-thirtieth as high as those in the intracellular water and do not accurately reflect the total body potassium stores. Yet only the serum level of potassium can be measured clinically. Unfortunately, the serum potassium frequently does not reflect the total body stores of potassium.

There are four general rules regarding potassium homeostasis that are true in common clinical settings: (1) The kidneys will conserve sodium and water to protect volume even if such conservation leads to large potassium losses in the urine. Thus, a patient may lose a large amount of his total body potassium in the urine at a time when he has a total body potassium deficit. (2) If a patient has a normal serum pH, a serum potassium below the normal range indicates a total body potassium deficit of at least 300 mEq. This deficit may be five times the total extracellular potassium content. (3) For each change in serum pH of 0.1, there is a reciprocal change in the serum potassium of approximately 0.6 mEq/liter. For example, if a patient has acidemia with a plasma pH of 7.2, the serum potassium will be increased by 1.2 mEq/liter. Conversely, with an elevation of plasma pH to 7.6, the potassium in the serum will be depressed 1.2 mEq/liter. (4) A patient with a normal creatinine clearance and chronic metabolic acidosis or chronic metabolic alkalosis of several days duration has a deficiency in total body potassium of at least several hundred milliequivalents.

HYPOKALEMIA

Patients with serum potassium values below the normal range may have muscle weakness, ileus, polyuria, and ventricular arrhythmias, especially if they are receiving digitalis.[17,22] Severe hypokalemia may present as respiratory paralysis or tetany. There are many non-potassium-related causes for these symptoms. The critically ill patient frequently has several obvious explanations for each. The critical care physician must think of hypokalemia in order to make the diagnosis. The most common causes of hypokalemia are listed in Table 5-11. Inadequate potassium intake is rarely the sole cause of hypokalemia. Gastrointestinal losses are usually relatively minor in terms of total body potassium content. However, volume-depleted states associated with hypochlor-

TABLE 5-11

Hypokalemia—Common Causes

Decreased dietary intake
Gastrointestinal losses
  Vomiting
  Diarrhea or fistula losses
  Chronic laxative use
Kidney losses
  Diuretics
  Mineralocorticoid excess, including hyperadrenal states
  Renal tubular acidosis
  Metabolic alkalosis
  Acute hyperventilation
  Starvation
  Ureterosigmoidostomy
  Antibiotics by differing mechanisms, e.g., carbenicillin, gentamicin,
    amphotericin
  Metabolic acidosis, especially with poorly absorbed anions as ketone
    bodies
  Acute leukemia
Cellular shift
  Alkalosis
  Insulin administration
  Periodic paralysis
Postresuscitative hypokalemia
  Massive blood transfusions
  Inappropriate cellular function
Potassium shifts and imbalance
  Undefined cellular changes
  Functional extracellular volume deficits

---

emic alkalosis may lead to further large potassium losses in the urine. This potassium loss might seem "inappropriate" were it not occurring as part of the sodium retaining mechanism to protect volume.

Patients with large gastrointestinal fluid losses may be kept in proper potassium balance by (1) administration of sufficient potassium to replace the amount known to be present in the type of lost fluid (see Table 5-12) and (2) administration of chloride containing solutions in sufficient amount to maintain a normal intravascular volume. The latter step decreases the potassium losses from the kidneys.

Patients who are given diuretics, especially if already taking digitalis, should have their serum potassium levels carefully monitored since hypokalemia related arrhythmias are common in such patients.

Although it is a rare problem, patients suspected of having primary or secondary aldosteronism should similarly be observed, especially if they are undergoing a voluminous diuresis. Any clinical state in which

TABLE 5-12

Electrolyte Content of Body Fluids Lost in Critically Ill Patients

Fluid	Na$^+$ (mEq/liter)	K$^+$ (mEq/liter)	Cl (mEq/liter)
Gastric juice*	60	9	84
Bile	149	5	101
Pancreatic juice	141	5	77
Ileal fluid	129	11	116
Cecal fluid	80	21	48
Sweat	45	5	58

* A simple equation usually is helpful; $K^+ + Na^+ + H^+ = 140$. If sodium and hydrogen ions are normally excreted, K^+ rarely exceeds 10 mEq/liter. However, the relationship between Na^+ and H^+ is extremely variable and therapy should be directed to replace these losses.

a large amount of a poorly reabsorbable anion is present in the urine may lead to potassium deficiency. Thus, bicarbonaturia of proximal renal tubular acidosis, large amounts of organic acids in the urine of a poorly nourished patient, presence of an antibiotic, such as carbenicillin, in the urine, urinary ketone bodies of diabetic ketoacidosis, and lysozymuria of acute leukemia may lead to heavy potassium loss.

In the intensive care patient, hypokalemia is an extraordinarily common finding. No complex endocrinologic or balance studies can usually be implicated to explain the findings. There are, however, specific clinical entities of such frequent occurrence that corrective therapy should be instituted. Although "banked" blood often can contain extremely high potassium levels, this represents the effects of storage—the red cells use all available oxygen contained in the vehicle in which it is stored. Pco_2 levels can approach 200 torr—the resulting acidosis and decreased red cell membrane function in this profound anaerobic state translocates potassium into the plasma in the transfusable blood. However, after infusion, the excess co_2 is immediately eliminated in the lungs and the potassium returns to its normal intracellular position.

Metabolism of the anticoagulant eventually releases excess bicarbonate and postresuscitative hypokalemic metabolic alkalosis is the rule. Potassium supplementation should be quantitated depending upon (equilibrated) potassium deficits. Since refractory arrhythmias may result, corrections of low potassium concentrations (< 3.0), especially if ventricular arrhythmias are produced, should be rapid (15 to 20 mEq/hr or even bolus infusion of 10 to 20 mEq potassium in 10 to 15 minutes) in order to correct the arrhythmias. In most cases, 10 to 15 mEq/hr prove adequate to restore normal potassium levels.

If cellular function is not normal, potassium supplementation may invigorate membrane function. The urgency to correct potassium deficits can be correlated to the serum level. If severe arrhythmias are noted,

40 to 50 mEq may be administered in 30 to 60 minutes. If no cardiac effects are noted, 10 to 15 mEq/hr are sufficient to correct serum abnormalities.

When functional extracellular volume is depleted, serum potassium is often lower than expected. Replenishing this deficit with balanced electrolyte solutions usually suffices, although potassium supplements are necessary if serum levels are reduced below 3.5 mEq/liter.

Treatment of Hypokalemia Careful replacement of potassium losses as they occur can prevent hypokalemia. Treatment of hypokalemia may be extremely difficult if the potassium losses continue during therapy. Consequently, correction of the underlying problem is as important as administering potassium to correct the loss. In hypochloremic states, chloride must be replaced in order to normalize the serum potassium. Potassium administered in the gluconate, bicarbonate, or citrate form will be lost in the urine if administered to such patients. Potassium chloride is not well tolerated by the gastrointestinal tract. The new potassium supplement Slo-K, a waxy, nonirritating tablet containing 8 mEq of potassium, is more palatable.

Intravenous potassium replacement by infusion control devices may be given in amounts up to 50 mEq per hour. This replacement rate is necessary only in extreme cases of potassium deficiency where there is life-threatening ventricular irritability, uncontrolled by antiarrhythmic therapy. At this rate of replacement, the patient must have constant ECG monitoring.[23] It is much safer to administer 10 to 20 mEq per hour of potassium through a peripheral vein. Remember, even patients who are potassium depleted may develop fatal arrhythmias if intravenous fluid with high potassium content is infused directly into the heart. This concentration may cause venous irritation or thrombosis.

HYPERKALEMIA

Patients with hyperkalemia may have clinical findings similar to those ascribed to hypokalemia.[22] They may have muscle weakness, ileus, and respiratory paralysis. The correct diagnosis of hyperkalemia must be considered before the proper laboratory test is ordered to confirm it. Frequently, the daily electrolyte "screen" will detect this problem before the patient is symptomatic. If a patient is acidotic, he may be comatose as a result of hyperkalemia alone. Arrhythmias, particularly atrial standstill and ventricular fibrillation, may occur when the serum potassium value exceeds 7 mEq/liter.[23] The initial electrocardiographic abnormalities of peaked T waves, elevated ST segments, and broadened QRS complexes are indications for rapid treatment of this problem. Serum potassium determinations at 1- to 2-hour intervals are necessary until this value is normal and remains so for 4 to 6 hours.

Table 5-13 lists the more common causes of elevations of serum

TABLE 5-13
Hyperkalemia—Common Causes

Pseudo hyperkalemia
    Hemolysis during blood collection
    Hematologic disorders with increased white blood cell or platelet counts
Exogenous excess potassium
    Administered KCl in intravenous infusions
    Potassium containing drugs, e.g., potassium penicillin
    Transfusions
Cellular shift of potassium
    Tissue destruction—trauma, ischemia, burn rhabdomyolysis, tumor lysis with
        therapy
    Digitalis overdose
    Acidosis
    Hyperosmolality
    Succinyl choline
Decreased renal potassium excretion
    Acute and chronic renal failure
    Potassium sparing diuretics
    Mineralocorticoid deficiency

---

potassium. Tissue breakdown, which may have not been previously detected, may lead to dangerously high levels of serum potassium in a matter of several hours. This is especially true if there is *any* degree of renal function impairment. Renal function that is less than 25 percent normal may lead to hyperkalemia, even if the potassium load to be excreted is normal. Potassium-retaining diuretics must be avoided if the serum creatinine is greater than 2 mg%.

Treatment of Hyperkalemia   A patient with a serum potassium value of greater than 6.5 mEq/liter must be treated emergently. Rapid treatment is especially needed if the patient does not have the protective antiarrhythmic influence of a low serum pH. The absence of classic electrocardiographic findings associated with severe hyperkalemia does not lessen the importance of prompt therapy. If the serum potassium is rapidly rising, a patient may initially have a normal ECG, only to develop fatal arrhythmias several minutes later.

   The following list is a proven series of therapeutic maneuvers to be used in the order given when treating severe hyperkalemia:

1. Calcium gluconate, 10 percent solution, 10 to 30 ml I.V. slowly—repeat in 8 to 10 minutes if necessary; or calcium chloride, 10 percent solution, 5 to 10 ml I.V. slowly—repeat in 10 minutes if necessary. This therapy reconstitutes the normal electrical distance between the resting potential and threshold at which myocardial cells depolarize.

Thus, the hyperirritability of the heart is decreased. Hypercalcemia may occur if the treatment is repeated more than 3 or 4 times.

2. Glucose, 50 percent solution, 50 ml I.V. with regular insulin, 10 U I.V. This therapy causes transport of potassium into cells as glucose crosses cell membranes. This effect may last only a few hours.

3. Sodium bicarbonate, 7.5 percent solution, 50 to 150 ml I.V. push. Potassium moves into cells as hydrogen ions move out to be buffered by the administered sodium bicarbonate. The sodium contained in 150 ml of this concentrated solution (132 mEq) is almost as much as that contained in 1 liter of normal saline (154 mEq).

4. Sodium polystyrene sulfonate, 50 gm in 100 ml/hr of a 70 percent sorbitol solution in retention enema. This is the first manuever mentioned on this list that removes potassium from the body. The enemas should be repeated until the serum potassium is normalized.

5. Saline diuresis plus I.V. Lasix 40 mg every 3 to 4 hours. This is a useful, but less effective method for decreasing total body potassium in a patient with (a) normal kidney function and (b) no significant danger of developing left ventricular failure with saline infusions.

6. Hemodialysis, or peritoneal dialysis (one-fifth as effective per hour as hemodialysis) may be needed if the patient has renal insufficiency. Both forms of dialysis should be used only after all of the first five steps have been implemented.

While performing steps 1 through 6 as needed, the patient must be monitored with a standardized ECG limb lead. The initial subtle changes of elevated T waves and elevated ST segments may be missed on a monitor recording from chest electrodes.

As hyperkalemia is being treated, the physician must rapidly review the list of the causes of this electrolyte abnormality. In many instances, the removal of the source of excess potassium, such as a dead limb or necrotic loop of bowel, may be necessary to save the patient's life. Serum potassium values must be determined every one to two hours for four to six hours until stable. It is only after this period of stability with the diagnosis of the etiology of the hyperkalemia established, that the therapeutic program may be relaxed slightly.

SODIUM AND WATER

At the beginning of this chapter, the role of the kidneys in salt and water balance was reviewed in the clinical context. It should be obvious that in order to retain or excrete large amounts of salt and water, the kidneys must be adequately perfused and glomerular filtration and tubular function from Bowman's space to the end of the collecting ducts must be normal. In addition, there must be normal hepatic, pituitary, thyroid, and adrenal function. The adrenal cortex and medulla must release appropriate levels of glucocorticoid and mineralocorticoid, respectively, for each physiologic and pathophysiologic state. Antidiuretic hormone levels in the blood must be appropriate for both serum osmolality and changing states of intravascular volume.

The kidneys of a normal 70-kg human will maintain a total body water volume of 42 liters. This is equal to approximately 60 percent of the total body weight. Twenty-eight liters of this water (1) is intracellular, (2) contains potassium as its principal cation, and (3) has an osmolality equal to that of the extracellular water. The 14 liters of extracellular water is composed of intravascular plasma water as well as interstitial water around cells. Sodium is the principal cation in the extracellular water or fluid (ECF). For clinical purposes, sodium as well as the other important ECF electrolytes will be discussed as having the same concentration inside and outside of blood vessels. Only the presence of plasma proteins allows one to distinguish between plasma water and the rest of the ECF.

In the critically ill patient, the principal abnormalities in the fluid and electrolyte contents of the body occur in the extracellular fluid compartment. Therapy is directed toward normalizing the volume of this compartment, thus assuring normal intravascular volume. If the osmolality of the ECF is also normal, the intracellular osmolality and volume will remain close to normal. Suffice to say, the electrolyte content inside of cells does not change greatly even if there are marked changes in ECF volume, osmolality, or electrolyte content. Instead, the cells behave as osmometers, gaining or losing water with changes in the extracellular fluid osmolality or tonicity.

If the previously described conditions for normal kidney function are met, a critically ill patient will rarely have a fluid and electrolyte problem. Exact daily requirements of sodium chloride, potassium, and water may be calculated by measuring correct output volumes of urine, stool, fistula drainage, and nasogastric aspirate. Using Table 5-12, one can then calculate the amount of electrolyte lost in the measured volumes. In more difficult cases, electrolyte content of each body fluid may be measured for more precise replacement. In addition to replacing measurable losses from the patient, insensible losses must be estimated and sequestration of fluid in the extravascular or interstitial space anticipated. In a patient who is breathing normally, afebrile, and not hyperactive (agitated or seizing), the insensible loss will be approximately 500 ml per day. This fluid loss is very dilute since it is composed of sweat and water vapor in expired air. It should be replaced with a solution such as 5 percent dextrose in water. This adds no solute to the body since the dextrose is quickly metabolized. If a critically ill patient is extremely agitated, markedly febrile, and not breathing humidified air, he may, in extreme cases, lose 6 to 8 liters of unmeasurable fluid per day. In this case, direct measurement of cardiac filling pressures and cardiac output is the only reliable method of being certain of adequate fluid replacement.

Patients may sequester large amounts of fluid in the skin, bowel, peritoneal cavity, or extremities. This fluid will have an electrolyte composition similar to the plasma. Again, this type of fluid loss is difficult to measure or even estimate. For example, a patient developing congestive heart failure may retain 8 to 10 lb of salt and water before becoming edematous. Again, measurement of cardiac filling pressures and cardiac output may be necessary to assess such a patient's volume status. Remember, a patient who is massively edematous as a result of extensive burns, hypoproteinemia, or blockage of the inferior vena cava may have concomitant intravascular volume depletion. The edema fluid of such a patient is not available to the circulation. Additional salt and water may have to be administered to such a patient to assure good cardiac output.

Fluid and electrolyte therapy need not be performed with complex solutions. Calculated replacement amounts of normal saline or half-normal saline will be excreted or retained appropriately by normal kidneys. On occasions, a patient may need more electrolyte-free water. In this case a 5 percent dextrose in water solution is useful. Ringer's lactate may be used if a patient can benefit from the alkalinizing effect of this solution. In general, the commercially available intravenous solutions with complex content are not necessary and may lead to electrolyte imbalance. Unless a critically ill patient has marked tissue destruction and potassium release from cells, he will need 40 to 80 mEq of potassium chloride per day to maintain normal serum potassium levels.

No mention thus far has been made of volume replacement using colloid-containing solutions. Studies performed in many clinical settings have shown that colloid-containing solutions, such as albumin in saline or plasma, are no better than crystalloid-containing solutions for volume replacement. Although colloid-containing solutions are much more expensive than crystalloid- or electrolyte-containing solutions, such as normal saline or Ringer's lactate, they may be of some use in patients who are extremely hypoproteinemic. Since criticially ill patients are often very catabolic, administered plasma proteins may be quickly degraded and thus, lose their colloid osmotic effect.

The following schematic may be used to evaluate a patient's fluid and electrolyte needs or excess. If a patient has a markedly abnormal volume status, there is no good formula for the precise addition or removal of volume needed to correct the abnormality. However, recognition of such an imbalance should clearly indicate the direction of therapy. Proper monitoring of the cardiovascular status will indicate a return to normalcy. The end result of all fluid and electrolyte therapy is to assure adequate cardiac filling pressures and consequent good cardiac output and tissue perfusion.

Volume measurement
  Input volumes
    Oral or enterostomy
    Intravenous
  Output volumes
    Measurable
      Urine

Stool
Fistula drainage
Nasogastric aspirate
Chest tubes
Other tubes or 'ostomies
Not measurable
Insensible, such as skin and respiratory losses
Sequestered fluid
Estimation or measurement of electrolyte intake and losses considering
insensible losses as water only and sequestered fluid losses as plasma
Review of daily weights for fluid and electrolyte trends undetected by
measurable intake and output volumes
Examination of the patient for evidence of intravascular and interstitial
volume excess or depletion
Suggestive of volume excess
Increased jugular venous pressure or directly measured pressures
Tachycardia and cardiac gallops
Hypertension
Pulmonary congestion
Hepatomegaly
Edema
Suggestive of volume depletion
Decreased jugular venous pressure (as above)
Tachycardia and distant heart sounds
Hypotension or orthostatic fall in blood pressure
Decreased skin turgor
Absence of axillary sweat
Region of massive sequestration of fluid, e.g., severe burn, massive
ascites, swollen thigh with fractured femur
Replacement of fluid losses in volume and concentration equal to ongo-
ing losses
Evaluation of the success of fluid and electrolyte therapy
Urine output greater than 1 liter per day
Stable blood urea nitrogen and serum creatinine
Stable cardiovascular status
Good arterial blood oxygenation and a normal AV—O_2 difference
Apparent excellent peripheral perfusion including good mentation
Absence of acidosis
Placement of a Swan-Ganz catheter if any goal of therapy is not fulfilled
or uncertain

ABNORMALITY IN SERUM SODIUM CONCENTRATION

Many patients have abnormalities in both total body fluid volume and
osmolality (tonicity). A patient may have any combination of hypoosmo-
lality, normal osmolality, or hyperosmolality and hypovolemia, euvole-
mia, and hypervolemia.[5] Thus, therapy will often be directed toward

correcting volume and osmolality abnormalities at the same time. Volume replacement has been discussed above. In the following paragraphs, different hyponatremic and hypernatremic states will be classified by variations in intravascular and extracellular fluid (ECF) volume. By careful assessment of the patient's volume status and application of a modest basic knowledge of the pathophysiologic states leading to an abnormal sodium concentration, one can quickly eliminate most of the possible causes of such an abnormality. The exact diagnosis may then be made using one or two additional laboratory tests.

Hyponatremia It is important to remember that the serum osmolality is, in a steady state, the same as the osmolality of the rest of the extracellular fluid. Similarly, it must be identical to the osmolality of the intracellular water, despite the fact that the osmotically-active particles in cells are very different from those outside of cells. In the extracellular fluid (14 of 42 liters of total body of water in the 70-kg person), sodium, urea, and glucose are the common osmotically active particles. The serum osmolality may be calculated as follows:

$$\text{serum osmolality} =$$
$$(2 \times \text{Na conc}) + (\text{BUN [mg\%]} \div 2.8) + (\text{glucose [mg\%]} \div 18)$$

Other osmotic particles which may appear in the extracellular fluid include mannitol, glycerol, and ethanol. By dividing their concentrations in mg% by 18, 9, and 4.6, respectively, one can calculate the number of milliosmoles they contribute to the plasma osmolality.

The most common cause of hyponatremia in the critically ill patient is overadministration of dilute fluids such as 5 percent dextrose in water. Once the dextrose in the solution is metabolized, a patient may have difficulty excreting any remaining solute-free water in excess of his needs. Although such a patient frequently has normal renal function and renal plasma flow, his kidneys may be experiencing an excessive antidiuretic hormone effect. Increased sensitivity to or increased secretion of this hormone may be caused by pain, emotional upset, or treatment with numerous drugs. These drugs are listed in Table 5-14. Consequently, the urine may not become sufficiently dilute to excrete water in excess of solute and thus prevent a hypoosmotic state; hyponatremia will then ensue. This common setting for hyponatremia is further discussed in the following section dealing with hyponatremia with a modest excess of ECF volume without edema.

If, conversely, the patient is hypovolemic, the kidneys will be further hampered in their ability to excrete a water load and the likelihood of hyponatremia will be even greater.

Less clear cut cases of hyponatremia are best classified by the patient's volume status, using the urinary sodium concentration to further focus on the correct diagnosis. The following paragraphs outline this approach.[5]

TABLE 5-14
Drugs Affecting Water Excretion

Diuretic drugs increasing renal water excretion[24]
Alcohol
Diphenylhydantoin
Lithium
Demeclocycline
Acetohexamide
Propoxyphene
Colchicine
Vinblastine
Antidiuretic drugs decreasing renal water excretion
Nicotine
Chlorpropamide
Tolbutamide
Clofibrate
Cyclophosphamide
Morphine
Barbiturates
Vincristine
Carbamazepine
Acetaminophen
Amitriptyline
Thorazine
Indomethacin

Hyponatremic States Associated with ECF Volume Depletion In Table 5-15 hyponatremic states associated with ECF volume depletion are categorized by the presence or absence of sodium in the urine. On physical examination, such patients should have evidence of volume depletion manifested by (1) low jugular venous pressure or central venous pressure, (2) poor tissue turgor, (3) orthostatic changes in blood pressure or hypotension, and (4) weight loss. A careful review of the data regarding the case in question should suggest one of the processes listed. Treatment of this group of patients includes correction of the underlying pathophysiologic process and return of extracellular fluid volume to normal with isotonic saline. Once this is accomplished, the balance between salt and water will be normally adjusted by the kidneys. Once again the kidneys will be able to excrete an excess of water if the patient remains or becomes slightly hyponatremic.

Hyponatremic States Associated with ECF Volume Excess Without Edema Table 5-16 lists states of hyponatremia associated with modest extracellular fluid volume excess without edema. All of these conditions are associated with abundant sodium in the urine and are best treated with water restriction unless the patient is dangerously hyponatremic.

TABLE 5-15
Hyponatremia with ECF Volume Depletion

Hyponatremia with Volume Depletion and U Na > 20 mEq/liter
  Excess diuretic
  Salt losing nephritis
  Mineralocorticoid deficiency
  Excess urinary anion loss—bicarbonaturia or ketonuria
Hyponatremia with volume depletion and U Na < 20 mEq/liter
  G.I. loss—vomiting, diarrhea, fistula drainage
  "Third space losses" with muscle trauma, burns, pancreatitis, or post surgery

---

Included in this category is the syndrome of inappropriate antidiuretic hormone secretion. This is a diagnosis made by excluding other causes of hyponatremia in this group. Importantly, it is defined as a hyponatremic state occurring in the absence of cardiac, liver, renal, thyroid, adrenal, or pituitary abnormalities. A patient with this syndrome has a low serum sodium and a urine that is less than maximally dilute. The urine osmolality need not be greater than the serum osmolality. If the patient is ingesting sodium, there will be abundant sodium in the urine. The patient will not be edematous. The blood urea nitrogen and serum uric acid values are usually in the low normal range. Many central nervous system disease processes and most major intrathoracic infections or tumors may cause this syndrome. In addition, drugs (Table 5-14) may be antidiuretic and cause this syndrome.

Three treatment approaches may be used for patients in this category:

1. If the serum sodium is greater than 125 mEq/liter and the patient is asymptomatic with regard to hyponatremia, simple water restriction to less than 1 liter of total fluid per day will correct the serum sodium concentration in several days.
2. If a patient in this category of modest ECF volume excess has a serum sodium of less than 110 mEq/liter but is not comatose or seizing, he may be treated with the infusion of normal saline and diuretics with

TABLE 5-16
Hyponatremia With Modest ECF Volume Expansion Without Edema

  Glucocorticoid deficiency
  Hypothyroidism
  Pain or emotional upset
  Drugs increasing ADH release or its renal effect
  Syndrome of inappropriate antidiuretic hormone secretion

---

careful weight and fluid intake and output management. Such a maneuver can lead to an exchange of ECF volume at a rate of approximately 1 liter every 2 hours. In this situation, a patient's serum sodium concentration may be increased to a value of 120 mEq/liter or slightly higher before slowing the rate of fluid exchange. Too rapid a rise in serum sodium is dangerous. The associated changes in cell volume with the change in extracellular osmolality may lead to cell damage as cells shrink.

3. If a patient has a dangerously low serum sodium of 110 mEq/liter and associated significant neurologic disturbances, 3 percent saline may be administrered intravenously to raise this value to 120 mEq/liter. The patient must be able to tolerate the volume in which saline is contained. In addition, the ECF volume will further expand as H_2O is osmotically drawn from cells. Clearly, hypertonic saline alone cannot be given to a patient with edema or questionable left ventricular function.

Remembering that water will be removed from cells as the ECF osmolality increases, one must calculate the number of mEq of Na needed to raise the serum saline concentration assuming the sodium is being added to the total body water. Saline does not enter cells but, instead, attracts water from them as the osmolality of the ECF is raised. If the total body water is 42 liters, the patient will need 10 mEq Na/liter times 42, or 420 mEq of sodium, to raise the serum sodium from 110 to 120 mEq/liter. For this calculation we assume a normal total body water and ignore the volume in which the 3 percent saline is contained.

Hyponatremic States Associated with Extracellular Volume Excess and Edema   Table 5-17 lists the causes of gross total body salt and water excess. Edema usually is associated with at least 8 to 10 lbs of extra salt and water in the body. Once again these conditions are separated into those with high and low urinary sodium concentrations. It is clear that appropriate therapeutic approaches for the specific underlying states must be used. Salt, and more importantly, water restriction are of paramount importance but often frustratingly slow in effecting a rise

TABLE 5-17
Hyponatremia with ECF Volume Expansion and Edema

Hyponatremia, edema, and U Na < 10 mEq/liter
   Nephrotic syndrome
   Liver failure
   Congestive heart failure
Hyponatremia, edema, and U Na > 30 mEq/liter
   Acute renal failure
   Chronic renal failure

---

in serum sodium. In the case of nephrotic syndrome, cirrhosis, and cardiac failure, the judicious use of diuretics may be helpful. Intravascular volume depletion must be avoided when using diuretics.

Table 5-18 lists signs and symptoms frequently seen in patients with hyponatremia. Many of these findings are very nonspecific and may even mimic localized neurologic deficits. These findings will disappear with the return of the serum sodium concentration to normal.

Table 5-14 lists pharmacologic agents that alter water excretion and may lead to hypo- or hypernatremia. These drugs affect water metabolism by accentuating or impairing the effect of ADH at the level of the distal tubule and collecting duct of the kidney. They may also affect ADH release. It should be obvious from the previous discussion that drugs may be only one of several additive conditions leading to hyponatremia.

Pseudohyponatremia In states of severe hyperlipidemia, the total water content of plasma is less than the usual 94 percent. Consequently, the serum sodium determination will be low. However, measurement of serum osmolality in these states should be normal unless a second pathophysiologic process is present. In states of severe hyperglycemia, the serum sodium will be low because of the attraction of water from the intracellular to the extracellular space by the osmotic influence of glucose molecules. For each 100 mg% rise of glucose in the serum, one can expect a 1.6 mEq/liter decrease in serum sodium concentration. Clearly, a normal serum sodium in the face of a markedly elevated serum glucose represents a large total body water deficit. This becomes evident with correction of the glucose value, since the patient will become markedly hyponatremic and may have apparent ECF volume depletion as water moves back into cells.

TABLE 5-18
Clinical Findings Frequently Associated With Hyponatremia

Symptoms
Lethargy, apathy
Disorientation
Muscle cramps
Nausea, anorexia
Agitation
Signs
Abnormal mentation
Depressed tendon reflexes
Cheyne-Stokes respiration
Hypothermia
Pathologic reflexes
Pseudo bulbar palsy
Seizures

TABLE 5-19
Hypernatremia with ECF Volume Depletion
(Low Total Body Sodium)

With low urinary sodium concentration and hypertonic urine
  Excess sweating
  Diarrhea
With normal urinary sodium concentration and isotonic or hypotonic urine
  Renal losses with osmotically active agents, e.g., mannitol, glucose, urea, and
    glycerol

Hypernatremia Hypernatremia may also be categorized by the extracellular and intravascular volume status of the patient.[25] Again the history and physical examination can be helpful in finding likely causes of this electrolyte abnormality. Table 5-19 lists states of ECF depletion frequently associated with hypernatremia. They are subcategorized by the presence or the absence of sodium in the urine. In these conditions, the patient usually becomes hypernatremic by losing water in excess of sodium. The patient has physical findings compatible with volume depletion. Treatment with hypotonic saline to replenish both sodium and water deficits in the body is appropriate. A planned reduction in serum sodium concentration of approximately 10 to 12 mEq/liter per 24 hours is appropriate if the patient is severely hypernatremic.

Table 5-20 lists two subgroups of patients who have simply lost water but retained a normal amount of sodium in the body.[25] Here the tonicity of the urine may be helpful in distinguishing between the two subgroups, since extrarenal water losses will always be associated with a hypertonic urine. The urinary sodium is variable and depends on the response of the kidneys to intravascular volume needs. The patient's volume status, rather than the high serum tonicity, influences the amount of sodium in the urine. In this group of patients with presumed normal renal function, correction of the underlying pathophysiologic state, and water re-

TABLE 5-20
Hypernatremia with Low Normal ECF Volume
(Normal Total Body Sodium)

Renal losses with hypo-, iso-, or hypertonic urine
  Central diabetes insipidus
  Nephrogenic diabetes insipidus
  Hypodipsia
Extra renal losses with hypertonic urine
  Respiratory
  Skin insensible losses

placement to dilute a normal amount of total body sodium, should be sufficient therapy.

If a patient has become hypernatremic from sweating, he has lost little salt from the body. If, for example, he has raised his serum sodium from 140 to 160 mEq/liter, he has lost one-seventh of his extracellular fluid volume. (The sodium concentration has increased by 20/140 or one-seventh.) His plasma or ECF osmolality has increased by 40 mOsm. Since water moves freely in and out of cells, the intracellular fluid must be similarly concentrated and have the same elevated osmolality. Thus, approximately one-seventh of the intracellular water has also been lost. To correct the serum sodium and, consequently, the total body water osmolality to normal, a 70-kg patient would need replacement of one-seventh of his 42 liters of total body water. Six liters of solute-free water, given in 18 to 24 hours, will safely correct a serum sodium abnormality.

Less commonly, patients develop hypernatremia due to an increased amount of sodium in the body. Table 5-21 lists the clinical states in which this may be seen. It is important to note that several of the items on the list represent physician mismanagement of sodium intake. If the kidneys are normal, the urinary sodium will be high as the body attempts to rid itself of excess volume. Clearly, a vigorous therapeutic approach with diuretics and water replacement will return both the patient's ECF volume and serum sodium concentration to normal.

TABLE 5-21
Hypernatremia with Increased Total Body Sodium and
Isotonic or Hypertonic Urine

Hyperaldosteronism
Cushing's syndrome
Hypertonic dialysis
Sodium bicarbonate or sodium chloride tablet ingestion

ACID-BASE BALANCE

The initial pages of this chapter outline normal renal function which includes hydrogen ion excretion. Each day the kidneys excrete 50 to 100 mEq of hydrogen ion. This hydrogen ion load is derived in equal parts from (1) inorganic acids in the diet, (2) tissue breakdown with release of hydrogen ion with sulfate and phosphate, and (3) bicarbonate loss in the stool. The lungs cannot excrete hydrogen ion produced from these sources. If one loads an individual (with normal kidney function) with progressively larger doses of hydrogen ion each day, in a week's time he can increase excretion to 400 to 500 mEq of hydrogen ion daily; he does so by increasing the production rate of ammonia in the kidneys. When the hydrogen ion-excreting ability of the kidneys or lungs is impaired, a patient will develop acidemia.

An excess of bicarbonate in the body is easily excreted by normal kidneys when the serum level is greater than 25 mEq/liter. To excrete bicarbonate in this fashion, an individual must have a normal intravascular volume and normal renal perfusion.

When bicarbonate is retained by the kidneys or carbon dioxide blown off in excess by the lungs, the result is alkalemia, and the following section will describe a functional approach to the diagnosis and treatment of acidemia and alkalemia.

ACID—BASE DISTURBANCES

The plasma of extracellular fluid hydrogen ion concentration is influenced by all the acid- and base-producing processes in the body. This plasma value is measured in pH units and is defined as the negative log to the base 10 of the hydrogen ion concentration in nano equivalents per liter (nEq/liter). The normal pH of the plasma is 7.4 + 0.05 units. The range of pH compatible with life is 6.8 − 7.8 (160 − 16 nEq/liter of hydrogen ion). Thus the pH change (1 unit) is translated into a tenfold change in H^+ concentration—far greater than sodium, potassium, or any other electrolyte (e.g., Na = 14 to 140 or K = 4 to 40). Yet we rarely assess changes in hydrogen ion in this perspective.

NORMAL ACID—BASE VALUES

$$
\begin{aligned}
\text{pH} &= 7.40 \pm 0.05 \text{ units} \\
H^+ &= 40 \pm 4.0 \text{ nEq/liter} \\
P_{CO_2} &= 40 \pm 4.0 \text{ torr} \\
HCO_3 &= 25 \pm 2.0 \text{ mEq/liter}
\end{aligned}
$$

Hydrogen ions are removed from the body by the lungs and kidneys. Immediately protection from an excess of hydrogen ions is supplied by buffer systems. These systems are composed of weak acids and their salts which reversibly bind hydrogen ions and effectively neutralize them. Thus, there is little change in the body fluid pH as hydrogen ions accumulate. In the 14 liters of extracellular fluid, the carbonic acid-bicarbonate pair accounts for 80 percent of the buffering that occurs. A quantitatively equal amount of buffering occurs in the intracellular fluid, a compartment twice as large as the extracellular fluid space. The nature of the intracellular buffer systems is poorly understood.

Formula 1 delineates the buffering of hydrogen ions by bicarbonate which is a base or proton (H^+) acceptor. Carbonic acid, a proton donor, is formed. Carbonic acid can form water and carbon dioxide gas, the latter being easily removed from the body by normal lungs. The kidneys can generate bicarbonate by combining carbon dioxide and water to form carbonic acid. This reaction is facilitated by the enzyme carbonic anhydrase. The hydrogen ion of carbonic acid is excreted by the kidneys while the bicarbonate ion is returned to the extracellular fluid.

$$HCO_3^- + H^+ \leftrightarrows H_2CO_3 \xrightarrow{\text{carbonic acid}} H_2O + CO_2 \qquad (1)$$

It is apparent that an excess of retained carbon dioxide gas forces this formula to the left causing an increase in bicarbonate production. Conversely, a decrease in the partial pressure of carbon dioxide gas (P_{CO_2}) causes the equilibrium to shift to the right with a decrease in serum bicarbonate.

DEFINITIONS

Acidemia: an extracellular fluid (plasma) pH less than 7.35.
Alkalemia: an extracellular fluid (plasma) pH greater than 7.45.
Acidosis: a metabolic process which can result in acidemia if not corrected by a compensatory mechanism or opposed by a primary counter balancing alkalosis.
Alkalosis: a metabolic process which can result in alkalemia if not corrected by a compensatory mechanism or opposed by a primary counter balancing acidosis.

RESPIRATORY ACIDOSIS

The 15,000 mEq/liter of carbon dioxide formed during fat and carbohydrate metabolism each day are easily excreted by normal lungs. This amount of acid excretion is enormous when compared to the 50 to 100 mEq/liter of hydrogen ion from nonvolatile sources that can and must be excreted by the kidneys. Failure to eliminate carbon dioxide results in a rise in concentration of this substance in the blood (increased P_{CO_2}) and a fall in serum pH.[26] This constitutes a respiratory acidosis. The alkalinizing effect of the compensatory increase in extracellular fluid bicarbonate prevents severe *acidemia* from occurring. In acute carbon dioxide retention, the bicarbonate will rise 1 mEq/liter for every 10 mm Hg increase in P_{CO_2}. If kidney function is normal, chronic carbon dioxide retention of greater than three days' duration will result in a bicarbonate rise of 4 mEq/liter for every 10 mm Hg rise in P_{CO_2}. Increases of bicarbonate greater than these values indicate the existence of an independent metabolic alkalosis. Absence of an increase in bicarbonate concentration of these dimensions suggest an independent metabolic acidosis.

All acid-base compensatory processes incompletely correct pH changes of the primary acid-base abnormality. This principle must always be considered in interpreting the critically ill patient's signs; if P_{ACO_2} is elevated *and* pH is also elevated, compensatory relation of bicarbonate cannot be the total explanation, since a compensating mechanism would reduce pH towards normal. An above-normal value necessitates consideration of a second etiologic process, metabolic alkalosis, in association with respiratory acidosis. The more severe the primary acid-

base process, the less effective the compensatory mechanism in normalizing the pH. If the pH is normal despite an obvious primary acid-base
disturbance, at least one additional acid-base disturbance, independent
of the first detected disturbance, must be suspected and elucidated.[27]

Figure 5-2 may be useful in diagnosing an acid-base disturbance
where there is only one primary process.[28] The acid-base data of a patient
with one disturbance will indicate a point on one of the confidence bands
shown. Points lying outside of the confidence bands indicate laboratory
error or the presence of more than one primary acid-base disturbance.

RESPIRATORY ALKALOSIS

Hyperventilation from any cause frequently results in respiratory alkalosis. The plasma P_{CO_2} falls and the serum pH rises in this condition.
In acute respiratory alkalosis, the plasma bicarbonate falls approxi-

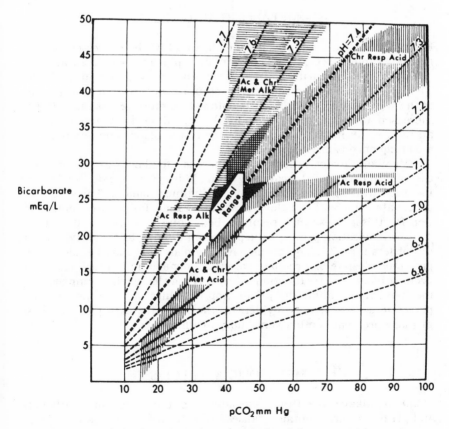

Fig. 5-2. In vivo nomogram showing bands for defining a single respiratory
or metabolic acid-base disturbance. (CMA Journal 109:291, 1973)

mately 2 mEq/liter for each 10 mm Hg decline in the P_{CO_2}. This decline in bicarbonate value may be better understood by reviewing formula 1 (p. 294). It is clear that the fall in bicarbonate is due to a shift from left to right in this formula as carbon dioxide is eliminated. As P_{CO_2} diminishes, more bicarbonate combines with hydrogen ion to form carbonic acid which dissociates to CO_2 and water. Less bicarbonate remains as a result of the physiochemical principles always operating.

In chronic respiratory alkalosis of at least 3 days' duration, the plasma bicarbonate will fall approximately 5 mEq/liter for each 10 mm Hg decline in P_{CO_2}. If the bicarbonate changes are not of this magnitude, the pH of the blood will rise sharply with hyperventilation. Failure of the bicarbonate to decline suggests an existing independent metabolic alkalosis. Conversely, if the bicarbonate decrease is greater than mentioned for the acute and chronic compensatory states, an independent metabolic acidosis should be suspected.

METABOLIC ACIDOSIS

Metabolic acidoses are best classified by dividing the processes into two groups (Table 5-22). The normal anion gap group is defined as those acidoses associated with no increase in abnormal anions in the blood. The difference between the serum sodium concentration and the sum of the serum chloride and bicarbonate values must be less than 16. The increased anion gap group includes those acidoses known to exist with an increase in negatively charged ions in the blood. The anion gap as a consequence is greater than 16.

Metabolic acidosis occurs when there is a total body load of nonvolatile acid in excess of the capacity of the kidneys to excrete this H^+ and its anion while concurrently regenerating bicarbonate.[7] The serum bicarbonate value will be below the normal range. Pulmonary compensation for this process may result in P_{CO_2} values as low as 10 mm Hg. This compensation prevents the pH from plunging to seriously low values of less than 7.0. The pulmonary compensation may be adequately protective despite bicarbonate values as low as 6 to 8 mEq/liter. Compromise of pulmonary function in any way may lessen this compensatory mechanism and allow the pH to drop to values of less than 7.0. This principle is most acutely evident in the intensive care patient whose primary problem is often ventilatory insufficiency.

METABOLIC ALKALOSIS

Metabolic alkalosis, with its associated rise in both serum bicarbonate and pH has several common causes.[29] The most frequent causes of this acid-base disturbance are: (1) the administration of alkali—either bicarbonate initially directed to the correction of acidosis or the metabolism

TABLE 5-22
Causes of Metabolic Acidosis

Normal anion gap
  G.I. loss of HCO_3^-:
    1. Diarrhea
    2. Small bowel or pancreatic fistula
    3. Ureterosigmoidostomy, ileal loop conduit
    4. Cholestyramine therapy with poor renal function
  Renal loss of HCO_3^-:
    1. Carbonic anhydrase inhibitors
    2. Renal tubular acidosis
    3. Hyperparathyroidism (?)
    4. Early chronic renal failure
  Miscellaneous:
    1. "Expansion" acidosis
    2. Administration of HCl, NH_4Cl, arginine HCl, etc.
    3. Hyperalimentation
Increased anion gap
  Increased acid production:
    1. Diabetic ketoacidosis
    2. Lactic acidosis
    3. Alcoholic (beta-hydroxy-butyric) acidosis
    4. Starvation
    5. Hyperosmolar nonketotic coma
  Ingested toxin acidosis
    1. Salicylate
    2. Paraldehyde
    3. Methanol
    4. Ethylene glycol
  Renal failure
    1. Acute
    2. Chronic

---

of administered lactate or citrate as resuscitating fluids in the form of balanced electrolyte solutions or banked blood, (2) chloride depletion most commonly from loss of gastrointestinal fluids, or (3) volume and potassium depletion with diuretic therapy. With chloride depletion and volume loss, a greater than normal fraction of sodium will be reabsorbed in the distal rather than proximal tubule of the kidney. Consequently, a greater than normal amount of potassium and hydrogen ion will be excreted in the distal tubule due to the electrochemical gradient established there·during sodium reabsorption. As the plasma pH increases, the patient will tend to hypoventilate, raising the serum Pco_2 as high as 55 mm Hg.[30] This compensatory process prevents severe alkalemia. If the Pco_2 is greater than this value, one should suspect an independent respiratory acidosis. If the Pco_2 does not rise, a condition associated with chloride depletion, hypovolemia, and a metabolic alkalosis, one should suspect an independent respiratory alkalosis.

DIAGNOSIS AND TREATMENT OF ACID-BASE DISTURBANCES

Having discussed the laboratory values associated with the four primary acid-base disturbances, the primary importance of using other clinical information must now be stressed. Careful history and physical examination plus review of non-acid-base laboratory data may allow the unravelling of complex disturbances. For example, the use of all available data may allow the diagnosis of diabetic ketoacidosis, metabolic alkalosis due to loss of gastrointestinal fluid, and respiratory acidosis due to chronic obstructive pulmonary disease in the same patient.

The goal of the treatment of acid-base disturbances is to maintain the pH of the total body fluid in a range compatible with life.[31] Rapid treatment is often necessary to accomplish this. Once the pH has been returned to the range of 7.2 to 7.55, slower changes in acid-base treatment are indicated. This slowing of the rate of therapy allows compensatory mechanisms to abate. This is particularly important in the case of the metabolic compensation for a respiratory disturbance. The excretion of extra bicarbonate or the regeneration of depleted bicarbonate may take 24 to 48 hours once a primary respiratory abnormality is corrected. Similarly the equilibration of the cerebral spinal fluid bicarbonate with the serum bicarbonate is a slow process and may take more than a day. A rapid change in the plasma P_{CO_2} will quickly be reflected in a similar change in the cerebral spinal fluid. A rapid change in the CSF pH will occur because of the inability of rapid adjustment of bicarbonate. Thus, a central nervous system acid-base disequilibrium will ensue.

Respiratory alkalosis and respiratory acidosis are obviously treated by effecting change in pulmonary excretion of carbon dioxide. Sophisticated ventilatory manipulations are dealt with in detail in other I.C.U.-related texts. Prompt treatment of altered P_{CO_2} values brings about gratifying correction of abnormal pH values. If metabolic compensatory processes are well established, complete correction of the P_{CO_2} must occur gradually in order not to convert an acidemia to an alkalemia or vice versa. This would leave the patient with only the compensatory process which is no longer needed, but which takes time to reverse. The first and most important steps in the treatment of metabolic acid-base disturbances is the diagnosis of the specific metabolic abnormality —or abnormalities—underlying the problem and the subsequent employment of therapy specifically directed to correct the diagnosed abnormality.[32,33] If the metabolic acid-base disturbance is severe, therapy with alkali or acid may be necessary to return the pH to a safe range.

Metabolic acidosis may be treated with sodium bicarbonate by the oral or intravenous route. The amount of bicarbonate needed to totally correct a metabolic acidosis is determined by the formula:

total bicarbonate deficit (mEq) =
   total body weight (kg) $\times$ 0.4 $\times$ (25 − actual serum bicarb [mEq])   (2)

This equation assumes no further H^+ will be produced or excreted. This is usually not the case. It is safest to administer one-half of the needed amount of bicarbonate with reevaluation of the plasma pH and bicarbonate 1 to 2 hours later. If bicarbonate value has improved by 50 percent, then a much slower rate of bicarbonate administration is indicated. In critical situations, the time frame must be accelerated, correction more rapidly instituted, and the frequency of testing plasma pH and bicarbonate levels accelerated to provide updated information every few minutes until the values are within "life" limits. The pH and plasma bicarbonate should be normalized in 24 to 36 hours. If correction of the bicarbonate value has not been accomplished after the initial treatment, the rate of administration of bicarbonate may have to be increased to neutralize a large acid load from an ongoing acidosis.[34] This, too, is common in the I.C.U. patient and implicates that effective therapy represents correction of the underlying cause of acidosis—not always possible but always desirable.

Metabolic alkalosis with alkalemia represented by a pH of greater than 7.55 may be treated with volume replenishing intravenous solutions containing both chloride and potassium. This therapy will allow renal correction, if possible, of the alkalemia. If the plasma pH is dangerously high, or renal function significantly impaired so that rapid correction of the process seems unlikely, a solution of 0.1 percent normal hydrochloric acid may be given intravenously. Formula 3 may be used to calculate the amount of hydrogen ion needed to completely correct a severe alkalosis.

total hydrogen ion deficit =

$$\text{total body weight (kg)} \times 0.4 \times \qquad (3)$$
$$\text{(actual serum bicarb [mEq/liter]} - 25)$$

As in metabolic acidosis, half of the needed hydrochloric acid dose should be given and the patient reassessed in several hours. If correction of the alkalemia is progressing well, the rate of therapy must be lowered in order to allow compensatory processes to readjust and to prevent central nervous system acid-base disequilibrium.

These combined and extreme problems are most commonly seen in the I.C.U. patient and will receive special consideration with respect to therapy.

DRUG THERAPY IN AN INTENSIVE CARE UNIT

Normal kidney and liver function is extremely important for normal metabolism and excretion of drugs used in the critical care setting. The kidneys, in particular, excrete many important drugs and their active metabolites. If renal function is depressed for *any* reason, a dangerously high level of a drug *or* its degradation product may occur. Since many patients do not have functionally normal kidneys, this consideration must always be remembered. Additionally, the level of kidney function often varies daily; so virtual day-to-day determination of proper drug dosage becomes a necessary reality when dealing with the patient suffering multisystemic critical illness. If a patient is edematous and has modest renal function impairment, there may be slower absorption of drugs administered by the gastrointestinal tract. Once absorbed, the drug will have a greater volume of distribution in the body. Nausea, vomiting, and diarrhea due to kidney failure makes the oral administration of drugs undesirable; in fact, most common I.C.U. conditions eliminate consideration of oral medications. With decreased creatinine clearance, protein binding of drugs in the plasma is also decreased. This is usually due to decreased levels of serum albumin and decreased binding sites on this protein. Albumin may either undergo structural changes or have fewer drug binding sites available, due to the accumulation of endogenous inhibitors in the blood during renal failure. These inhibitors then occupy some of the binding sites. The consequences of decreased protein binding are an apparent increase in the volume of distribution of an administered drug and decreased total plasma or blood levels of that drug. Because of decreased protein binding, the free drug level may be normal or even increased. Thus, there is the possibility of either increased drug activity or loss due to faster metabolism and excretion of the more available unbound form of the drug. It is clear, then, that the critical care physician must look carefully at the following issues when giving drugs to seriously ill patients with impaired renal function:

1. What percentage of the drug is normally protein bound?
2. What percentage of the drug is normally excreted by the kidneys?
3. What toxic metabolites may accumulate if the drug is administered in its conventional dosage to a patient with impaired renal function?
4. Is there an accurate assay for blood levels of the drug?
5. What is the toxic-to-therapeutic ratio of blood levels of the drug?
6. What are the consequences of toxicity from this drug?
7. Do the toxic manifestations of the drug correlate well with blood levels of the drug?
8. Are there clinical parameters that may be safely followed to assure therapeutic but nontoxic levels of the drug?
9. If the drug seems ill-advised for use in a patient with renal function impairment, is there a safer alternative?

With impaired renal function, most drugs are administered using a normal loading dose (equivalent to that ordered for a patient with normal kidney function). Subsequent doses may be given at the usual interval but in smaller amounts, thus keeping the blood level of the drug relatively constant. Alternatively, increasing the dosage interval allows the use of conventional doses of a drug, but allows wider variation in blood level.

Most drugs reach a steady blood level at 3.3 times the drug half-life. If a drug has a long half-life and is dependent on the kidney for excretion, any change in glomerular filtration necessitates a change in the amount of drug given. Digoxin, for example, has a half-life of 1.5 days in the normal individual. In a patient with severely impaired renal function, the half-life is almost five days. Thus, the time to effect total equilibration after the drug is initially given, changes from less than 5 days in the normal to almost 15 days in the uremic individual. Thus, digitalis toxicity or underdigitalization may become apparent several weeks after changing the dose of this drug.

Numerous drugs are oxidized by hepatic microsomes. Chronic renal failure may accelerate this metabolic process. Examples of medications rapidly degraded in this fashion are diphenylhydantoin, pentobarbital, propranolol, and antipyrine.

With impaired renal function, metabolites of drugs degraded by the liver at a normal rate may accumulate in the blood. Many of these substances are pharmacologically active and dangerous to the patient. Drugs included in this category are meperidine, procainamide, azathioprine, and propranolol.

Table 5-23 lists drugs commonly used in the critical care setting.[4,35] The main route of excretion and normal dose intervals are indicated. Also listed is a suggested change in dosage for patients with varying degrees of impaired renal function. Serum creatinine values may be misleading when estimating a patient's level of kidney function.[1,2] A three or four hour urine specimen, if accurately collected, can be used to calculate a creatinine clearance. The serum creatinine is a valuable indicator of the stability of change in renal function but will not accurately predict the actual creatinine clearance, since the level varies greatly with body build, muscle mass, and catabolic state of each patient.

Table 5-9 (p. 276) lists the metabolic load or consequence of many of the drugs listed in Table 5-23. These consequences are often not anticipated, since they have nothing to do with the primary pharmacologic effect of the individual drugs.

Table 5-24 lists important drug-drug interactions that may occur in a critical care setting. The chances of such interactions may be heightened if any of these drugs are retained in the body in abnormal amounts due to decreased renal or hepatic excretion.[36]

Hepatic necrosis may occur with numerous medications, listed in Table 5-25.

DIURETIC THERAPY

Earlier in this chapter the use of diuretics was discussed in the context of acute renal failure. Most critically ill patients should receive diuretics by the intravenous route. Strong diuretics such as furosemide and etha-

TABLE 5-23

Drug Therapy in Patients with Abnormal Renal Function

Drug	Excretion	Normal Dose Interval (hr)	Dose Change (hr) or % Dose Creatinine Clearance (ml/min)		
			>50	10–50	<10
Antibiotics					
Aminoglycosides					
Amikacin	Renal	8–12	12–18 hr	24–36 hr	36–48 hr
Gentamicin	Renal	8	75–100% or 8–12 hr	50–75% 12–24 hr	25–50% 24–48 hr
Tobramycin	Renal	8	75–100% or 8–12 hr	50–75% 12–24 hr	25–50% 24–48 hr
Kanamycin	Renal	8	24 hr or 75%	24–72 hr 50%	72–96 hr 25%
Neomycin	Renal	8	6 hr	12–18 hr	18–24 hr
Streptomycin	Renal	12	24 hr	24–72 hr	72–96 hr
Cephalosporins					
Cephalexin	Renal	6	6 hr	6 hr	6–12 hr
Cephalothin	Renal (hepatic)	6	6 hr	6 hr	8–12 hr
Cefazolin	Renal	8	8 hr or 100%	12 hr 50%	24–48 hr 25%
Chloramphenicol	Hepatic (renal)	6	unchanged	unchanged	unchanged
Clindamycin	Hepatic (renal)	6–8	unchanged	unchanged	unchanged
Colistimethate	Renal	12	75%	50%	25%
Erythromycin	Hepatic	6	unchanged	unchanged	unchanged
Lincomycin	Hepatic (renal)	6	6	12	24
Penicillins					
Amoxicillin	Renal	8	8 hr	12 hr	16 hr
Ampicillin	Renal (hepatic)	6	6 hr	9 hr	12–15 hr
Carbenicillin	Renal (hepatic)	4	4 hr or 100%	6–12 hr 75%	12–16 hr 25–50%
Cloxacillin	Hepatic (renal)	6	unchanged	unchanged	unchanged
Dicloxacillin	Renal (hepatic)	6	unchanged	unchanged	unchanged

Methicillin	Renal (hepatic)	4	4 hr	4 hr	8–12 hr
Nafcillin	Hepatic	6	unchanged	unchanged	unchanged
Oxacillin	Renal (hepatic)	6	unchanged	unchanged	unchanged
Penicillin	Renal (hepatic)	8	100% or 8 hr	100% 8 hr	50% 8–12 hr
Ticarcillin	Renal	4–6	100% or 4 hr	50–75% 8 hr	50% 12 hr
Sulfisoxazole	Renal	6	6 hr	8–12 hr	12–24 hr
Tetracyclines					
Tetracycline	Renal (hepatic)	6	8–12 hr	12–24 hr	24 hr
Doxycycline	Renal (hepatic)	12	unchanged	unchanged	unchanged
Minocycline	Hepatic	12	12 hr	18–24 hr	24–36 hr
Analgesics (non-narcotic)					
Acetaminophen (Tylenol)	Hepatic	4	4–6 hr	6 hr	8 hr
Acetylsalicylic acid	Renal (hepatic)	4	4 hr	4–6 hr	avoid
Phenazopyridine (Pyridium)	Renal	8	8–16 hr	avoid	avoid
Narcotics and narcotic antagonists					
Codeine	Hepatic (renal <16%)	4	unchanged	unchanged	unchanged
Meperidine (Demerol)	Hepatic (renal <10%)	4	unchanged	unchanged	unchanged
Methadone	Hepatic (renal <21%)	4	unchanged	unchanged	unchanged
Morphine	Hepatic (renal <12%, G.I. <10%)	6–8	6 hr	8 hr	8–12 hr
Naloxone (Narcan)	Hepatic	4 bolus	unchanged	unchanged	unchanged
Pentazocine (Talwin)	Hepatic (renal <12%)	4	unchanged	unchanged	unchanged

(continued)

TABLE 5-23 (continued)

Drug	Excretion	Normal Dose Interval (hr)	Dose Change (hr) or % Dose Creatinine Clearance (ml/min)		
			>50	10–50	<10
Central Nervous System Drugs					
Barbiturates					
Pentobarbital	Hepatic	8	unchanged	unchanged	unchanged
Phenobarbital	Hepatic (renal)	8	8 hr	8 hr	8–16 hr
Secobarbital	Hepatic	24	unchanged	unchanged	unchanged
Benzodiazepines					
Chlordiazepoxide (Librium)	Hepatic	6–8	unchanged	unchanged	unchanged
Diazepam (Valium)	Hepatic (renal, G.I.)	8	unchanged	unchanged	unchanged
Flurazepam (Dalmane)	G.I. (renal)	24	unchanged	unchanged	unchanged
Haloperidol	Hepatic (renal, G.I.)	8	unchanged	unchanged	unchanged
Phenothiazines					
Chlorpromazine	Hepatic	6–12	unchanged	unchanged	unchanged
Cardiovascular					
Antiarrhythmic agents					
Lidocaine	Hepatic (renal <20%)	bolus 0.5–1; constant infusion 16	unchanged	unchanged	unchanged
Procainamide	Renal (hepatic 7–24%)	3–4	4 hr	6–12 hr	8–24 hr
Propranolol	Hepatic	6–8	unchanged	unchanged	50%
Quinidine	Nonrenal (renal 12–36%)	6	unchanged	unchanged	unchanged

Antihypertensive agents					
Diazoxide	Renal (nonrenal 20–70%)	bolus	unchanged	unchanged	unchanged
Hydralazine	Hepatic (renal 7–58%, G.I.)	?	unchanged	unchanged	8–16 hr (fast); 12–24 hr (slow) 12–24 hr
Methyldopa	Renal (hepatic 18–48%)	6	unchanged	9–18 hr	12–24 hr
Minoxidil	Nonrenal	8	unchanged	unchanged	unchanged
Nitroprusside	Nonrenal	constant I.V. infusion	unchanged	unchanged	unchanged
Prazosin	Hepatic (renal 5%)	8–12	unchanged	unchanged	unchanged
Cardiac glycosides					
Digitoxin	Hepatic (renal)	24	unchanged	unchanged	50–75%
Digoxin	Renal (nonrenal 15–40%)	24	100%	25–75%	10–25%
Diuretics					
Chlorthalidone	Renal (nonrenal)	24	24 hr	24 hr	48 hr
Ethacrynic acid	Hepatic	6	6 hr	6 hr	avoid
Furosemide	Renal	6	unchanged	unchanged	unchanged
Metolazone	Renal	24	unchanged	unchanged	unchanged
Thiazides	Renal	12	unchanged	unchanged	unchanged

(continued)

TABLE 5-23 (continued)

Drug	Excretion	Normal Dose Interval (hr)	Dose Change (hr) or % Dose Creatinine Clearance (ml/min)		
			>50	10–50	<10
Miscellaneous					
Anticoagulants					
Heparin	Nonrenal	4	unchanged	unchanged	unchanged
Neurologic drugs					
Diphenylhydantoin (Dilantin)	Hepatic (renal)	8	unchanged	unchanged	unchanged
Neostigmine	Nonrenal	6	6 hr	6 hr	12–18 hr
Hypoglycemic agents					
Insulin, regular	Hepatic (renal)	6	100%	75–100%	50–75%
Neuromuscular blocking agents					
Gallamine	Renal	intravenous bolus	unchanged	avoid	avoid
Succinylcholine	Nonrenal	intravenous bolus	unchanged	unchanged	unchanged
Tubocurarine	Renal	intravenous bolus	unchanged	unchanged	unchanged

TABLE 5-24
Drug—Drug Interactions of Commonly Used Critical Care Drugs

Antibiotics

Aminoglycosides (gentamicin, kanamycin, etc.) and curariform drugs—neuromuscular blockade with possible respiratory paralysis

Aminoglycosides and ethacrynic acid—additive effect of individual ototoxicities

Cephalosporins and aminoglycosides or ethacrynic acid or furosemide—increased chance of nephrotoxicity

Tetracycline (oral) and antacids—decreased tetracycline absorption from the gastrointestinal tract

Tetracycline and barbiturates—decreased antibiotic level in the blood

Diuretics

Diuretics and corticosteroids—increased potassium loss in the urine

Diuretics and curariform drugs—increased curariform effect due to hypokalemia

Diuretics and digitalis—increased digitalis toxicity due to hypokalemia, hypomagnesemia, or hypercalcemia (the latter with thiazides only)

Antacids

Aluminum or magnesium and chlorpromazine—decreased chlorpromazine absorption from the gastrointestinal tract

Antacids and digitalis—decreased digoxin absorption from the gastrointestinal tract

Barbiturates

Barbiturates and corticosteroid or quinidine or tetracycline—decreased effect of corticosteroids, quinidine, or tetracycline due to increased degradation by hepatic microsomes

Anticonvulsant

Diphenylhydantoin and oral anticoagulants, or chloramphenicol or isoniazid—increased diphenylhydantoin toxicity

Diphenylhydantoin and corticosteroid or quinidine—decreased corticosteroid or quinidine effect

Diphenylhydantoin and insulin—unpredictable high or low blood glucose

Diphenylhydantoin and halothane—increased halothane toxicity

Miscellaneous

Insulin and propranolol—hypoglycemia without the usual clinical signs if only endogenous insulin is present; hyperglycemia if the patient requires exogenous insulin

TABLE 5-25
Critical Care Drugs Frequently Associated with Hepatic Necrosis

Acetaminophen	Furosemide*
Salicylate	Azathioprine*
Halothane	Mecaptopurine*
Sulfonamide	Methotrexate
Diphenylhydantoin	Phenothiazine
Methyldopa	

* May also give a cholestatic picture

crynic acid are often needed. If a diuretic is being given to increase urine output and sodium excretion in a patient with normal kidney function, modest doses of furosemide 20 mg or ethacrynic acid 50 mg every 4 to 6 hours will suffice. Administration of these powerful diuretics, which block the chloride pump in the loop of Henle, must be monitored carefully to prevent volume depletion. A large diuresis from either of these diuretics is usually associated with substantial losses of potassium and calcium in the urine. Consequently, the serum values of these two electrolytes must be determined on at least daily basis. Potassium levels require even closer monitoring, since the magnitude of potassium excretion may cause substantial—and dangerous—decreases in serum potassium, with a potential for serious arrhythmias. Analysis of a urine aliquot for potassium concentration in conjunction with serum potassium determinations can be used to direct appropriate potassium supplementation. Hyperglycemia and hyperuricemia may also occur. Since furosemide is chemically dissimilar from ethacrynic acid and, in addition to its effect on the loop of Henle, also blocks carbonic anhydrase in the proximal tubule, one may see a response to this diuretic in patients who have not responded to ethacrynic acid. On occasion, the converse may also be true.

In patients who are grossly salt and water overloaded and refractory to low dose therapy of these two diuretics, as much as 120 to 160 mg of furosemide or 200 mg of ethacrynic acid may be needed twice a day to achieve an adequate diuresis. Doses of this size should be used only when the physician is certain that the blood flow to the kidneys has been maximized. Both furosemide and ethacrynic acid are ototoxic: the latter has caused many cases of permanent hearing loss, especially those with impaired renal function.

Because of the effect on the loop of Henle, both of these diuretics will paralyze the kidney's ability to concentrate or dilute the urine. Consequently, a waterload will not be excreted normally. A patient given large amounts of dextrose in water may become severely hyponatremic while on diuretic therapy induced by these two drugs.

Other diuretics such as the thiazides and potassium-sparing spironolactone and triamterene have no real place in the management of the critically ill patient. They are not powerful diuretics. The potassium sparing effect of the latter two only is manifest after many days of therapy.

ANTIHYPERTENSIVE THERAPY

Patients in the intensive care setting with diastolic blood pressure of greater than 115 mm Hg frequently require rapid lowering of their blood pressure. This is particularly true if the patient has (1) left ventricular failure, (2) coronary artery or cerebral artery disease, or (3) recent vascular surgery. Patients with marked elevations of blood pressure may even develop hypertensive encephalopathy in one or two days if diastolic blood pressures remain greater than 130 mm Hg. Several therapeutic agents are available to effect acute lowering of the blood pressure.

Diazoxide is one of the few drugs that must be administered in a rapid I.V. bolus to be effective. A 300 mg intravenous dose given in less than one minute may return the blood pressure to normal. The drug effect may last from 4 to 12 hours and may be repeated as often as every 4 hours. On occasion a patient will have moderate hypotension associated with administration of this drug. Blood pressure must be constantly monitored and the initial dose given only after a previously mixed intravenous infusion of a pressor, such as dopamine, is available.

Nitroprusside (see pp. 233–43), administered as a constant intravenous infusion, can be used to titrate the blood pressure. An intravenous infusion of 10 mg/liter may be administered at a rate of 0.5 to 8 μg/kg/min using an infusion pump. The blood pressure must be followed constantly with direct arterial pressure monitoring. Thiocyanate levels must be followed if the drug is continued since this substance reaches toxic levels in 48 hours, especially in patients with any degree of impaired renal function. If a patient has liver disease, cyanide produced from the metabolism of the drug cannot be converted to thiocyanate. In addition, lactic acidosis has been reported in patients receiving this drug.[37]

Trimethaphan camsylate may be administered in a constant intravenous infusion. This drug is as effective as nitroprusside in lowering blood pressure quickly but frequently must be given in increasingly higher doses each day due to the development of tachyphylaxis.

A maintenance program of antihypertensive drugs which will lower the diastolic blood pressure to less than 90, can include apresoline 10 to 25 mg every four hours intravenously or intramuscularly up to a total dose of 200 mg per day. If the usual reflex tachycardia occurs, intravenous propanolol in a dose of 1 to 2 mg every four hours may be helpful to controlling both the heart rate and hypertension.

Methyldopa, in a dose of 250 mg to 500 mg intravenously every 4 to 8 hours, may be effective but less predictably so. The onset of action is slower than apresoline making it a less desirable drug to use in weaning a patient off intravenous nitroprusside.

There are two instances in which lowering the blood pressure to normal may have undesirable effects. If a patient has malignant hypertension with retinopathy and azotemia, the normalization of the diastolic blood pressure to less than 90 may make the patient anuric and in need of dialysis. If a patient has retinal abnormalities and hypertensive encephalopathy, this temporary loss of glomerulofiltration is warranted in order to protect the vascular beds in the heart and central nervous system from further damage. However, in many instances it is wisest to lower the diastolic blood pressure to between 100 and 110 and reassess the patient over the next several days.

If a patient has localized narrowing of a critical vessel, such as one of the carotid, renal, or mesenteric vessels, lowering the blood pressure to normal after months or years of elevation may bring about severe symptoms of hypoperfusion in the area served by the narrowed vessel. In this instance, it may be wisest to allow the blood pressure to remain slightly elevated in order to prevent tissue ischemia or infarction.

Once blood pressure is acutely controlled, the patient must be evaluated for the cause of hypertension. The most common finding will be that of an exacerbation of longstanding hypertension. However, moderate fluid excess, severe pain, or drugs with moderate vasoconstrictive effects in the presence of left ventricular failure may all cause hypertension. Review of the patient's record for historical or physical evidence of primary aldosteronism, Cushing's disease, renal artery stenosis, coarctation of the aorta, or pheochromocytoma may suggest the diagnosis of a curable form of hypertension. In the case of a pheochromocytoma, a misdiagnosis may lead to repeated hypertensive crises since the patient has constant or intermittent outpouring of catecholamines associated with the stresses of his illness.

CONCLUDING REMARKS

The kidneys interact in a variety of ways in critical illness. Elimination of wastes, excretion of drugs, acid-base balance, and electrolyte problems are variously affected by the normal or abnormal kidney, and especially compounded by disorders in organ, system, and cellular function. A most important priority in the critically ill patient becomes accurate and ongoing assessment of renal function, always mindful of these extraordinarily complex and important interactions.

REFERENCES

1. Corkcroft DW, Gault MH: Prediction of creatinine clearance from serum creatinine. Nephron 16:31, 1976
2. Bennett WM, Porter GA: Endogenous creatinine clearance as a clinical measure of glomerular filtration rate. Br Med J 4:83, 1971
3. Miller TR et al: Urinary diagnostic indices acute renal failure. Ann Intern Med 89:47, 1978
4. Appel GB, Neu HS: Nephrotoxicity of antimicrobial drugs. N Engl J Med 296:663, 1977
5. Berl T et al: Clinical disorders of water metabolism. Kidney Int 10:117, 1976
6. Morris RC et al: Renal acidosis. Kidney Int 1:322, 1972
7. Oh MS et al: The anion gap. N Engl J Med 297:814, 1977
8. Flamenbaum W: Pathophysiology of acute renal failure. Arch Intern Med 131:911, 1973
9. Anderson RJ: Nonoliguric acute renal failure. N. Engl J Med 296:1134, 1977
10. Levinsky NG, Alexander EA: Acute renal failure. In Brenner B, Rector F (eds): The Kidney. Philadelphia: Saunders, 1976

11. Harwood TH: Prognosis for recovery of function in acute renal failure. Arch Intern Med 136:916, 1976
12. Lordon RE, Burton JR: Posttraumatic renal failure in military personnel in Southeast Asia. Am J Med 53:137, 1972
13. Koffer A et al: Acute renal failure due to nontraumatic rhabdomyolysis. Ann Intern Med 85:12, 1976
14. Gutman RA et al: The immune complex glomerulonephritis of bacterial endocarditis. Medicine 8:342, 1972
15. Deftos LJ, Neer, R: Medical management of the hypercalcemia of malignancy. Ann Rev Med 25:323, 1974
16. Goldsmith RS: The differential diagnosis of hypercalcemia. N Engl J Med 274:674, 1966
17. Relman AS, Schwartz WB: Nephropathy of potassium depletion: clinical and pathological entity. N Engl J Med 255:195, 1956
18. Kjellstrand CM et al: Hyperuricemic acute renal failure. Arch Intern Med 133:349, 1974
19. Van Zee BE: Renal injury associated with intravenous pyelography in nondiabetic and diabetic patients. Ann Intern Med 89:51, 1978
20. Kleinknecht D et al: Uremic and nonuremic complications in acute renal failure: Evaluation of early and frequent dialysis on prognosis. Kidney Int 1:190, 1972
21. Abel RM et al: Improved survival from acute renal failure after treatment with intravenous essential 1-amino acids and glucose. N Engl J Med 288:695, 1973
22. Kunau RT, Stein JH: Disorders of hypo- and hyperkalemia. Clin Nephrol 7:173, 1977
23. Fisch C: Relation of electrolyte disturbances to cardiac arrhythmias. Circulation 47:408, 1973
24. Singer I, Forrest JN: Drug induced states of nephrogenic diabetes insipidus. Kidney Int 10:82, 1976
25. Feig PU, McCurdy DK: The hypertonic state, N Engl J Med 297:1444, 1977
26. Rastegar A, Thier SO: Physiologic consequences and bodily adaptations to hyper- and hypocapnia. Chest 62(suppl):28S, 1972
27. McCurdy DK: Mixed metabolic and respiratory acid base disturbances: diagnosis and treatment. Chest 62(suppl):35S, 1972
28. Arbus GS: An in vivo acid base nomogram for clinical use. Can Med Assoc J 109:291, 1973
29. Kurtzman NA: Pathophysiology of metabolic alkalosis. Arch Intern Med 131:702, 1973
30. Tuller MA, Mehdi F: Compensatory hypoventilation and hypocapnea in primary metabolic alkalosis. Am J Med 50:281, 1971
31. Mitchill JH: The effects of acid base disturbances of a cardiovascular and pulmonary function. Kidney Int 1:375, 1972
32. Felig P: Diabetic ketoacidosis. N Engl J Med 290:1360, 1974
33. Heird WC et al: Metabolic acidosis resulting from intravenous alimentation mixtures containing synthetic amino acids. N Eng J Med 257:943, 1972
34. Garella S et al: Severity of metabolic acidosis as a determinant of bicarbonate requirement. N Engl J Med 289:121, 1973
35. Bennett WB et al: Guidance for drug therapy in renal failure. Ann Intern Med 86:754, 1977
36. Adverse interactions of drugs. Med Lett Drugs Ther 19:5, 1977
37. Mitchill JH: Drug induced liver injury. Hosp Pract 13:95, 1978

SIX

Metabolism and Nutrition

George H. Rodman, Jr.

Metabolic derangements when encountered in I.C.U. patients are rarely single or isolated abnormalities but frequently present as multiple disturbances with complex interrelationships. Such abnormalities may result from as well as cause interactive organ dysfunctions. For instance, the acidosis and hyperkalemia of uremic renal failure may have a deleterious effect upon cardiac function which results in further renal damage because of decreased perfusion. Descriptions of "normal" metabolic profiles for the I.C.U. patient must take into account expected compensatory responses to injury or any stress. Furthermore, the I.C.U. population does not have a "normal distribution" in terms of age, body habitus, nutritional status, magnitude of stress, and functional status of physiologic reserve. Since heterogenous patient groups manifest many clinical forms of the same metabolic abnormality, metabolic therapy must be deeply rooted in physiologic mechanisms regulating water and electrolyte balance, energy substrate utilization during stress and starvation, and disturbances of acid-base homeostasis. With such knowledge effective therapeutic goals can be based on (1) surveillance guidelines affecting *preventive* therapy, (2) cooperating with homeostatic mechanisms, and (3) safe, rapid, and maximum therapy designed to limit the duration of established metabolic disorders. The following review of metabolic problems in the I.C.U. is designed to form a framework of knowledge to meet the above therapeutic goals (Table 6-1).

TABLE 6-1
Goals of Metabolic Therapy

Surveillance of body composition
Prevention of major disturbances
Serve homeostasis
Limit and reverse established disorders

BODY COMPOSITION:
WATER AND ELECTROLYTES

Our understanding of body composition and alterations in disease states has been aided greatly by dilution techniques using radioactive isotopes.[1-3] Measurements of total body water, red blood cell volume, plasma volume, intracellular water, total exchangeable sodium, potassium, and chloride are feasible. Although some imprecision still exists in the absolute definitions of the spaces delineated, comparison of results obtained from repeated observations in the same patient have aided our understanding. Other experimental techniques have been developed which measure interstitial and intracellular constituents in vivo in skeletal muscle[4] and kidney, and in vitro studies of tissue slices of brain and liver.[5] Extrapolation to common metabolic problems seen in critically ill patients has improved our clinical care based upon increased physiologic knowledge.

Direct measurements of total body water have been done with dilution techniques utilizing heavy water and various tracer substances. When these substances are injected, they diffuse rapidly throughout the body and across cell membranes, establishing equilibrium within two to three hours (Fig. 6-1). Measuring the resultant concentration allows calculation of the total volume of distribution, in this case, total body water:

$$\text{injectate counts} \times \text{injectate volume} = \text{final counts} \times \text{total body water}$$

or

$$\text{total body water} = \frac{\text{injectate counts} \times \text{injectate volume}}{\text{final counts}}$$

These methods have added basic knowledge particularly to the changes in the extracellular fluid compartment following operation, trauma, or hemorrhage.

Body water is distributed between two compartments, the intracellular and extracellular compartments. The intracellular compartment is twice the size of the ECF, representing about 40 percent (32 liters in an 80-kg adult) of body weight. Thus, the total ECF in this same adult would contain about 16 liters which is divided into plasma water and interstitial water. About 20 percent of the extracellular fluid is plasma

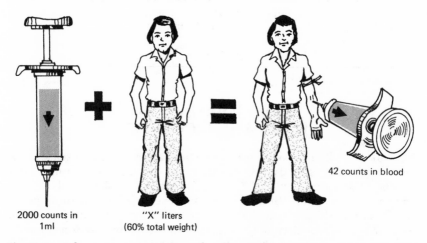

2000 counts in
1ml

"X" liters
(60% total weight)

42 counts in blood

Fig. 6-1. A known concentration of radioactivity in a known volume is injected. After total body equilibration, a blood sample (final sample) is withdrawn. Total volume can be calculated. In the 80-kg patient, total body water would be 48 liters.

volume (3 to 3.5 liters) and 80 percent is interstitial volume (12 to 13 liters). Thus, rapid calculation of plasma volume for adults can be made by estimating plasma volume as 4 percent of ideal weight:

$$0.04 \times 80 \text{ kg} = 3200 \text{ ml of plasma volume}$$

Intravascular fluid exchanges across capillary walls with the interstitial fluid (Fig. 6-2). Interstitial fluid may be pictured as the medium in which the cellular mass is swimming with constant exchange of minerals and nutrients between the intracellular environment and the interstitial compartment. Thus, the delivery or removal of metabolic products from the intracellular space is based on a bidirectional transfer of constituents across the interstitial space sandwiched between the circulation and the cell mass of the body. Such divisions of the body water compartments are arbitrary and best serve as visual aids in interpreting changes in body composition, since they can only represent a static image of a continuously changing medium.

Estimates have been made for exchangeable quantities of total body sodium and potassium.[2] The term "exchangeable" in this instance means the amount of a substance which will participate in the exchange for a radioactive substance. For inactive portions of the body, this amount might be small since active cell mass and extracellular fluid are the most important constituents in terms of pathophysiologic change; exchangeable sodium and potassium *can* be used to represent these areas. Inactive sodium and potassium need not be included in the measurement technique since their activity bears little or no relationship to cell mass and extracellular fluid changes. Calculation of total body sodium in the average 70-kg adult yields about 4000 to 4200 mEq. Of this quantity, about 50 percent is extracellular, 40 percent is associated with bone (of which only one-half is exchangeable), and 10 percent is intracellular. Total body potassium on the other hand can be estimated at about 3200 mEq but its distribution is 98 percent intracellular and only 2 percent extracellular. Thus, the ECF-ICF concentration of the

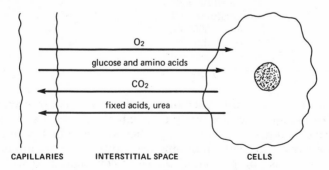

Fig. 6-2. A diagrammatic representation of the interplay of forces across the capillary membrane and the function of the interstitial fluid.

body's two major cations (sodium and potassium) are roughly reversed, sodium being the major extracellular cation and potassium the most abundant intracellular cation. Unlike sodium, almost all potassium is exchangeable and thus, major reductions in total body potassium can occur but are camouflaged by the movement of intracellular potassium to the extracellular fluid compartment without significant changes in measured concentrations of potassium in the plasma compartment of the ECF.

A similar ratio exists for the body's two most abundant anions (chloride and phosphate). Chloride is the principal extracellular anion, with concentration in plasma at approximately 103 mEq/liter while phosphate is the major intracellular anion (140 mEq/liter). Intracellular chloride and extracellular phosphate both measure approximately 2 mEq/liter. Bicarbonate is the other major extracellular anion; it is equally distributed between ECF and ICF and is freely exchangeable (Table 6-2).

TABLE 6-2
Body Composition

Water (60%)
    Extracellular—approximately 20 to 25%
      Intravascular—4 to 5%
      Interstitial—16 to 20%
    Intracellular—40%
Sodium (4000 to 4200 mEq)
    Extracellular—50%
    Bone—40%
    Intracellular—10%
Potassium (3200 mEq)
    Extracellular—2%
    Intracellular—98%
Chloride (2000 mEq)
    Extracellular—99%
    Intracellular—1%
Phosphate (3000 mEq)
    Extracellular—1%
    Intracellular—99%

Such differences in transcellular ionic gradients are present even though cell membranes are freely permeable to these ions. Thus, active ion transport against concentration gradients exists which requires some form of energy to drive the pumping mechanism to maintain ionic gradients. Sodium is pumped out of the cell to evacuate that which leaks in by passive diffusion. This outward pumping of sodium is linked to the inward pumping of potassium. *The maintenance of ionic gradients by energy dependent pumps is vital for the normal metabolic functions of cells.* Certain specialized cellular and organ functions depend on ionic gradients (i.e., gastric HCl production, skeletal muscular contraction, cardiac cell pacemaker activity). Cellular function is impaired when the pumping mechanism is inhibited. Hypoxia and hypothermia (shock) are common inactivators of the sodium/potassium pump.[4]

REGULATION OF FLUID EXCHANGE

Even though the ECF and ICF differ substantially in electrolyte concentration, the concentration of osmotically-active particles is roughly equal between the two compartments. The tendency to maintain osmolar equilibrium has been used therapeutically since changes induced in the plasma osmotic pressure will be mirrored by similar intracellular changes. Osmotic concentration is expressed in terms of osmolarity, i.e., the number of osmotically active particles per liter of solution. Osmotic effect is dependent upon the number of particles, not on their charge or their valence. Thus, plasma proteins, although they are large molecules, exert minimal osmotic effect compared to electrolytes because the number of molecules is so much smaller. Osmotic pressure is measured in osmols. An osmol represents 1 gm molecular weight (mole) of a nondissociating substance such as glucose. Clinically, the unit of concentration employed is the milliosmol (mOsm = 1/1000 osmol).

For electrolyte solutions, osmotic pressure is proportional to the ionic concentration. Thus, for sodium chloride (NaCl) which is completely dissociated and contains two active ions (Na and Cl), one mole exerts an osmotic effect of two osmols when dissolved in 1 liter of water. Since the freezing point of a solution will be depressed proportional to the number of active particles (osmolarity) of the solution, the osmolarity is measured by determining the freezing point depression of body fluids.

Other osmotically active substances normally found in the serum include glucose and urea. One may also calculate serum osmolarity in determined concentrations of sodium, glucose, and urea by the following formula:

$$\text{Serum osmolarity} = (\text{Na} \times 1.86) + \frac{\text{BUN}}{2.8} + \frac{\text{glucose}}{18}$$

when Na is expressed in mEq/liter, BUN and glucose as mg%.

The range of normal osmolarity in the healthy state is 280 to 295 mOsm/liter of water. At the low level (280), ADH release is completely inhibited and urine is maximally diluted (less than 100 mOsm/liter). At the highest (295), maximum urinary concentration occurs in response to ADH release ($\geq$800 to 1000 mOsm/liter of water).

Fluid and electrolyte exchange occurs freely across the capillary walls through pores of a size too small to allow free passage of protein molecules. With a large protein concentration gradient established between the intravascular and the interstitial spaces, total osmotic (electrolyte plus protein) pressure is higher in the plasma than in the interstitial fluid. This tendency to rob the interstium of its water volume is almost exactly counterbalanced by the larger hydrostatic pressure in the capillary. Thus, fluid movement of the capillary level depends on a balance of hydrostatic and osmotic forces across the capillary membrane. Predictions about the net movement of water and ions, but not protein, can be made only if the membrane maintains its selective permeability characteristics. Inflammation, whether local as in cellulitis or systemic as in septicemia, typically disrupts selective permeability of capillary walls with a loss of intravascular water, ions, and protein into the interstitial space until a new equilibrium is reached. In such circumstances, lymphatics which drain the interstitial spaces have an increase in total lymph flow with an increase in protein content. Furthermore, even if the membrane coefficient is changed for permeability, predictions as to direction of water movement must still be based on differences in both plasma as well as interstitial pressure forces—hydrostatic and osmotic. Unfortunately, no clinical assessment exists to measure interstital pressures or osmolarity.

Both the volume and the composition of body fluids is regulated under fairly tight physiologic control. Body water is lost continuously by vaporization from the skin and lungs, as well as in gastrointestinal discharges. The insensible loss (nonsweating) through the skin averages 300 to 500 ml per day for adults, with a similar volume through the lungs. As bodily metabolism increases, so does the rate of insensible water loss (7 percent per degree F increase). Water is supplied to the body by both the intake of food and liquids as well as from endogenous production of metabolic water secondary to oxidation of foodstuffs. Metabolizing 100 calories produces about 10 to 12 gm of water.

To review briefly, the kidney serves as the final regulator of water excretion. It forms about 100 ml of ultrafiltrate each minute while receiving blood flow about 50 times that rate. Of this glomerular filtrate volume, 75 to 85 percent is reabsorbed isosmotically in the proximal renal tubule, thus markedly reducing the volume of filtrate by the time it reaches the loop of Henle. The counter current mechanisms of the medullary interstitium allow for a slight reduction in volume, but more importantly, sodium is actively reabsorbed, thus rendering the tubular fluid hypotonic with respect to plasma. Final control over the ultimate elaboration of dilute versus concentrated urine is governed by the distal renal tubule under hormonal control of antidiuretic hormone (ADH) secreted by the posterior pituitary gland. Variations in osmolarity of extracellular fluids sensed by the osmoreceptors signal ADH secretion. Hyperosmolar conditions (osm ≥ 295) trigger release of ADH resulting in the elaboration of concentrated urine to conserve water and return the osmolarity to normal. Excess water in the ECF (hypotonicity − osm ≤ 280) inhibits ADH release so that dilute urine is excreted. Furthermore, release of ADH is responsive to changes in the volume of the ECF. The hypovolemic state results in an ADH effect on the distal tubule to concentrate urine. Likewise, increases in ECF volume (hypervolemia) allow formation of dilute urine by decreased ADH release. Thus, both *tonicity* and *volume* of the ECF determines ADH secretion; however, tonicity is selectively preserved over volume. Thus, ADH effect on the distal tubule attempts to maintain serum osmolarity in a fairly narrow range of 270 to 285 mOsm. To accomplish this task, urine osmolarity may range from less than 100 to 1400 mOsm. Water excretion, however, is limited by solute delivery, i.e., solute in tubular fluid must be present to allow water excretion. This feature of limiting free water excretion has been translated into a principle which guides fluid management in postoperative patients. Giving large quantities of D5W to postop patients (i.e., solute-free water), can exceed the limits of distal tubule water excretion with serious reductions occurring in the tonicity of ECF.

Sodium excretion varies with the amount of salt filtered by the glomerulus and the amount reabsorbed by the renal tubule. Aldosterone elaborated by the adrenal cortex regulates sodium-potassium exchange in the distal tubule. The adrenal cortex secretes aldosterone when (1) serum potassium is increased, (2) blood pressure is decreased, (3) ACTH is increased, and (4) renin production is increased, secondary to a decreased blood flow to the renal juxtaglomerular apparatus. Any of these stimuli affect the distal tubule by increasing sodium reabsorption in exchange for extruding potassium to the tubular fluid. Of particular clinical relevance is the tight control of water and sodium excretion mediated through aldosterone and ADH secretion and signaled by decreased blood volume or blood pressure. Even though the ECF volume and sodium concentration are regulated carefully by renal tubular mechanism, potassium homeostasis seems to have little priority. Depriving the patient of all potassium intake will not initiate renal potassium conservation. Instead, continued potassium secretion occurs (10 to 20 mEq/liter) in the face of no potassium intake, with the result that significant depletion to the total body potassium stores may occur (Table 6-3).

TABLE 6-3
Fluid Exchange

Osmotic equilibrium across cell membranes but different electrolytes important
Oncotic gradient across capillaries
    Albumin most active but gradient not alterable by therapeutic measures
Antidiuretic hormone inhibited at low osmolarity; therefore, diuresis of free water is provided
Antidiuretic hormone released at high osmolarity; therefore free water conserved
Aldosterone released signals "need" to conserve sodium—shock, fluid losses, renin release, ACTH release
The kidney is the ultimate regulator

METABOLIC ALTERATIONS OF SHOCK

The planned correction of the rearrangement of body fluids and electrolytes in various body departments which occurs in response to injury forms the basis for the modern fluid therapy of shock. When the magnitude of injury is sufficient to produce shock, i.e., 10 percent reduction in blood volume, autoregulatory changes in the peripheral circulation are designed to reestablish circulating blood volume. Transcapillary refill of plasma volume from available interstitial volume partially explains the reduction in ECF which has repeatedly been shown to occur in man in hemorrhagic shock. However, measurements of ECF in shock by analysis of radiosulphate dilution curves also suggest that the decrease in interstitial fluid volume occurring during hemorrhagic shock could not be explained solely by transcapillary refill.[5] By combining ultramicroelectrode measurements of membrane potential with the interstitial fluid analysis of electrolytes, a 10 percent increase in the intracellular volume was found as well. A 10 percent change in intracellular volume means interstitial volume must have been reduced 25 to 30 percent. Subsequent measurements have elucidated the cell membrane dysfunction associated with shock. The cell membrane is permeable to sodium and the energy-requiring, sodium–potassium, ATP-linked pump continuously evacuates sodium from the intracellular environment (Fig. 6-3). But as shock progresses, the pump seems to be unable to keep up with the leakage of sodium in and potassium out of the cell. Furthermore, the transport of substrates, particularly in the form of glucose and normally enhanced by the action of insulin at the cell membrane level, is significantly blunted during shock.[6] Transport is not increased until one adds a dose of insulin equal to 200 times normal. This is termed a relative "insulin resistance."

The high energy phosphate compounds in the liver and kidney decrease substantially in early shock.[5] The skeletal muscle, however, seems to be more resistant; ATP levels do not decrease until the later stages of shock. ATP is regenerated slowly and forms a measure of adequate resuscitation. Thus, hypovolemic shock seems to induce major changes in cellular function in terms of electrical potential, electrolyte concentration, energy, and metabolism. These changes are reversible with appropriate resuscitation. The cell membrane alterations which allow isotonic swelling along with the leakage of potassium are probably related to a reduction in the efficiency of the energy-dependent cell membrane

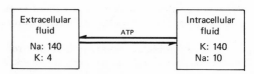

Fig. 6-3. The extracellular environment must be kept separate from the intracellular environment; this can only be maintained by ATP-linked reactions.

pump. Thus, the insult of shock begins at the cell membrane level with an alteration of membrane potential associated with an inability of the sodium–potassium/ATPase pump to keep sodium pumped out of the cell. As energy is wasted by the inefficient pump, cylic AMP and ATP levels decrease. Eventually, mitochondrial swelling occurs with further decrease in ATP production. This reduction in metabolic capability leads to lysosmal breakdown with subsequent cellular destruction. Intracellular products from a single cell may then damage adjoining cells.

Thus, the repair of damaged biochemical functions should be a main objective of shock therapy. The changes which occur in the energy capabilities of subcellular organelles during shock may be totally reversed if shock is not prolonged and resuscitation is complete.

ECF REPLACEMENT

Complete restoration of the ECF deficit produced in the shock state is the most important goal of shock therapy.[7] Total ECF replacement requires replacing interstitial fluid losses as well as normalizing blood volume. Since the magnitude of the ECF deficit correlates most directly with the depth and duration of shock, these patients should require much larger quantities of resuscitative fluid if shock has been prolonged. Rarely do our estimates of fluid requirements correlate with actual quantities ultimately required. An accurate notion of the volume required for resuscitation includes measured ECF losses, internal redistribution of ECF into injured or inflamed areas, intracellular fluid accumulation, as well as the reduction of functional ECF which represents no true anatomic loss. Nevertheless, anatomic overexpansion of the ECF (i.e., weight gain) is a physiologic necessity if the functional ECF deficit is to be completely corrected. Correction of the functional ECF deficit, in addition to replacing shed blood, correlated with improved survival from experimental hemorrhagic shock, when compared to shed blood replacement alone.[8] Furthermore, similar reductions of ECF have become apparent when careful monitoring techniques have been applied to patients in shock from nonhemorrhagic causes, i.e., acute myocardial infarction and sepsis.

ALBUMIN-CONTAINING SOLUTION VERSUS SALT SOLUTION

The choice of balanced electrolyte solution (Ringer's lactate) versus normal saline has never been shown to influence survival from shock as long as adequate quantities of either are given.[8] Controversy arises, however, when discussions turn to the necessity for protein (albumin replacement).[9] Volume for volume, protein-containing solutions will restore intravascular volume to a greater extent than balanced salt solutions. Thus, resuscitation to precise physiologic endpoints with either solution requires a volume of salt solution four to five times greater than contained in protein solutions. Resuscitation with protein-containing solution has been suggested to minimize the accumulation of interstitial pulmonary edema and the occurrence of respiratory insufficiency associated with resuscitation from the shock state. Both clinical and experimental studies fail to demonstrate a protective pulmonary effect of albumin-containing solutions when compared to balanced salt solutions.[10,11] Albumin's apparent advantage, its ability to stay in the intravascular space, actually creates two disadvantages: (1) it will not correct functional ECF deficits and (2) it may result in increased intravascular pressures and so enhance the formation of pulmonary edema, unless invasive cardiovascular monitoring and careful and cautious administration of fluid volumes are employed. This may be difficult in the emergency room and during the initial stages of surgery. By demonstrating no clear physiologic advantage of albumin solutions and some disadvantages, a rational choice of resuscitative fluids based on economics clearly favors balanced salt solutions. Albumin-containing solutions cost $280.00 per liter. Balanced salt solutions cost $10.00 per liter. Thus, the use of balanced salt solutions combined with red cell replacement can be considered the best available means for correcting circulatory failure and restoring the functional extracellular fluid deficit associated with shock.

INTRACELLULAR METABOLISM ENHANCEMENT

Newer advances with the drug therapy of shock include infusions of substances designed to enhance the altered intracellular metabolism and overcome the energy crisis of shock. Associated with the changes in cell membrane potential difference in the shock state is the development of insulin resistance at the cellular membrane.[6] This further limits intracellular substrate utilization and energy production in an otherwise substrate-depleted cell. Ischemic cell damage is thus compounded by relative cell starvation. Salvaging ischemic cells is the goal of glucose-insulin-potassium (G-I-K) infusions.[12] Transcellular migration of glucose and potassium should aid in restoring depleted energy substrate as well as normalizing the intracellular to extracellular ionic gradient. Improvement of cell metabolism and organ function are difficult to demonstrate with such therapy. Nevertheless, enhancement of myocardial contractility has been demonstrated when G-I-K is added to standard resuscitative measures.[13] Although this improvement in myocardial performance has been demonstrated in patients being resuscitated from hemorrhagic and septic shock, clear correlation with improved survival has not been demonstrated. In patients with acute myocardial infarction, the ischemic cells at risk are those in the peri-infarct area of the myocardium. Since survival from infarction-induced cardiogenic shock is determined by the viability of the peri-infarct tissue, attempts made at salvaging these critical myocardial cells with G-I-K therapy has a sound rationale. In experimental animals following coronary artery ligation, G-I-K infusions result in increases in cellular ATP and glycogen content, as well as reduction of the areas of necrosis and ischemia.[14] Thus, the ultimate clinical utility of G-I-K may be limited to those clinical situations in which myocardial function alone determines survival, i.e., acute myocardial infarction. Maximum amounts of G-I-K that could be safely infused in a group of septic patients with circulatory failure, did indeed improve myocardial function.[15] Cardiac index improved and patients were able to be weaned from other cardiotonic agents (dopamine, isuprel, and epinephrine) following 24 hours of G-I-K therapy. Nevertheless, ultimate mortality rates were still excessive (80 percent).

More direct attempts to solve cellular energy crisis of shock by infusing high energy compounds (ATP—$MgCl_2$) have been shown to result in improved survival from hemorrhagic shock in experimental animals.[16] Furthermore, ATP infusion favorably influenced measured energy levels as well as correcting the cellular insulin resistance associated with shock.[17] These same improvements in energy levels and survival occurred after severe sepsis was induced in another experimental situation in which resuscitation included ATP as well as standard resuscitative measures.

Although no clinical application of those energy substances is as yet available, such encouraging results reinforce the concept of shock as a state of energy deprivation. All efforts to support the injured cells in shock, utilizing biochemical manipulations, must be employed at the first signs of failure of more standard forms of resuscitation if they are to be effective (Table 6-4).

TABLE 6-4
Temporal Relationships in Shock Therapy

Immediate—cardiovascular collapse
  Goal—restore intravascular volume
  How—asanguinous balanced electrolytes; replenish red cell mass if necessary
  Monitor—cardiovascular system; assessment indirect if healthy
Continued instability
  Goal—must also resuscitate interstitial volume and replace sodium
  How—balanced electrolyte solutions
  Remember—30–40% deficit may exist = 5–6 liters
  Monitor—Cardiovascular parameters; invasive monitoring preferred; urine volume and sodium; overall clinical assessment
Prolonged insult
  Goal—ischemic cell salvage; enhance intracellular metabolic functions
  How—glucose-insulin-potassium (approximately 400–800 gm of glucose); start with 10 gm per hr and advance; insulin infusion to regulate sugar, potassium supplements
  Monitor—dextrostix/blood sugars every hr; add 10 U insulin/100 mg blood sugar; reduce sugar load if 100 U of insulin cannot control blood sugar (> 500 mg/dl) in 4–6 hours
  Potassium—4.5–5; caution should be used if renal function is poor or expected to worsen

DISORDERS OF SODIUM HOMEOSTASIS

Cell membranes are more or less impermeable to most solutes but freely permeable to water. Therefore, ECF and ICF osmolarity equalizes despite very different solute composition. Major osmotic solutes in the ICF are potassium, magnesium, organic phosphates, and protein. In the ECF, sodium, and its anions, chloride and bicarbonate, are the major osmotic constituents. The intracellular compartment contains about two-thirds of all the body's osmotic solutes, whereas one-third is in the ECF. Water distributes to equalize osmolarity between these two compartments. It follows, therefore, that two-thirds of body water is ICF and one-third is ECF. Thus, ICF volume is determined by ECF tonicity.

Hypertonic states have an increased concentration of impermeable ECF solutes and net ICF volume depletion. Thus, increases in the ECF osmolarity result in dehydration of the intracellular fluid compartment. High urea levels and ethanol may raise plasma osmolality but do not cause a decrease in ICF since they distribute evenly in total body water and exert no lasting osmotic pressure gradient across cell membranes. Nevertheless, they are common causes of increased osmolarity. Mannitol-induced hypertonicity is not due to mannitol itself, but to the hypernatremia which results from hypotonic diuresis.

The brain is structurally vulnerable to the acute dehydration that may result from acute increase in ECF osmolarity. Severe shrinking of the brain moves it away from the calvarium and can tear surface vessels with resulting hemorrhages. However, the brain ICF will reverse outward water flow, increasing intracellular solutes over time, i.e., an *adaptation*. During acute hypernatremia, brain shrinking develops initially but is reversed in seven days. In acute hyperglycemia, on the other hand, the response occurs within hours. Thus, if adaptation has occurred in the face of increased plasma osmolarity, returning plasma to normal suddenly by rapid infusion of hypotonic solutions may result in sudden expansion of intracellular fluid water. Deterioration of the sensorium or the appearance of neurologic signs during rapid correction of hypertonic states strongly suggests that this mechanism has been activated.

Hypertonicity can occur from either net water loss or net gain of impermeable solutes. Both are associated with hypertonicity of all body fluids and intracellular fluid volume depletion. Clinically, however, water loss or solute addition rarely occur as isolated events. For example, hyperglycemia caused by addition of glucose as an extra solute also causes osmotic diuresis and excessive losses of both water and sodium. Hyperglycemia dehydrates most cells and produces a predictable hyponatremia due to the intracellular fluid to extracellular water shift. Sodium should fall 1.3 to 1.6 mEq/liter for every 100 mg% glucose present in the plasma.

The treatment of the hypertonic state has three objectives: (1) to replace deficits, (2) to match intercurrent losses, and (3) to decrease the losses as soon as possible. Estimates of the total body water deficit which must be corrected can be approximated closely enough by the following formula to initiate therapy:

$$\text{water deficit} = 0.6 \times \text{TBW} \times \left(1 - \frac{140}{\text{Na}}\right)$$

where TBW = 60 percent body weight; normal plasma Na = 140 mEq/liter. The water deficit should be corrected depending on the severity of the dehydration and the patient's response, since replacing water losses too rapidly runs the risk of producing "isotonic water intoxication." Rapid correction should be attempted only in extreme deficits and the neurologic response must be closely monitored. For example, normal total body water is 40 liters. If a patient has already lapsed into coma with plasma sodium at 180 mEq/liter, one could calculate that the theoretical water loss is 9 liters. One could initiate therapy by rapidly replacing the first half of the deficit. Full correction should only be attempted in one to two days. If neurologic impairment initially improves but then suddenly deteriorates, cerebral edema should be suspected even if the plasma sodium and osmolality remain above normal. If signs of increased intracranial pressure (funduscopic exam) are detected, the water administration should be stopped. One might even recreate the hyperosmolar state by the addition of hypertonic saline or mannitol until signs of cerebral edema improve (Table 6-5).

Hyperglycemia can occur secondary to total parenteral nutrition (TPN): the syndrome of hyperosmolar, hyperglycemic nonketosis (HHNK). This may also occur in some diabetics without the development of true ketoacidosis (DKA).[18] Glucose normally spills into the urine when plasma glucose exceeds 160 to 180 mg%. In this syndrome, plasma glucose has been measured as high as 2000 mg%. Therapy for HHNK differs from DKA primarily in the insulin dosages required. Since ECF loss is significant, treatment should include ECF expansion and low dose insulin therapy. The initial insulin dose rarely exceeds 50 U for the first 24 hours.

Increased antidiuretic hormone (ADH) activity results in a number of important clinical situations in critically ill patients. Bioassay measurements have demonstrated a prompt increase in ADH activity in blood of patients undergoing major surgery.[19] In hyponatremic patients with congestive heart failure, excess ADH activity has been demonstrated to seriously limit free water formation in response to water loading. Furthermore, alcohol may suppress ADH activity resulting in a massive—and physiologically "appropriate"—postoperative diuresis if emergency surgery has been performed in a patient who has ethanol intoxication.

A serum sodium concentration ≤120 mEq/liter can cause many symptoms, including anorexia, nausea and vomiting, irritability, personality changes, and confusion. A serum sodium of 100 mEq/liter is associ-

TABLE 6-5
Hypertonic State

Causes
  Water losses—evaporation, burns, dehydration, G.I. losses
  Solute accumulation—diabetes, TPN, inappropriate fluid-electrolyte therapy,
    failure to conserve water in kidneys, excess load location content of antibiot-
    ics, hypertonic tube feedings
Objectives for Treatment
  Replace deficits
  Match intercurrent losses
  Decrease further losses
Calculations
  Assume total body water = 60% body weight
  Normal serum Na = 140 mEq/liter

$$\text{Deficit} = 0.6 \times \text{TBW} \times \left(1 - \frac{140}{\text{Na}}\right)$$

Correction
  Rapid—planned only with neurologic changes; one-half deficit over 3–6 hr; full
    correction in 2 days
  Prolonged—no neurologic, cardiovascular, or renal impairment; 1–2 days
Monitor
  Na and osmolarity every 4 to 6 hr; invasive cardiovascular monitoring may
    be necessary in multisystem illness
Caution
  Cerebral edema may result from excessively rapid corrective measures

---

ated with advanced neurologic abnormalities such as decreased reflexes,
positive Babinski sign, stupor, and convulsions. Simultaneous reduction
in serum chloride also occurs.

Patients with inappropriate ADH syndrome (IADHS) often do not
correct the decreased serum sodium even when large quantities of sodium are administered (400 to 800 mEq/day).[20] Prompt renal excretion
of sodium follows slight increases in serum sodium and this therapy—
sodium administration—usually produces only transient correction. Increased ADH excretion has been associated with malignant tumors
(lung, duodenum, pancreas) as well as head injuries and intracranial
tumors.[20] A urine, less than maximally dilute, in the presence of plasma
hypotonicity, provides clear evidence that there is a defect in free water
excretion. In patients with head injury, as the acute phase of the disease
has subsided or disappeared, the syndrome of inappropriate ADH excretion also promptly disappears.

Unfortunately, most severe reductions in serum sodium (hyponatremia) in the I.C.U. patient still occur as a result of inappropriate fluid
management (Fig. 6-4). Severe sodium restriction in patients with compromised cardiovascular, renal, and hepatic function is frequently advo-

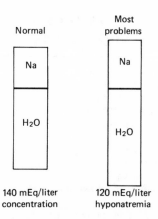

Fig. 6-4. The most common abnormality is dilutional hyponatremia with increased total body sodium and markedly increased total body water.

cated during acute illness. Consequently, sodium-free I.V. solutions (D5W) when given in volumes usually considered moderate (2 to 3 liters/ day) produce dilutional hyponatremia and progressive signs of water retention. The compromised kidney has difficulty effecting an appropriate free water diuresis in response to plasma hypotonicity, even if plasma volume is increased. The mistaken belief that elevated *total* body sodium (cirrhosis, CHF) demands complete sodium restriction *under all* circumstances, confuses daily maintenance of the ECF in the "compensated" state with the obligatory requirement to *replace* ECF losses after injury or stress. Complete restoration of ECF deficits in these patients requires balanced electrolyte solutions—*not* sodium restriction—particularly if ECF losses have been considerable (i.e., pancreatitis, trauma, UGI hemorrhage, shock, prolonged intra-abdominal surgery). A decrease in functional extracellular space produces a hypovolemic response which entails water conservation. Activation of the renin-angiotensin mechanism via release of aldosterone results in renal retention of sodium and water. Renal water retention is also induced because of increased ADH activity, reflecting the response to decrease ECF volume despite a decrease in plasma osmolarity. Hypotonic infusions of D5W or D5½NS further aggravate this situation. An infusion of balanced salt solution does not increase renal sodium retention.

Furthermore, the simultaneous administration of vasopressin and water can produce a syndrome exactly similar to IADHS. Since peripheral vasopressin is commonly employed to control gastrointestinal bleeding in portal hypertension and sodium intake is usually restricted in these same patients who often have coexisting ascites, the incidence of iatrogenic "inappropriate ADH syndrome" is probably many times greater than the naturally occurring phenomena (Table 6-6).

TABLE 6-6
Hypotonic State

Causes
Inappropriate I.V. orders (free water excess)
Cirrhosis, ascites, and water loading
Inability of kidney to excrete free water
Isotonic losses/hypotonic replacement
"Inappropriate ADH"
Objectives for treatment
Raise osmolarity by decreased input
Encourage free water clearance
Restore concentration (sodium) if symptomatic
Calculations
Assume total body water = 60% body weight
Normal serum sodium = 140 mEq/liter
Estimate normal body weight

$$\text{Excess} = 0.6 \times \text{NBW} \times \left(1 - \frac{140}{\text{Na}}\right)$$

Correction
Restrict fluid input; use small volumes of normal saline
Encourage hypotonic urine diuresis
    Mannitol 12.5 to 25 gm
    "Loop" diuretics—hypotonic urine usually will result (urine Na ≤ 70 mEq/
        liter)
Administer 3% NaCl (approximately 500 mEq/liter); restores concentration of
    sodium by increasing total body sodium relative to increased water
Monitoring
Serum and urine electrolytes every 4 to 6 hours during acute therapy
Serum and urine osmolarity to check effectiveness of therapy
State of consciousness and invasive cardiovascular monitoring in severe states
    and multisystem disorders
Cautions
Hypertonic saline may overload intravascular volume
Rapid changes can produce severe cerebral fluid shifts and neurologic changes
Hyponatremia, untreated, will further impair renal function and lead to frank
    renal failure

PHYSIOLOGIC RESPONSE TO STRESS

The metabolic and endocrine factors in the physiologic response to stress
or injury are closely interrelated and are subject to complex influences
which must be studied at the cellular level if mechanisms are to be
manipulated effectively when severe alterations in the metabolic cellular functions occur. The metabolic response to trauma, as the clinical
model of the body's response to acute severe stress, has been studied
extensively and is one of the most complex pathophysiologic events that
can occur in the human organism. Early studies of gross changes in

the body as a whole have been replaced by a modern approach which elucidates disordered cellular processes. Understanding the endocrine and metabolic consequences of injury or any severe stress lays the framework for developing a sound approach for treatment of disordered cellular metabolism.

The effects on energy pathways may be the common denominator to all types of human injury or stress. Understanding alterations of energy balance in I.C.U. patients is based on understanding (1) the body's response to acute starvation, (2) the body's response to acute stress, and (3) the combinations of the two which produce some of the more serious metabolic cellular alterations that limit complete restoration of organ function in the critically ill patient.

The body cell mass which constitutes 40 percent of the total body weight includes the lean body tissues active in energy metabolism. The remaining 60 percent is fat, ECF, transcellular water, and extracellular solids. This latter component functions to support the body cell mass.

The unstressed 70-kg adult requires about 1800 calories per day to maintain vital physiologic functions.[21] All cellular functions are dependent on the body's ability to take fuel substrate and convert potential energy to stored energy in the form of high energy phosphate bonds (ATP). Energy expended during the biochemical and mechanical activities of daily living is then provided by ATP.

$$\text{fuel substrates} \xrightarrow{\text{oxidation}} \begin{array}{c}\text{ATP energy}\\\text{and heat}\end{array} \longrightarrow \begin{array}{c}\text{physiologic}\\\text{functions}\end{array}$$

The three available fuel substrates are carbohydrate (glucose), fat (fatty acids), and protein (amino acids). Body stores of these three major fuel substrates form an emergency energy supply. The common pathway for the conversion of foodstuffs to energy is the TCA (tricarboxylic acid) or Krebs cycle. The adult patient has about 1200 calories of carbohydrates stored as glycogen, whereas stored fat and protein represents approximately 140,000 and 25,000 calories of potential energy, respectively. Since the unstressed daily requirements for energy is 1800 calories per day, it is obvious that the storage forms of carbohydrates provide energy for only a short period. During starvation, an alternate energy source is required. Triglycerides may be hydrolyzed to glycerol and free fatty acids. Glycerol is primarily converted to glucose in the liver but accounts for only a small fraction of daily energy requirement. Oxidation of fatty acids yields both abundant energy (9 cal/gm) and ketone bodies—a marker for adapted starvation. Thus, simple starvation is basically a protein-conserving state where body tissues are maintained as long as possible while satisfying the demands for energy fuel for vital functions. Protein, of course, is present as a structural and functional component of body cell mass. A perfectly efficient metabolic system would entirely utilize fat and preserve protein in times of starvation when the glycogen storage has been depleted.

However, due to metabolic "imperfections," structure and function are sacrified for energy. Thus, the clinical manifestation of simple starvation progressively shows the effects of body cell mass erosion, i.e., protein depletion. Musculature is depleted and intercostal and diaphragm muscles are wasted which leads to hypoventilation and ultimately to pneumonia. Furthermore, protein-depleted systems, such as antibody synthesis, are impaired. With the continued protein drain associated with simple starvation, it is clear that a previously healthy patient with reasonable protein stores tolerates this daily protein depletion longer than the poorly nourished patient subjected to starvation. Unfortunately, the I.C.U. patient often is drawn from the latter group (Table 6-7).

TABLE 6-7
Stress Response

Energy balance depends upon
Response to starvation
Stress response
Metabolic adjustments
Calorie sources
Carbohydrate stores—1200 cal
Fat stores—140,000 cal
Protein stores—25,000 cal
Limitations
Fat mobilization impaired
Carbohydrate stores limited
Protein burning wastes body cell mass

THE REGULATORS

The regulation of utilization (combustion versus storage) of the three fuels described above is determined by a complex interrelation of various hormones. Insulin seems to be the central hormone initially because it controls glucose for the utilization and production of energy—but it also exerts effects on fat cells and liver cells to promote the storage of glucose in the form of glycogen or fat. Insulin favors anabolic functions encouraging the incorporation of amino acids into protein. The insulin-deficient state, on the other hand, causes the reverse effects and rather than augmenting substrate storage and protein synthesis, the insulin-deficient environment is the body's signal to mobilize its substrates. Insulin deficiency favors *proteolysis*. Some by-products of protein oxidation at skeletal muscle level, like alkaline, may be shunted to the liver where deamination of alanine yields pyruvate, which by "reverse" glycolysis, forms new glucose. This process of glucose formation from protein is called *gluconeogenesis* (new formation of glucose). The insulin-deficient state also promotes *lipolysis* so that fat oxidation of fatty acids becomes the main energy-yielding mechanism.

Affected Tissues	Insulin's Blocking Functions	Insulin's Enhancing Functions
Fat cells	↓ Lipolysis	↑ Fat synthesis
Liver	↓ Glycogenolysis	↑ Glycogen storage
Lean body mass	↓ Gluconeogenesis	↑ Protein synthesis

The metabolic marker of the insulin deficient state is the appearance of ketones in the blood and urine. Therefore, when no carbohydrate is being consumed, insulin levels in the blood fall and the body must utilize its abundant fat stores to supply its energy requirements (except for the necessity of glucose to satisfy those cells which cannot immediately convert to fat utilization—brain, RBCs, WBCs, macrophages, fibroblasts). In the starvation-induced insulin deficiency state, the body will still use exogenous glucose and gluconeogenesis is no longer needed. If the glucose or calorie load is sufficient to meet the stress state and still provide extra calories, the proteolysis stops altogether and protein synthesis begins again. Thus, the starving man solves the energy crisis which results from inadequate exogenous substrate provision by shifting to the utilization of endogenous energy stores. The metabolic regulator which signals this "adaptation" process seems to be low circulating insulin levels.

Thus, insulin may be viewed as having a dual function, i.e., "feeding and fasting," which are dose-dependent. Exerting *feeding* function at normal or elevated insulin levels, glucose is transported across cell membranes and simultaneously discourages lipolysis, proteolysis, and glycogenolysis. As insulin levels fall, associated with carbohydrate deprivation (fasting function) some degree of lipolysis and gluconeogenesis begins. However, since insulin levels in the blood never get to "0" levels, some "rate control" of proteolysis and gluconeogenesis still exists. In other words, only a few microunits per ml of insulin stand between widespread catabolism and mild but well-tolerated catabolic protein destruction. Thus, the diabetic (severe insulin deficiency) loses the regulatory balance of feeding and fasting. This, basically, is the definition of ketoacidosis, the rapid catabolism which occurs in the diabetic due to insulin deficiency that is not regulated to within tolerable limits. The simulation of this state is the nondiabetic nonstressed person. The stressed patient does not "obey" these rules.

THE STRESS RESPONSE

After severe stress (injury or infection) afferent stimuli are transmitted to the brain to indicate that tissue damage and/or microbiologic invasion has occurred. These signals set into motion an integrated neurohormonal response that results in metabolic alterations programmed to aid host defense and facilitate tissue repair. The magnitude of these signals depends primarily on the extent of stress; the tissue response may be modulated by physiologic and nutritional reserves as well as the underlying disease processes.

A variety of circulating substances may mediate the hypermetabolic response associated with stress. Bacterial exo- or endotoxins, cell breakdown products and endogenous pyrogens, are capable of providing the initial metabolic signal which leads to substrate mobilization and the energy alterations which characterize the stress response.

The hormonal pattern of severe stress dictates the regulation and choice of metabolic fuels for the energy needs of the body. After injury, hormones that stimulate the mobilization of body fluids are increased relative to circulating insulin levels which normally regulates storage of body fuels. Increased levels of glucagon, corticoids, and growth hormone signal, along with catecholamines, a pattern of mobilization of substrates with a strong stimulus toward gluconeogenesis by the liver.

Catecholamine levels are elevated with stress and seem to correlate with the hypermetabolic state.[22] In burn patients who are severely stressed, α- and β-blockade or β-blockade alone result in a consistent decrease in the metabolic rate. In fact, further evidence stresses the importance of autonomic mediators. Autonomic reserves in the form of catecholamine stores can act as neurotransmitters, if necessary, if the body can continue to maintain the required metabolic level in the face of continuing challenges of repetitive stresses (infection and hemorrhage). In patients dying from severe stress or injury, catecholamine stores have been depleted from the adrenal medulla, sympathetic nerve endings, sympathetic ganglia, and heart stores of catecholamine. Energy replenishing is thus more important than suggested by mere body energy requirements.

Although all the hormonal interactions are important, the primary regulatory substances that determine mobilization or storage of body fuels appear to be catecholamines and insulin.

Insulin appears central to the regulation of skeletal muscle protein metabolism; relative changes of plasma insulin levels are associated with either amino muscle acid uptake or release. Consequently, low circulating insulin levels combined with the high circulating catabolic hormones dictate that skeletal muscles must mobilize amino acids.

Studies of thyroid hormone in severely catabolic, critically ill patients show a pattern of decreased T4 (thyroxin) and decreased T3 (triiodothyronine) while reverse T3 concentrations were elevated.[23] All of these responses occurred while TSH levels remained normal. The appearance of reversed T3 in patients with complicated illnesses suggests that it is associated with the catabolic process and, along with its precursor amino acids (tyrosine and phenylalanine), serves as a metabolic marker of body catabolism.

The mechanism and mediators of increased glucose flux after severe stress have been clarified recently. Cahill's studies show that glucose-dependent tissue gets glucose from transport of alanine to the liver as well as from gluconeogenesis.[24] Because glycogen stores are limited and fatty acids cannot be converted to new glucose, this flow of alanine provides an ongoing supply of glucose at the expense of body protein. The same sequence occurs with infection and any physiologic stress; the only difference is the magnitude of stress, gluconeogenesis, and protein depletion.

Fibroblasts, leukocytes, and new epithelial cells are all glycolytic. Thus, increased hepatic glucose production resulting from injury serves as a primary fuel source for healing wounds. When glucose is oxidized, it must be replaced by amino acids that are mobilized from the skeletal muscle and transported to the liver to serve as additional gluconeogenic precursors (Fig. 6-5). Alanine is an important precursor. The nitrogen residue thus formed (when alanine is converted to pyruvate) is processed in the liver to form urea, which is subsequently secreted in the urine. Therefore, the rate of gluconeogenesis is related closely to ureagenesis.

The observed glucose intolerance after severe stress of trauma or surgery, even in nondiabetic subjects, is not due to decreased glucose utilization or availability. The glucose pool size and glucose turnover have been shown to be doubled in severely stressed patients studied by Long.[25] Increased growth hormone and cortisol levels and glucagon levels as well as catecholamine levels result in an increased rate of gluconeogenesis. This amounted to a loss of 60 gm of lean body mass protein per day. This loss occurred despite the infusion of 200 gm of glucose I.V. per 24 hours—unlike the situation in normal nonstressed subjects in whom similar glucose infusions almost completely stops gluconeogenesis. Maximal suppression of gluconeogenesis can only be realized when portal vein insulin levels are adequate to suppress hepatic gluconeogenesis (directly related to peripheral insulin levels), lipolysis, and proteolysis. The therapeutic implication of this as a guideline for nutritional management is clear. Glucose and amino acids introduced

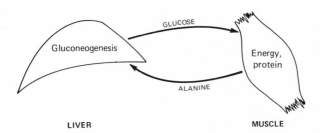

Fig. 6-5. The mobilization of skeletal amino acids and then subsequent transformation into glucose mediated by hepatic cells. Protein oxidation results in an energy salvage mechanism whereby the products of oxidation (alanine) are converted to "new" glucose in the liver. This new glucose is then available as energy substrate for muscle.

into the plasma by the intravenous route produce a much smaller rise in insulin than when the same amount is supplied orally.

Thus, differences between starvation and the metabolic sequences associated with adaptation versus the metabolic responses mediated by stress become very clear. The stress response of injury, mediated through catecholamine secretion, suppresses insulin release as well as creates a peripheral insulin resistance at the skeletal muscle. Although the energy fuel deficit created after injury in the starving man is similar to starvation in the sense that a relative insulin deficiency is created, he cannot call upon the same mechanisms used in true starvation. In simple starvation, the depressed glucose levels result in insulin suppression. In the immediate stress response, elevated catecholamine levels promote the insulin deficient environment. Furthermore, unlike the simple starvation state, the stress state of massive injury is not altered by minimal glucose loading. Proteolysis, fat oxidation, and the lack of protein synthesis are all immediate stress responses governed by the hormonal profile of stress. Catecholamines and glucagon provide a strong glycogenolytic stimulus and oxidation of fat is increased secondary to the lipolytic effects of catecholamines. Glucocorticoids and growth hormone antagonize the peripheral action of insulin leading to a sacrifice of lean muscle tissue in favor of maintaining adequate levels of free amino acids for visceral protein synthesis and energy fuel substrates. This hormonal interplay results in peripheral protein catabolism and gluconeogenesis. Thus, the other hormones secreted as part of the stress response do, in these very high levels, just what insulin does at very low levels. The net effect of this hormonal environment after stress results in raising circulating substrates, although they are inefficiently utilized.

The cumulative effect of proteolysis and gluconeogenesis which occurs after injury depends on the amount and the duration of insulin

TABLE 6-8
Stress Versus Starvation

Catecholamines continue to be released
Insulin response diminished
Peripheral insulin resistance
Increased cortisol
High growth hormone levels
Increased glucagon
Fat mobilization impaired
Increased proteolysis and gluconeogenesis
Magnitude of stress quantified by extent of proteolysis (negative nitrogen balance); in severe stress, there is substrate selection—glucose preferred; protein sacrificed; fat stores unavailable

suppression, which is proportional to the magnitude and duration of the stress. Those events which maintain elevated catecholamine levels (hypovolemia and infection) thus lengthen the duration of the acute protein catabolic state. If proteolysis continues, protein depletion exerts its widespread effects by promoting weakness, impairment of wound healing, impairment of bowel function, and probably most importantly the promotion of infection by interfering with immune mechanisms. In time, if the stress abates and catecholamine levels diminish, the body begins to adapt just as in simple starvation to a more efficient utilization of endogenous fat stores as its main energy source. The preference for glucose burning associated with stress, give way to the fat-burning state. Thus, the acute phase characterized by an obligate protein catabolism utilizing small quantities of fat for energy source, converts to the adaptive phase characterized by fat catabolism and minimal protein catabolism (Table 6-8).

The fact that the body can make these adjustments to solve its energy problems immediately after injury, prevents a quick death. But the rate-limiting step which allows this protein-conserving state to develop depends upon the catecholamine level which, in turn, depends upon the magnitude and duration of the physiologic stress. Thus, the biggest difference between simple starvation and that complicated by stress may be considered to be the failure to adapt to a more efficient protein-conserving state of endogenous fat burning as a major source of energy (Fig. 6-6).

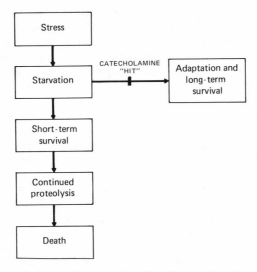

Fig. 6-6. The metabolic and hormonal milieu dictated by the perceived bodily stress determine the primeval but also antiquated bodily response: an unalterable metabolic "fact of life" in the I.C.U. patient.

QUANTIFICATION OF ENERGY AND PROTEIN BALANCE

One clinical measure of the energy crisis of massive stress is to estimate the magnitude of proteolysis by nitrogen balance. If there is no nitrogen intake, then the excreted nitrogen reflects the amount of proteolysis. True calculation of nitrogen balance requires careful analysis of total collections of all excreted body fluids. But for clinical use, an estimate can easily be made by quantitating the amount of urinary nitrogen excretion. In this sense, the amount of urea nitrogen excreted for 24 hours can be an indicator of the severity of hypermetabolism in stress conditions. One gm of nitrogen is derived from 6.25 gm protein; 1 gm protein can be derived from 32 gm of muscle. If the patient excretes 16 gm of nitrogen over a 24-hour period with no nitrogen intake, he has lost 512 gm or 1.1 lb of muscle ($16 \times 32 = 512$). Excreted urinary nitrogen, chiefly in the form of urea, comprises 70 percent of the body's total daily excretion. Ammonia, uric acid, creatinine, amino acids, and some peptides make up the rest. A close approximation of daily nitrogen losses can then be made by measuring a 24-hour urine volume and concentration of urea. Multiplication of volume and urea concentration yields 24-hour urinary urea output. By adding a constant (3.5 gm) to account for nonurinary nitrogen losses (gut), total daily nitrogen losses can be quantified. It is not unusual to find nitrogen losses after moderate injury or stress to be 10 gm/day. If stress is severe, these losses reflect an increased protein catabolism and may reach levels of 15, 20, and even 25 gm nitrogen loss/day.

The attributing of positive nitrogen balance to protein synthesis, however, is limited by the interpretation of "clinical" nitrogen balance. As a rule, nitrogen intake is overestimated and output underestimated. In the majority of instances, nitrogen balance calculations represent relatively small differences between large intake and large output; therefore, small errors in intake and output result in large errors in balance measurement.

Kinney has shown that a reasonable approximation of energy expenditures can be predicted based on clinical state and body size.[26] For the 70-kg adult, resting caloric expenditures are about 1800 kcal/day. Energy requirement increases no more than 10 percent after elective surgery (herniorrhaphy, cholecystectomy, gastrectomy). However, the *mild* catabolism of trauma which is represented by multiple fractures results in a 25 percent increase (2200 kcal) above baseline. *Moderate* catabolism (peritonitis) accounts for a 50 percent incremental increase (2700 kcal) while *severe* catabolism of large surface thermal injury may result in doubling (3600 kcal) of resting energy expenditures (Fig. 6-7).

Kinney's studies analyzed the rate of metabolic expenditure by analyzing the production of CO_2 and oxygen utilization. His reports indicate that severe stress impairs those very mechanisms which could minimize protein breakdown and nitrogen excretion. He found that nitrogen excretion increased dramatically even when fat mobilization should have

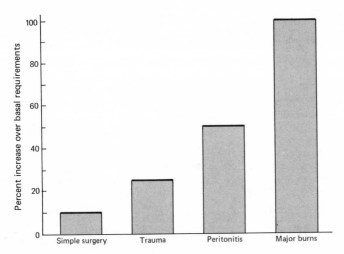

Fig. 6-7. Energy requirements above basal (1800 cal/day) in stressed patients. These figures can be used as baseline determinations in calculating caloric administration.

been adequate for the energy demands of the body. Thus, the increase in protein catabolism is not primarily generated to meet the energy needs, but to provide precursors for hepatic gluconeogenesis which persists at a high rate despite elevated blood glucose. In prolonged unstressed fasting, substrate availability appears to be the major factor determining the rate of proteolysis and hepatic gluconeogenesis. Provision of exogenous glucose will suppress gluconeogenesis in normal patients, but not in the severely stressed.

The basic distinction, therefore, between stress and simple starvation may be defined as substrate selection based on hormonal balance—significant immediately, but not for long-term survival. Where anti-insulin hormones predominate, proteolysis, gluconeogenesis, lipolysis, and glycogenolysis prevail (Fig. 6-8). During the stress response, cells respond by creating nutrients from endogenous sources instead of taking them up to continue basic metabolic functions. Teleologically, this response seems acutely appropriate because it is designed to meet sudden increase in substrate requirements during brief emergency situations. For the I.C.U. patient, the duration of the stress response exceeds metabolic reserves; although this response is initially helpful, the continuation of the stress-metabolic profile becomes a considerable liability. Unrelenting proteolysis eventually takes a serious toll on important functional as well as on structural components of the body.

If stress remains severe, then the loss of secretory or visceral proteins occurs fairly rapidly (Fig. 6-9). Serum albumin and transferrin, the iron-binding protein, have been suggested as markers of severity of this protein depletion process.[27] Albumin concentrations <3.5 gm% and transfer-

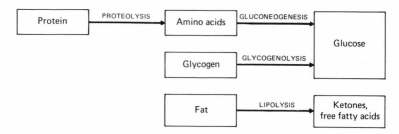

Fig. 6-8. Anti-insulin hormone milieu promotes creation of nutrients from endogenous substrates. This affects short-term survival. Energy requirements of prolonged stress state make this mechanism a form of "internal cannibalism."

rin levels of <220 mg% represent values lower than normal. Likewise, delayed cutaneous hypersensitivity to recall previously "identified" antigens may reflect a significant decrease in visceral protein functions. Inability to respond (anergy) with a 15 mm skin enduration after the placement of a variety of antigens—PPD, mumps, Candida, Varidase (streptokinase and streptodornase), and Trichophyton—correlates with high sepsis rates and high mortality.[28] Functional neutrophil defects (chemotaxis) coexist with anergy when immune testing is performed in surgical patients.[29] Reversal of anergy, when possible, correlates with return of neutrophil function to normal. Lymphocyte (anergy) as well as neutrophil (chemotaxic) functions, even have clearly separable immune functions. Nevertheless, the absence of one (anergy) correlates with defects in the other (neutrophils) in critically ill persons.

How severe stress interferes with the immune responses has not been clearly identified. However, infection appears to be the specific responsible factor for sequential organ system failure and death in I.C.U. patients—and would seem to be linked to the deficit immune response.

The degree of the immune impairment associated with severe stress can be directly correlated with the magnitude of injury or the nutritional

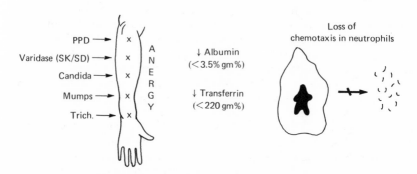

Fig. 6-9. Markers of severe depletion in stress. Note anergy to five common skin antigens—usually 2 to 3 positive. Decrease in certain proteins and loss of chemotaxis can be determined in the laboratory.

defect.[29] It is also possible that severe bacterial sepsis aggravates the nutritional deficit by increasing catabolism, decreasing tissue macrophage activity, and further decreasing resistance to infection, therefore potentiating a vicious cycle of nutritional drain and advancing sepsis.

By understanding the hormonal pattern of severe stress, it becomes easier to see how anabolism can be induced by exogenous infusions of protein and calories in the form of carbohydrates, despite continuing stress. By endogenously inducing or exogenously providing a hyperinsulin state, the stress response can be effected. Under insulin effect, amino acids are taken up instead of mobilized in gluconeogenesis.

INDUCTION OF ANABOLISM

Rx	Effect
Glucose	↑ Energy
Amino acids	↑ New protein
Insulin	↓ Gluconeogenesis,
	↑ glucose utilization,
	↓ lipolysis

Hyperinsulinemia during a stressful period, necessary to counterbalance the sum of anti-insulin hormones, will go unopposed if the stress is suddenly relieved with the rapid decrease of endogenous anti-insulin hormones; exogenous insulin requirements will decrease as the stress decreases and must be adjusted accordingly if severe hypoglycemia is to be avoided.

The importance of insulin as a regulator of the rate of gluconeogenesis, in addition to its primary role of promoting glucose utilization, was highlighted in studies of patients who were moderately to severely catabolic (≥ 15 gm urea production/day).[30] These patients all received the same amount of protein per day (10 gm of nitrogen in the form of essential amino acids). Glucose alone was marginally more protein sparing than a regimen containing Intralipid. For those who excreted less than 15 gm of urea per day, i.e., mild-to-moderate catabolism, the addition of insulin did not affect nitrogen excretion. Therefore, insulin has an important protein-sparing effect in the severely ill patient but little effect when the catabolic rate is not increased.

In addition to the types of calories and insulin effects, gluconeogenesis may also be regulated by the nitrogen source itself. Branch-chained amino acids (valine, leucine, and isoleucine) are unique, in that they represent a direct source of energy for muscle. This energy source is vital for skeletal muscles after glycogen has been depleted and particularly in light of the ill-defined intracellular block to utilize carbohydrates effectively (sepsis). Furthermore, branched-chain amino acids may somehow regulate the rate of muscle breakdown of protein. It has been possible in both animals and humans to demonstrate a decreased release of endogenous amino acids by providing a solution high in calories and, especially, with increased quantities of branched-chain amino acids.[31,32] Fischer further suggests that utilization of branched-chain amino acids in muscles is increased in sepsis, while associated hepatic dysfunction results in an accumulation of the aromatic amino acids. Whereas glucose does not influence gluconeogenesis in sepsis, the administration of branched-chain amino acids decreases gluconeogenesis by offering muscle an alternate energy substrate and thereby inhibiting amino acid efflux from the muscle.[33]

Thus, a physiologic approach to total care of the I.C.U. patient must include attention to nutritional needs. The catabolic phases of the stress state can be viewed as an energy crisis which, if left unsolved, can lead to severe protein depletion. If immune impairment is a consequence of this erosion, sepsis and multiple organ failure result. Reducing the original stress and limiting its total metabolic impact by complete cardiovascular resuscitation is the first therapeutic step. Control of sepsis prevents recurrence of stress catabolic depletion. Likewise, a modern treatment plan, if sepsis is established, now includes nutritional support. Although it is difficult to stem this tide of metabolic erosion, a positive nitrogen balance can be achieved in septic patients by the continuous infusion of amino acids and glucose in amounts greater than those required by the same individual under nonseptic conditions. Provision of branched-chain amino acids in these septic patients may ultimately prove to further enhance nitrogen retention by decreasing gluconeogenesis rates and halting proteolysis (Table 6-9).

TABLE 6-9
Consequences of Stress State

Lean body mass sacrificed
Immune response blunted
Dependence upon carbohydrates which are unavailable
Healing delayed
Gut function diminished

NUTRITIONAL THERAPY FOR THE I.C.U. PATIENT

In times of severe stress, appetite is certainly decreased; in fact, for practical purposes gastrointestinal function ceases, as far as nutrient absorption is concerned. Nevertheless, the foremost principle of nutritional therapy for I.C.U. patients is to utilize the gastrointestinal route as much as possible (Fig. 6-10). Elemental diets have been introduced to provide an enteral food source free of residue and which can be virtually totally absorbed by necessary digestive functions. High-osmolar diets introduced into the stomach may cause gastric retention; when introduced into the small intestine, they may cause severe and limiting

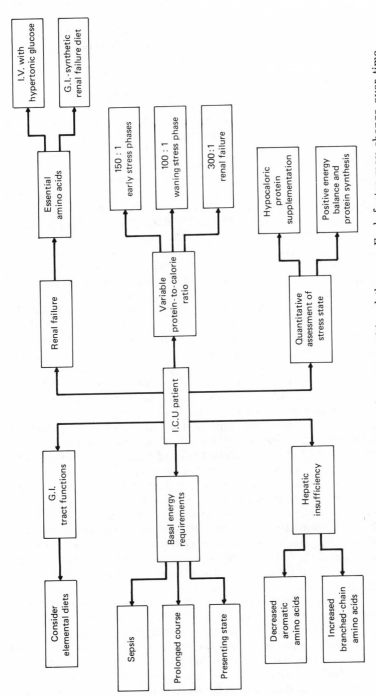

Fig. 6-10. Considerations necessary to provide adequate nutritional therapy. Each factor may change over time. Obviously, a "cookbook" formula cannot succeed.

diarrhea. On the other hand, nonelemental diets are available at less expense and can be utilized in some critically ill patients. Isocal, for instance, an example of a nonelemental diet, is a complete liquid diet. It contains 32.5 gm of protein per liter, 42.5 gm of fat, and 125 gm of carbohydrate per liter. This is a lactose-free formula providing 1 cal per ml and osmolality of only 350 mOsm per liter.

In patients with renal failure, defined formula diets, such as Aminade (McGaw Labs, Irvine, California), allow protein feeding to generally protein-intolerant patients—if gastrointestinal function permits. This solution contains a nitrogen source in the form of purified essential amino acids. A similar parenteral solution (Nephramine) exists which will be discussed in a later section.

Enteral feedings are best administered through a small (no. 8 French) silastic feeding tube. One such device (Dob-Hoff) incorporates a mercury-weighted tip which facilitates passage into the stomach.[34] Infusions of any enteral diet (low residue) should be initiated at 40 to 50 ml per hour of a half strength formula; gastric retention and diarrhea are avoided because the concentration of initial feedings approaches isotonicity (200 to 300 mOsm/liter). Continuous infusion is required. Elevation of the patient's head during infusion decreases the possibility of regurgitation and pulmonary aspiration. On subsequent days, the tonicity may be increased to full strength as tolerated. If no diarrhea develops, subsequent dose adjustments may be made by increasing the hourly volume. Rarely, can one reach levels of greater than 3000 to 3500 ml/day of a full-strength (1 cal/ml) enteral solution. Even this level will require slow and careful titration—at least 7 to 10 days from the initial feeding. Often parenteral hyperalimentation is started concomitantly to provide the necessary nutrients and avoid "forcing" the G.I. tract with "backstepping," necessitated by vomiting, stasis, and/or diarrhea. Addition of Lomotil (5 to 10 mg) to 1 liter of the solution may assist in control of stool frequency. Caution must be employed in the use of antidiarrheal agents. Profuse diarrhea may signal gastrointestinal intolerance of the solution. Excessive use of antidiarrheal agents can lead to severe ileus requiring complete cessation of enteral feedings.

Although enteral feedings are preferred over parenteral, some severely stressed patients, particularly those with sepsis, lack adequate gastrointestinal function. In these patients, parenteral nutrition is mandatory. The question remaining is the choice and amount of the calorie and nitrogen source.

From Gamble's original studies, we know that starvation ketosis can be prevented and nitrogen losses diminished by giving 100 gm of glucose daily.[35] We have, thus, extrapolated this information to the treatment of the starving patient. Since the energy requirements after minimal stress are only 1800 to 2000 cal a day, a hypocaloric solution utilizing peripheral administration of 10 percent glucose and amino acids may offset some of the calorie balance, while at the same time providing some nitrogen source. Although early studies[36] suggested that provision of small quantities of dextrose interfered with endogenous fat utilization by elevating insulin levels and thus, inhibiting protein-sparing effect, it is now clear that at constant levels of protein, infusion with the addition of more calories spares more protein than infusion of the protein source only in the form of amino acids.[37] Adding dextrose does not pose any obstacle to the utilization of amino acids and results in a less negative nitrogen balance than when using amino acids alone. Nevertheless, the provision of hypocaloric forms of nutritional therapy, irrespective of the total nitrogen load, cannot be advocated for treatment of the moderately to severely stressed individual in the intensive care unit. The goal must remain, insofar as it is possible to achieve positive energy as well as nitrogen balance. Nevertheless, one such role of hypocaloric forms of solution has been advocated as a cyclical form of parenteral nutrition therapy. Patients on long-term (two weeks or greater) total parenteral nutrition with concentrated dextrose and amino acid solutions, have been demonstrated to develop hepatic enzyme alterations suggestive of a cholestatic pattern (increase in bilirubin, alkaline, phosphatase, and transaminases).[38] Liver biopsies, done in those patients with enzyme elevations, have confirmed fatty depositions in the liver. Presumably, this is the histologic effect of prolonged, or perhaps, "excess" carbohydrate infusions. While preserving the protein load through peripheral infusions, smaller quantities of dextrose in the form of a hypocaloric solution, as mentioned above, may be utilized for 24 to 48 hours to allow clearing of the histologic fat deposits in the liver. Although, this procedure has some metabolic and physiologic justification, it is not at all clear that interruption of standard TPN solutions in severely stressed septic patients is (1) warranted or (2) safe, even though liver enzyme alterations may be present. Obviously, in such patients, hepatocellular dysfunction may result from a variety of causes (Table 6-10).

Basal energy requirements are related to a person's age, sex, and body surface area. In an adult male, average requirements are around 40 cal/sq m/hr or around 1700 to 1800 cal/day. Metabolic rate increases 7 percent for each 1° F increase in temperature; 13 percent per 1° C. But a number of factors independently increase energy expenditure in surgical patients.[39]

When total parenteral nutrition became a viable clinical concept, a protein hydrolysate solution was initially used. Federal regulation requires that protein need only be hydrolyzed 50 percent to component amino acids in such solutions. Therefore, most solutions are 55 percent hydrolyzed. Since peptides are not immediately utilized as a nitrogen source or for incorporation directly into the protein synthetic processes, 45 percent of the nitrogen source was generally wasted and excreted in the urine following administration, even when appropriate quantities of carbohydrate were given. Nitrogen equilibrium can be achieved with synthetic amino acid solutions at much lower infusion rates.[40] Concentrations of the synthetic amino acid in these solutions is similar to natu-

TABLE 6-10
Nutritional Therapy

Goals
  Reverse catabolism-negative nitrogen balance
  Supply needed glucose calories (resting plus stress)
  Provide all essential nutrients
    Vitamins
    Minerals
    Essential fatty acids
  Maintain fluid and major electrolyte balance
Sources
  Gastrointestinal absorption
    Preferred but not usually available
    "Elemental diets"—no digestive processes necessary
    Balanced caloric and osmotic loads
  Total parenteral nutrition
    Amino acid solutions
    Concentrated glucose (25%)
    Vitamin, mineral, electrolyte supplements
    Volume of infusions must be considered in multisystem disorders

---

rally occurring proteins of high biologic value, i.e., casein, fibrin, or egg albumin.

The impact of total parenteral nutrition is that it probably provides a calorie source that promotes protein synthesis. The calorie-to-nitrogen ratio required for a positive energy balance is generally estimated as between 150 to 250 nonprotein calories per gram of administered nitrogen. But this ratio is not constant and may vary at different times through the course of the I.C.U. patient as his basic disease processes either worsen or improve. For instance, in renal failure, the optimal figures for avoiding further increases in BUN may require a calorie to nitrogen ratio of 300:1 or even higher. In moderate catabolic states, a ratio of approximately 150 to 200:1 is probably adequate. As the severe catabolic state wanes, calorie-to-nitrogen ratios may be dropped to 100 to 125:1 to avoid fat accumulation in the liver. The demonstrable limit for glucose tolerance appears to be related to intravenous glucose administration; the oral route enables provision of 8,000 to 10,000 cal per day by combining both the enteral and parenteral route.

ADMINISTRATION OF NITROGEN

Nitrogen intake for normal man had been said to be 0.2 to 0.24 gm of nitrogen per kilogram per day.[21] In severely catabolic patients, this figure may need to be higher. Excessive nitrogen administration, however, may lead to an accumulation of one of the two nitrogen waste products, urea or ammonia, even if renal and hepatic function are normal. Nevertheless, clinical practice shows that modest elevation of BUN (up to 50 mg%) usually is not associated with symptoms or clinical problems.

Modifications of the amount and type of nitrogen source may be important to affect the nutritional goals in patients in the I.C.U. who develop hepatic or renal insufficiency. Originally, dietary therapy was used as a replacement for dialysis utilizing the Giordano-Giovanetti diet modified for intravenous use for central administration of essential amino acids and hypertonic dextrose.[41] In a group of surgical patients, the mortality decreased from 56 to 25 percent. The authors were able to document that BUN rose less rapidly if 26 gm of protein equivalent of the essential amino acid solution (Nephramine) per 24 hours was administered. Although it is not clear that this represents "urea recycling" as originally suggested by the authors, those receiving parenteral nutrition based on the essential amino acid formula clearly showed an ability to provide nitrogen loading, even in patients who had dialysis-dependent renal failure.

Patients with hepatic insufficiency are a clear example of the dilemma of nutritional requirements combined with nitrogen intolerance. Hepatic encephalopathy has been attributed to many things: protein loading, ammonia, and other serum factors. More recently, deficiency in CNS neurotransmitters has been implicated.[42] Perhaps alterations in CNS neurotransmission is partially a result of the alterations in plasma amino acid profile, particularly relative excesses of the aromatic amino acids (phenylalanine, tyrosine, tryptophan), which seem to be important in neurotransmitter synthesis due to a competition for blood-brain transmission sites with branched-chain amino acids. Nevertheless, patients with mild-to-moderate hepatic insufficiency will tolerate infusions of hypertonic dextrose and synthetic amino acid solutions which are commercially available; however, patients with hepatic encephalopathy usually do not. A solution with special concentrations (decreased aromatics and increased branched-chain amino acids) has been proposed for the comatose patient and is presently undergoing clinical trials (Table 6-11).[34]

ADMINISTRATION OF CARBOHYDRATES

The basic principle of parenteral nutrition is based on the recognition that providing adequate numbers of exogenous calories prevents the endogenous destruction of vital protein for a calorie source. The concept of nitrogen sparing is illustrated clearly by the requirements to achieve a nitrogen balance of zero when no additional calories or extra glucose calories have been given. Nitrogen balance may be zero if 2 gm/kg of a synthetic amino acid solution are given. But when glucose in the amount of 55 cal per kg is provided, only 0.5 gm per kg of parenteral amino acid is required for nitrogen equilibrium.[43] In addition, particu-

TABLE 6-11
Guidelines

Calories
  1800 resting state
  Add 10 to 100% depending upon severity of stress
  Add 50% if parenteral feedings used
  Avoid hyperglycemia
Protein
  1 gm/kg resting state
  Add additional amounts if severe catabolism exists
  Vary calorie/nitrogen ratio to achieve "negotiated nitrogen balance"
    150 cal/gm—normal
    300 cal/gm—renal failure
    Diminish ratio as catabolism wanes
  Consider special formulas
    Essential amino acids in renal failure
    High levels of branched chain amino acids in hepatic failure
Fat
  Essential fatty acids necessary
  Additional calories may not "spare" protein
  Use 5 to 10% of caloric requirements

---

larly after severe stress or in sepsis, new protein synthesis from endogenous protein breakdown (catabolism) proceeds efficiently only if an energy source is available in the form of exogenous carbohydrate. Therefore, one may consider provision of carbohydrate as not only protein sparing, i.e., reducing the rate of gluconeogenesis, but also as a provider of the energy for new protein synthesis from both the endogenous and exogenous nitrogen sources.

Carbohydrate sources in the form of fructose, xylitol, and sorbitol have been attempted as alternative sources of calories, but have serious limitations. Indeed, about 80 percent of these administered carbohydrates are converted to glucose prior to utilization. Furthermore, fructose, when metabolized, results in increased production of lactate which limits utilization in patients who are already acidotic. Xylitol, furthermore, has proven hepatotoxic.

ADMINISTRATION OF FATS

The role of exogenously administered fat, as either a major or supplemental form of calories, is not clearly defined for severely ill intensive care patients. Fat in the diet may not be essential except for a source of essential fatty acids (linoleic acid). Oddly enough, excessive carbohydrate and protein administration through the parenteral route may, in fact, end up as fat. Nevertheless, there may be some advantage to providing fat in the diet. It clearly provides more calories, yielding 9 cal per gram with complete oxidation as opposed to 3.4 to 4 cal per gram for glucose combustion. Fat is available now as a soybean-egg-phosphatide emulsion (Intralipid 10 percent solution); however, fat may not be protein sparing under all conditions. Gamble's classic work established the protein-sparing effect of small amounts of glucose. On the other hand, fat may not spare protein when administered without amino acids. In severe stress, fatty acid mobilization may be maximal but fat utilization is suboptimal. Thus, administering exogenous fat when endogenous fat is not being utilized (i.e., an overweight patient manifesting protein-calorie immunologic malnutrition), does not have an apparent rationale and may not be expected to have salutary effects. In studies which test the protein-sparing effects of fat versus carbohydrates in severe stress, carbohydrates seem to be superior. If fat is added to carbohydrates, no further protein-sparing effects have been shown.[43]

Essential fatty acid deficiency during total parenteral nutrition with amino acids and glucose may, nevertheless, be prevented by provision of 5 to 10 percent of the caloric requirement by fat emulsions. This amounts to giving approximately 500 ml of 10 percent solution of Intralipid twice weekly. Equally efficacious, if oral intake is possible, is the administration of 25 to 50 ml per day of any unsaturated (corn, safflower, sunflower) oil. Intralipid is isotonic, and therefore, has a theoretical advantage of sparing vascular endothelium and its consequent reduction in instances of phlebitis, when compared to isocaloric-dextrose infusions through peripheral veins.

It is commonly believed that fats may impair liver function; however, liver function abnormalities may improve when Intralipid is given. Recent evidence suggests that continuous infusions of Intralipid in experimental animals seem to suppress leukocyte chemotactic mobility in direct proportion to the blood levels of the fat emulsion.[44] This may indicate that exogenous lipid calories further impair the deficient immunologic state.

ADMINISTRATION OF SUGARS

The total dose of dextrose and amino acids as a protein source that can be provided parenterally is limited by the body's ability to metabolize them so that excesses do not occur. The limit of metabolism has been projected to be 1.5 gm/kg/hr in most adults but this depends on age, stress, glucose, and insulin resistance, as well as pancreatic function (Fig. 6-11). In practice, 56 (0.8 × 70) gm glucose per hour in a 70-kg adult is a reasonable goal. In a 24-hour period, the low tolerable limits of glucose infusion may then be 1344 (56 × 24) gm glucose/day. Since a standard solution of TPN contains about 25 percent dextrose solution (250 gm), as much as 5 liters could theoretically be given.

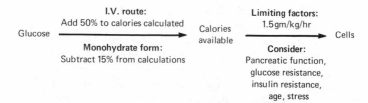

Fig. 6-11. Calculations of glucose calories must be modified when intravenous hyperalimentation is used. Limitations in uptake also influence the daily rate calculations.

Because glucose in the intravenous form is in a monohydrate, rather than an anhydrous form, one liter of 25 percent glucose solution actually contains 850 cal rather than 1000 cal (3.4 cal per gram rather than 4.0 cal per gram). Thus, a standard TPN solution containing 25 percent dextrose and 4.25 percent amino acids when administered at 150 ml/hr, offers a total of 3600 ml per day and 3000 cal. Two hundred milliliters per hour of TPN yields 4800 ml per day volume and 4000 cal (Table 6-12).

The exact amount of "calorie wastage" brought about by the intravenous administration of glucose has been estimated to be as much as 50 percent. Certain metabolic processes seem to be more efficiently carried out when the nutrient material enters the portal circulation via the enteral route rather than the systemic circulation as required by

TABLE 6-12
TPN Formulas

"Standard liter" supplies
  850 "glucose" cal
  42.5 gm amino acids
  1 to 2 ml vitamin supplements
  Added electrolytes
    Sodium—30 to 40 mEq/liter
    Potassium—20 to 40 mEq/liter
    Acetate—if chloride is high
    Phosphate—20 to 40 mEq/liter
    Calcium—4 to 5 mEq/liter
    Magnesium—10 to 20 mEq/liter
100 ml/hr supplies
  2000 cal; 100 gm amino acids—adequate for resting state
150 ml/hr supplies
  3000 cal; 150 gm amino acids—adequate for most stressed patients
200 ml/hr supplies
  4000 cal; 200 gm amino acids—adequate for most severe cases

---

parenteral administration. Translated into practice, intravenous calories should exceed estimated oral requirements by 50 percent.

Control of the blood sugar at such high glucose infusion rates in the severely ill, stressed patient, even though he has never been a diabetic, often requires the administration of exogenous insulin. Regular insulin, when given intravenously by continuous infusion, has been shown to control blood sugars in a more constant fashion when treating diabetic ketoacidosis.[45] This same principle when applied to the regulation of blood sugar for patients receiving TPN, is best accomplished by adding regular insulin to the TPN solution. Although some insulin may indeed be adsorbed on the glass and plastic surfaces in the I.V. bottle and tubing, the amount of insulin lost is constant and is rarely more than 15 percent of the total amount of insulin added to the solution.[46] Since insulin dosage is titrated based on blood sugar, and since a continuous infusion of dextrose occurs simultaneously, hypoglycemic reactions are extremely rare in these stressed patients. Maintaining blood sugar $\leq$ 250 mg% is a reasonable goal. Significant glycosuria (2^+ urine sugar) may lead to osmotic diuresis, but severe dehydration does not develop until urine sugar concentration approaches 3^+ or 4^+. Nevertheless, simultaneous measurements of blood sugar in these critically ill patients is preferable to relying on urine sugar determinations for supplemental insulin doses, since renal thresholds may vary hour-to-hour and concomitant renal impairment of filtration and absorption mechanisms destroy any predictable relationship between blood sugar and urine sugar determinations. Fluctuations in glomerular filtration rate, particularly in septic patients receiving TPN, may alter the renal tubular threshold for glucose. In our experience, it is not infrequent to see fractional urine analysis for a sugar yield of 1^+ even on serial determinations while blood sugar ranges from 300 to 400 mg%. Although no osmotic diuresis occurs in these patients, substantial intracellular dehydration may result with increases in the extracellular fluid space and plasma volume compartment of this space secondary to hypertonicity due to this level of hyperglycemia. In addition to the insulin contained in the TPN bottles if supplemental insulin has been required over a 24-hour period, preparation of new bottles of TPN should include some extra insulin. Our practice is to add two-thirds of the supplemental insulin dosage required in the previous 24 hours to the new 24-hour solutions being prepared. In some patients, it is not unusual for the total insulin dose, using the previously outlined scheme, to approach 100 to 150 units of insulin per day by continuous infusion in order to affect normal serum blood sugars. The alternative to glucose control in these patients, of course, is to significantly decrease the rate of TPN administration. This denies these critically ill patients an important adjunctive form of therapy. Furthermore, there is strong suggestive evidence that insulin infusions in these patients may, irrespective of the carbohydrate load as a primary energy source, have more to do with controlling the rate of gluconeogenesis than the absolute energy intake.[31]

HYPO- AND HYPERGLYCEMIA

Hypoglycemia is extremely rare in the stressed patient. Nevertheless, it may occur if stress factors wane and insulin supplementation is not decreased as the patient's condition improves. Hyperglycemia, on the other hand, is frequent and can be fatal. Otherwise stable patients receiving TPN infusion at constant dosage, who suddenly develop hyperglycemia, usually develop additional complications—usually sepsis, but also myocardial dysfunction or ischemic cellular changes, either localized (i.e., intestinal) or total body-deficient, energy-dependent metabolic functions. Diabetes mellitus is not a relative contraindication for TPN usage. It is merely another complicating factor. In fact, only a minority of patients on TPN who develop glucose intolerance are previously diagnosed as diabetics.

Hyperglycemia can lead to hyperosmolar diuresis as a result of spillage of serum sugar into the tubular filtrate. Severe water diuresis may result in a marked increase in serum osmolarity with rapidly developing signs of dehydration and hypertonicity (see p. 327).

When beginning TPN infusion for the severely septic patient, we initiate the infusion of the standard solution (25 percent dextrose) at 50 to 75 ml/hr. In addition, small quantities of insulin for severely septic, stressed patients, are added to each bottle (10 to 15 units) each succeeding 24-hour period. The TPN infusion is increased 25 ml/hr until total daily infusion approaches 4000 ml of the solution per day. Although this glucose load introduces a necessity for induced CO_2 excretion, this is rarely but occasionally a significant problem. Correction of severe hyperglycemia, particularly if substantial free-water diuresis has occurred, is based on correction of the hypertonic state in the plasma. Supplemental insulin (25 units) may be required if blood sugar is suddenly increased. Associated with insulin addition, correction of the water deficit with solutions containing free water (25 percent normal saline or D5W) results in appropriate distribution of both intracellular and extracellular water deficits. If the degree of water dehydration has been judged to be severe resulting in alterations of CNS function, water replacement should then proceed cautiously. Complete correction of the water deficit should be planned to occur over a 24-hour period at a minimum, even in the I.C.U. where dramatic changes are implicitly advocated.

SERUM ELECTROLYTE ADMINISTRATION

Frequent monitoring of serum electrolytes (sodium, potassium, chloride, combined with arterial blood gases for P_{CO_2} and pH measurements) are mandatory to avoid severe metabolic changes associated with TPN infusions.

$$\text{Negative nitrogen balance} \xrightarrow{\dfrac{\text{calories and protein}}{K^+, Mg^{++}, Ca^{++}, PO_4^{\equiv}}} \text{Positive nitrogen balance}$$

Serum sodium concentration is affected by increased levels of blood glucose. Sodium in the serum decreases 1.6 mEq/liter for every 100 mg% increase in blood sugar. This is apparently due to the hyperglycemic hypertonic effect which causes a shift of intracellular fluid water into the extracellular compartment. Likewise, marked hyperlipemia will falsely decrease sodium concentration because the lipid adds appreciable volume to the plasma sample.

Potassium A similar reduction in all intracellular cations and anions may also be seen if the effect of exogenous calorie and protein solutions results in restoration of depleted body cell mass. Since potassium is the major intracellular cation, infusions of concentrated dextrose and amino acid solutions may cause reductions in serum potassium, which suggests intracellular migration (a goal of TPN) but requires major potassium supplementation. Although as much as 40 to 50 mEq of potassium chloride may be added to each liter of TPN solution, periodic adjustments throughout the 24-hour period may be required. Remember, the creation of 1 new kilogram of body mass must sequester 150 mEq of potassium to provide the intracellular cation. This is best accomplished by hourly supplementation through the second intravenous site required in critically ill patients for administration of additional fluids, electrolytes, and/or antibiotics. For example, if serum potassium is determined to be only 3.0 mEq/liter despite continuous infusion of 40 mEq/liter of TPN infusion, supplementation may be accomplished by adding 10 mEq to 15 mEq potassium chloride per hour (with frequent serum potassium determinations to avoid hyperkalemia) until it approaches a high normal level of 4.5 to 5.5 mEq/liter. If there are no substantial potassium losses in fistula drainage or urine, which could be determined by sampling of both fluids, then only 4 to 6 hours of supplemental dosage, depending on total body potassium depletion, could result in the desired serum potassium determination. It is not unusual, however, for the critically ill patient in whom substantial weight loss has already occurred that adequate daily potassium supplementation may require 200 to 400 mEq/day (10 to 15 mEq/hr for 24 hours). If, on the other hand, fistula or urine losses of potassium are substantial, the maintenance potassium concentration must be calculated recognizing these known losses. A fistula output of 3 liters per day containing 25 mEq/liter of potassium would then require a minimum replacement of 75 mEq/day just to prevent further total body potassium depletion. Correction of potassium depletion would then be adjusted to provide potassium in addition to these maintenance losses.

Inadequate potassium replacement during periods of rapid intracellular replenishment is the cause of hypokalemia. Three milliequivalents of potassium are accumulated for every gram of nitrogen retained. Therefore, assuming normal renal function, 100 to 160 mEq potassium per day are required. In fact, if adequate potassium is not given, glucose intolerance may result. Since both potassium and phosphorus are required for intracellular reconstitution, potassium should be given as both chloride and phosphate salts.

Phosphorus   Phosphate depletion in patients on TPN infusions may appear after only 48 to 72 hours of concentrated dextrose/amino acid infusions. When protein hydrolysate solutions were used as a protein source ("early TPN"), serum phosphorus depletion was unusual since phosphorus was a "contaminant" in the preparation of the hydrolysate fractions. The more purified nitrogen forms (amino acid solutions), however, contain minimal quantities of phosphorus and, therefore, require substantial phosphate additions to the solution. As a rule of thumb, 25 mEq of phosphorus should be added for every 1000 cal. In addition to providing the required inorganic phosphorus as an important cofactor in the formation of high energy phosphate bonds (ATP), the important role of phosphorus in cell membrane (phospholipid) formation is equally significant. Hypophosphatemic states have been associated with altered red-blood-cell oxygen dynamics.[47] Phosphorus is a critical element for the required high levels of 2,3-DPG which maintains red blood cells' ability to offload oxygen in the peripheral tissues. Low serum phosphorus has been shown to result in substantial "left" shifts of the oxyhemoglobin dissociation curve. Decreases in serum phosphate correlate with total body phosphate.

Sodium   Some sodium is required to excrete the water load of TPN. Although the tonicity of the standard TPN solution is approximately 1400 to 1600 mOsm/liter, the bulk of this tonicity is supplied by the glucose molecule; therefore, rapid metabolism of the glucose molecule in vivo results in a substantial free water load. Minimum requirements of sodium to allow appropriate excretion of this water load is probably 25 mEq/liter. Although sodium administration in patients with limited cardiac reserves has traditionally been contraindicated, it is now apparent, paradoxically, that avoidance of any sodium administration while administering a free water load may result in severe overwatering hypotonicity, increased secretion of ADH, and a consequent inability to secrete the free water load, resulting in further hyponatremia and a vicious cycle. In some patients it may be necessary to administer diuretics to assist in the excretion of the free water load.

Magnesium   Magnesium supplementation (28 to 32 mEq/day) may be required for anabolism to be complete. If these magnesium requirements are met, it may be reflected by an ease with which total serum calcium levels are maintained, since calcium levels vary, dependent upon both magnesium and phosphate ions.

Magnesium is important in many enzymes critical to cellular metabolism and protein synthesis. Severe magnesium depletion can result in increased neuronal excitability manifested by muscle twitching and, in some cases, tetany. Calcium deficiency, likewise, is associated with the same clinical signs. Deficiencies in magnesium cause an apparent ineffectiveness of parathormone with resultant hypocalcemia that cannot be corrected by calcium administration alone. Unfortunately, serum depletion of magnesium can occur even though the intracellular magnesium content is normal and intracellular depletion may coexist with normal serum concentrations. It is the intracellular concentration which is an important determinant of tetany. Magnesium depletion may coexist with malnutrition, severe diarrhea, or any type of enteral losses, such as large fistula losses. Likewise, magnesium depletion occurs with ethanolism, delirium tremens, and cirrhosis. Digitalis intoxications in patients with normal serum potassium may well be related to a magnesium depletion state. Normal serum magnesium is 1.6 to 2.1 mEq/liter, although cellular deficiencies may still exist. Acute replacement of magnesium, for instance in tetany, may be based on replacing the extracellular fluid magnesium deficit over a 48-hour period by giving 10, 25, or 50 percent solution of magnesium sulphate intravenously at a rate that does not exceed 1.5 ml of a 10 percent solution per minute—or its equivalent. Magnesium sulphate has traditionally been administered to counteract the seizure tendency of eclampsia. The usual dosage of 1 to 2 ml of the 50 percent solution calculates to be a similar dosage (1 to 2 gm/hr). One must calculate administered dosage no matter what the "traditional" concentration or rate of administration! Remember that gm% = gm/100 ml gm% × 10 = gm/liter—then hourly rates can be calculated.

Calcium   Acute symptoms associated with decreased calcium may be treated with 10 to 20 ml of 10 percent calcium chloride solution over 10 to 15 minutes. In the plasma, 60 percent of calcium is protein bound, primarily to albumin, and the remaining fraction is ionized. A reciprocal relationship exists between serum levels of calcium and phosphate. When hyperphosphatemia is present, serum calcium falls. This becomes important when correction of severe hypophosphatemic states is undertaken with exogenous phosphate infusions. Subsequent increases in serum phosphate may be associated with sudden, precipitous decreases in serum calcium. Since the ionized fraction of calcium seems to be the important determinant of cellular metabolic function, sudden alterations in pH may disturb the ionized-to-unionized calcium balance. Hypocalcemic tetany may be produced by the rapid infusions of bicarbonate in an acidemic patient (Table 6-13).

TPN Infusions   Acidosis may be also seen in patients receiving high volume TPN infusions. In critically ill patients, particularly those with respiratory insufficiency requiring ventilatory support, this acidosis may

TABLE 6-13

Caveats and Complications

50% extra calories may be required
Blood sugars must be controlled!
　Urine sugars *not* reliable
　Insulin sliding scale (I.V.)—best coverage

Blood sugar	Insulin
200–250	5
250–300	10
300–350	15
350–400	20
> 400	individual dose

Consider continuous insulin
　Add to infusion based on previous day's requirements (2/3)
　Control high sugars with constant infusion
　Add extra required insulin to next day's order
　Do not diminish rate of glucose unless control is unattainable
Hypoglycemia—extremely rare
Hypophosphatemia and hypokalemia—expected if TPN works; new intracellular
　protein requires 140 mEq of each per kg
All possible electrolyte and fluid disturbances—simple arithmetic calculations
　of formulas relating intake to output usually suffice

---

appear to be a result of combined metabolic and respiratory factors. The metabolic acidosis seen may be easily explained as either an anion gap or non-anion gap form of acidosis. The hyperchloremic form suggests a non-anion gap type and has been ascribed to the administration of excess chloride during TPN infusion. Current amino acid preparations, however, contain small quantities of chloride ion (<20 mEq/liter). Should hyperchloremic acidosis in the reduced load be present, sodium acetate should be incorporated to correct any excess chloride administration. Likewise, potassium administration may be given in the form of potassium phosphate salts. On the other hand, the anion gap form of acidosis associated with normal serum chloride, suggesting that there is an unmeasured anion addition to the extracellular fluid, is harder to explain. Many of the amino acids are in the anion form in the prepared solutions. It has been presumed that the circulating levels of amino acids make up the unmeasured anion component. To correct an anion gap acidosis, administration of bicarbonate either added to the TPN bottle or as a second intravenous site supplement may result in normalization of the blood pH. However, the critically failing patient responds to *no* transient metabolic therapy; this may provide a delineation of treatment modalities. This does not imply initial therapeutic failure but that continued therapy may be to no avail.

It has become apparent recently that a respiratory component of the acidosis may be contributory in patients receiving high volume—and thus high glucose—TPN infusions. Glucose kinetics in normal and stressed man have been studied utilizing C-14.[27] In normal humans, the percentage of expired CO_2 which comes from glucose metabolism is about 29 percent—as much as 51 percent in injured and/or septic humans. Thus, it is possible during large glucose infusions that CO_2 production may double. In fact, high carbohydrate loads associated with TPN usage have been shown in Kinney's studies to increase CO_2 production over twice as much as the associated increase in oxygen consumption.[48]

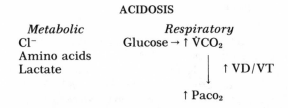

ACIDOSIS

Metabolic   *Respiratory*
Cl^- Glucose → ↑ $\dot{V}CO_2$
Amino acids
Lactate   ↓ ↑ VD/VT

                    ↑ $Paco_2$

Other Factors For patients with respiratory insufficiency, receiving some form of ventilatory support, measurements of the dead space to tidal volume ratio (VD/VT) has been suggested as a parameter which may quantitate severity of gas exchange and pulmonary dysfunction. Measurement of VD/VT requires information about 3 other variables: (1) minute volume of ventilation, (2) CO_2 production, and (3) alveolar (arterial) Pco_2. Kinney has further suggested that the use of the ventilatory equivalent (liters of air moved/liters of O_2 consumed or CO_2 produced) examines the relationship of two of the three variables needed for measuring VD/VT. Thus, by examining the ventilatory equivalent for CO_2, the parameter most useful in separating those patients whose increased minute ventilation due to a primary pulmonary pathology or a primary metabolic problem may be the minute CO_2 excretion. In our own practice, patients with respiratory insufficiency manifested by an inability to excrete CO_2 in response to an increased CO_2 load caused by an increased CO_2 production (TPN), develop hypercarbia when 3 to 4 liters of the standard TPN solution have been used. Measurements of CO_2 excretion have been performed documenting an increase in CO_2 production in these patients with compromised ventilatory reserve (Fig. 6-12). Since these rare patients have not been able to compensate by spontaneous increases in minute ventilation, they develop progressive increases in $Paco_2$. We have been reluctant to increase the component of mechanical ventilation in an attempt to increase alveolar ventilation since one disadvantage of positive pressure in mechanical ventilation is to increase VD/VT further. When lowering the TPN infusion, a decreased calorie load has been associated with a return toward normal of the arterial Pco_2 in most of these patients. The proper delineation

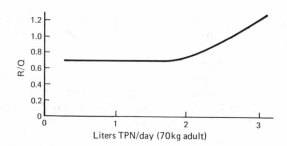

Fig. 6-12. Calculation of "optimal" TPN daily dosage must include consideration of the metabolic "cost" of increasing caloric utilization, i.e., an increased CO_2 production. This effect is important if ventilatory function cannot cope with the increased production.

of calorie load to the ventilatory capacity of the patient forms a new determinant of the maximal calorie load tolerated in these complex patients. Too often, the calorie load calculated exceeds the tolerable load, thus further compromising the desirable and effective nutritional therapy postulated to effect maximal survival in the most vulnerable patient population.

VITAMINS AND TRACE ELEMENTS

Vitamins are an integral part of diet since they serve as cofactors in metabolism. Although daily requirements are known for the healthy state, there is no similar data for the stress state. With respect to the water soluble, nontoxic vitamins B and C, we assume an increased requirement. Fat-soluble vitamins A, D, and E may be given in the usual supplemental formulas to the extent that the hypervitaminosis state may be created by TPN. The fat soluble vitamins are stored in abundance and should, therefore, be given only slightly above the minimum requirement. Standard vitamin supplements do not distinguish normal I.V. supplements and hyperalimentation regimes. As far as trace metals are concerned, there is little definitive knowledge to their requirements. We are learning more as deficiency states develop and are clinically identified when patients receive parenteral forms of nutritional therapy alone.[49] Zinc shortage has been associated with a deficiency in wound healing. This is not often seen in patients on short-term TPN (less than 3 to 4 weeks). Characteristically, zinc deficiency is associated with a perioral rash which also occurs in the extremity flexion creases. Copper deficiency has been associated with an anemia but, in fact, iron deficiency is the most important cause of anemia in this group of patients. Chromium deficiency is associated with the development of a diabetes-like state but has been identified only in patients with long-term parenteral nutritional use and no oral intake.

CATHETER CARE

Many cases of I.C.U. sepsis represent iatrogenic infections. Most catheter sepsis is related to breaks in technique and catheter care and is not due to hematogenous colonization of the catheter by bacteria. Nevertheless, in patients where bacteremias are frequent, as in burn patients, contamination by hematogenous seeding may be more common. The most common current practice suggests that approximately every 48 hours, the catheter insertion site must be cleansed with iodine-containing solution followed by application of an air-occlusive dressing. Catheter sepsis seems to result from skin contaminants growing along the catheter and being deposited in the fibrin sheath. Good catheter care has been rewarded by a decreased incidence of infection (Fig. 6-13). In Ryan's study, there was a seven-fold increase in catheter sepsis in a group of patients receiving TPN where a single violation of the technique occurred.[50] In the "proper care" group, catheter sepsis occurred in only 3 percent. Povidone ointment is of importance because it also kills saprophytic skin fungi. Although *Staphylococcus epidermidis* is considered a contaminant in most bacteriologic laboratories, this may be an important pathogen in catheter sepsis in patients who have central catheters. This organism is difficult to eradicate once established and is frequently only sensitive to vancomycin. Fungal growth has largely been controlled by better mixing and storage of the nutritional solution in defined preparation areas and use of iodine ointments. Although most organisms, including candida, proliferate rapidly in dextrose and protein solutions, contamination is virtually nonexistent when proper phar-

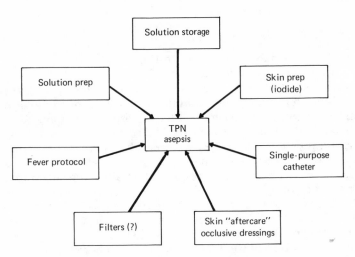

Fig. 6-13. Establishment of a strict protocol for TPN preparation and storage, catheter insertion techniques, and skin site "after care" has been shown to reduce the incidence of TPN-induced sepsis.

macy techniques are employed. No solution should be stored for longer than 24 hours; all storage should be done in a refrigerator at less than 4° C.

The length of time that an indwelling venous catheter is in place cannot be correlated with the incidence of sepsis in critically ill patients. However, the length of time the catheter is in place certainly increases the potential for contamination due to intermittent septicemic episodes. Thus, a necessity for standard rotation of the catheter site has not yet been proven. Ryan's study reported a 75 percent incidence of "unnecessary" catheter removal when catheter sepsis was suspected but not ultimately confirmed.[50] Yet, temperature "spikes" remain a clear signal when considering catheter removal since established catheter colonization (by means of peripheral and similar cultures) is usually associated with systemic effects—defined as catheter infection. Although the site may be anatomically distinct, i.e., an appendiceal abscess, the effect of a blood-borne septicemia may produce distant clinical illness.

Thus, a temperature work-up for these patients must be directed to search out other sites of infection. If a source cannot be immediately identified, the persistent fever would require catheter removal. A waiting period of 12 to 24 hours should precede the reintroduction of a new catheter at a new site, if possible. Hemodynamically unstable patients must still be treated by resuscitative principles.

The value of in-line filters for prevention of catheter sepsis has not been established.[51] Filters, on the other hand, may be regarded as a potential portal of entry for microorganisms, even when aseptic precautions are taken during filter changing.

THE DIABETIC

The adult onset diabetic still has fasting insulin function preserved, thereby inducing minimal catabolism. His problem is in generating an appropriate insulin feeding function with glucose loading. Pancreatic beta cells produce insulin in an amount that is inadequate to manage the substrate load induced by feeding. These patients are fairly well controlled on diet or perhaps hypoglycemic oral agents. During the stress of surgery, they tolerate stress and even glucose infusions fairly well. Monitoring blood sugar daily during the perioperative period is usually adequate to detect continuing insulinization since the substrate load is decreased, i.e., the patient is "NPO." Some glucose infusions are indicated for these patients to avoid starvation ketosis which may be confused with diabetic ketoacidosis. Such glucose infusions in the range of 100 to 200 gm of glucose per day may help spare some nitrogen loss if catabolic signals are weak and are not an excessive challenge to the mild diabetic.

The major problem is to differentiate starvation ketosis, which is not unexpected, from ketoacidosis, which represents catabolism totally out of control due to gross insulin deficiency. Steps must be taken to

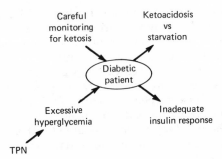

Fig. 6-14.   Special TPN and metabolic problems for the diabetic I.C.U. patient.

separate these two since therapy is radically different. Initially one may look at the amount of carbohydrate being infused. If less than 50 to 75 gm have been infused over the last 24 hours, then starvation is likely or partly responsible for ketone production. Fractional urine sugars should be 2+ or less in starvation; in the presence of ketonuria, and 3+ to 4+ sugar reactions, diabetic ketoacidosis is more likely. If acidosis is present when lactic acidosis from poor tissue perfusion can be excluded with an unmeasured anion (anion gap >19), diabetic ketoacidosis is most likely. Ketonemia also accompanies ketoacidosis but not starvation, contrasted with ketonuria with "trace or negative" serum reaction which is common in starvation.

Once the differentiation has been made, therapy may proceed according to necessity and expectations. If the starvation is temporary, then nothing must be done. If the starvation is expected to continue without the possibility of resuming oral intake, 150 to 200 gm per 24 hours of glucose are indicated. If the diagnosis of ketoacidosis has been made, then appropriate fluid and electrolyte therapy plus insulin supplementation must be administered. Glucose administration should not be started until the blood sugar has been controlled. The management of ketoacidosis is beyond the scope of this chapter. However, the principles of fluid resuscitation are always the same. This hypertonic electrolyte-depleted state requires administration of large volumes of fluids, sodium, chloride, bicarbonate, and potassium. Insulin appears most effective when given as a continuous infusion. Invasive cardiovascular monitoring is much preferred whenever ketoacidosis is severe, as in the elderly, or when it appears as a complication of other significant illnesses (Fig. 6-14).

SUMMARY OF NUTRITIONAL THERAPY FOR THE I.C.U. PATIENT

Human injury is followed by an immediate generalized depression of physiologic functions. Immediate resuscitation and general treatment, if successful, is associated with restoration of the blood volume, cardio-pulmonary function, and substrate mobilization from the body tissues.

It is the magnitude and duration of this phase which is geared toward metabolic and hemodynamic alterations associated with tissue repair. The effects of stress differ from simple starvation states in that there is a specific and selective drain on body and protein coupled with the increased energy demand of critically ill patients. Substrate is transferred from body stores to provide energy for the synthetic requirements essential to host defense mechanisms or to facilitate wound healing.

An understanding of the pathophysiology of starvation including quantification of body calorie reserves, coupled with guidelines for monitoring, leads to a rational approach to nutritional management of the intensive care unit patient.

ACID-BASE DERANGEMENTS

Maintaining blood pH within a normal range which is fairly narrow is accomplished by an elaborate system involving the action of body buffers, alterations in ventilation, as well as renal bicarbonate and hydrogen ion reabsorption and secretion. A general review of acid-base physiology can be found in Chapter 5 of this volume. As part of a total approach to metabolic management, a discussion follows of the severest acid-base derangements found in I.C.U. patients. Fundamental to accurate diagnosis and treatment in such patients is an understanding of the combined forms of acid-base disorders which may be derived from commonly available arterial blood gas data.

The major body acid (carbonic acid) is a volatile acid capable of physically varying between a gas and liquid state. As a volatile acid, its control is primarily by the ventilatory system. All other potential sources of hydrogen ion are nonvolatile acids (fixed) and are under renal regulatory mechanisms, with some help from hepatic regulation. Thus, the lung may compensate for an inability of the kidney and liver to maintain acid-base homeostasis by decreasing carbonic acid concentration via CO_2 exhalation. Likewise, for chronic states of hypercarbia, the kidney responds by conserving base (bicarbonate) to offset the respiratory system-induced acidosis. It is very unusual for either a renal or respiratory state to overcompensate for the other acid-base problem.

Major sources of fixed acids include lactic acid and keto acid as common causes of increased hydrogen ion concentration in the body. The kidneys' main role in acid-base balance is to add one bicarbonate ion to the blood for every hydrogen ion excreted. Thus, any disorder of the metabolic function of the body which causes an increased hydrogen ion excretion by renal tubular cells, in effect adds an equivalent amount of base to the blood. Likewise, the necessity for maintaining electrical neutrality may result in electrolyte changes when acid-base changes occur. For instance, since the sum of the cations must equal the sum of the anions to preserve electrical neutrality, any change in bicarbonate concentration may provoke a reciprocal change in chloride concentrations. Likewise, a decrease in chloride necessitates an increase in bicarbonate. Furthermore, when chloride is not available in sufficient quantity, cation exchange at the renal tubular level may be affected because of a lack of freely exchangeable anion. The meaning and importance of electrolyte changes are much easier to interpret when the acid-base status is known. Unfortunately, the clinical laboratories routinely include some measurement of bicarbonate ion when reporting serum electrolyte but, in fact, this is usually a measurement of standard bicarbonate and not actual bicarbonate. The necessity for basing therapy on *actual* bicarbonate rather than *standard* bicarbonate levels will be discussed thoroughly in this section.

CHANGES IN pH AND PCO_2

It is preferable to describe acid-base status of blood by reporting the actual data in terms of pH and Pco_2. Deviations of pH may be described as an alkalemia or an acidemia; hyper- and hypocapnia pertain to Pco_2 changes; thus, the terms acidosis and alkalosis describe the clinical entity and not the arterial or blood pH.

Deviations from the normal range indicate severe metabolic alterations; but these same deviations may cause a further derangement in organ system functions. Organ damage may develop particularly in the heart or the brain when the pH deviates from a range of 7.1 to 7.6. Severe acidosis (pH 6.8 to 7.2) causes depression of the contractile state of the myocardium. Unlike most other ions, CO_2 diffuses rapidly across the blood-brain barrier. Thus, Pco_2 of the blood determines pH of cerebral tissues. In addition, cerebral blood flow increases with an acute rise in Pco_2 and decreases with a fall in Pco_2, irrespective of blood pH. With chronic blood acid-base derangements, the interstitial pH may gradually approach that of blood, whatever the Pco_2 may be. To further complicate this system, it is known that changes in blood pH are poor indicators of pH in the brain or CSF. Rapid equilibration occurs between CSF and blood Pco_2. Thus, acidosis, diagnosed by blood gas measurement (which is generated by increased Pco_2—hypoventilation), is rapidly reflected by a corresponding acidosis in CSF. Reversal or normalization of blood Pco_2 and pH (mechanical ventilation), however, is not always associated with return of the patient's ventilatory response to normal. In other words, CSF acidosis may persist, resulting in hyperventilation despite normal blood Pco_2 and pH. Although the pH of both blood and brain provides the major chemical mechanisms for ventilatory control, the delayed adjustment of CSF and brain tissue pH back toward normal, after an acute change in acid-base balance, results in gradual modification of the ventilatory response to the new steady-state level.

GENERAL THERAPEUTIC PRINCIPLES

With this background, general therapeutic principles can be derived. One can, in general, predict that it is more dangerous to repair a chronic or subacute acidosis rapidly than slowly, and more dangerous to repair it through a respiratory pathway than through alkalai infusions. Infusions of bicarbonate solution will not be rapidly reflected in brain tissue so that cerebral alkalosis and vasoconstriction are less likely to occur than if alkalinization is achieved by rapidly lowering Pco_2 with hyperventilation.

Thus, respiratory alkalosis should be avoided. Respiratory alkalosis may be caused by hyperventilation of a patient on assisted ventilation, as a consequence of some primary central disorder or secondary hypoxic stimulation of peripheral arterial chemoreceptors. The resultant decrease in arterial Pco_2 causes constriction of cerebral vessels and reduction of cerebral blood flow. In addition, alkalosis causes impairment of tissue oxygen by impeding off-loading from red cells by shifting the oxyhemoglobin dissociation curve to the left. If, in the critically ill patient, a preexisting cerebral vascular disease or a poor cardiac output is present, significant cerebral ischemia may result from the acute hypocarbic state. Likewise, correcting arterial pH by increasing the inspired CO_2 concentration may be very dangerous unless one is certain the hyperventilation is not caused by decreased brain pH. A low CSF pH has been recorded in association with central hyperventilation and high blood pH in a variety of central nervous system lesions, such as meningitis and tumors as well as systemic sepsis.[52]

In spite of the dangers of accompanying rapid changes in blood pH, there are clinical situations in which rapid alkalinization is required. If acidosis persists (pH $\leq$ 7.2) following complete resuscitation from hemorrhagic shock, then bicarbonate infusions are indicated. Failure to treat the acidosis increases the risk of precipitating cardiac dysfunction as volume expansion occurs. Furthermore, acidosis may threaten survival by inducing hyperkalemia and ventricular fibrillation; both the heart and peripheral circulatory beds become less responsive to endogenous or exogenous catecholamines. A patient with progressive cardiogenic shock and severe acidosis may require a rapid correction of the pH before cardiac function can be improved. Cardiac inotropic agents (dopamine, dobutamine, epinephrine) may not be as effective as β-stimulators at pH $\leq$7.20.

ANALYSIS OF BLOOD GAS RESULTS

Many methods have been described by which one may come to an understanding of acid-base disturbances. The method we utilize is best characterized by its simplicity. All interpretations may be made and treatment rendered without having to resort to charts, tables, graphs, nomograms, or slide rules. Basically, one simply looks at the reported value for arterial Pco_2 to diagnose and quantitate the respiratory disturbance while using the reported value of bicarbonate to diagnose and quantitate metabolic disturbances. It must be stressed that the bicarbonate value to be employed is the *actual* bicarbonate and not the standard bicarbonate. Actual bicarbonate is derived by solution of the Henderson-Hasselbach equation using determined values for pH and Pco_2 and is reported as such by most microprocessor blood gas analyzers (Corning-175, IL 913, etc.)

$$pH = 6.1 + \log \frac{HCO_3^-}{Pco_2 \times 0.03}$$

Utilizing other methods (standard bicarbonate, base excess, body buffer base) for expressing acid-base dysfunction implies certain inherent inaccuracies. All of these methods are based on in vitro testing of blood or plasma with CO_2. Titration of CO_2 in vitro varies from that which occurs in vivo; CO_2 in vivo equilibrates not only with blood but also with the interstitial fluid—a compartment which of course is not present during in vitro CO_2 titration. Such errors in calculating acid-base changes using in vitro techniques have resulted in substantial therapeutic miscalculations when these expressions are used.

If actual bicarbonate concentrations reflected only the metabolic acid load, then acid-base corrections would be as simple as making manipulations based on the absolute expression of bicarbonate. Unfortunately, bicarbonate varies not only with the *metabolic* status, but also with the *ventilatory* status. The following series of reactions demonstrates why increased CO_2 results in increased bicarbonate and vice versa.

$$H_2O + CO_2 \rightleftharpoons H_2CO_3 \rightleftharpoons H^+ + HCO_3^-$$

Increased CO_2 will tend to "push" the equation to the right and ultimately creates both an increased H^+ concentration and increased HCO_3^-. Thus, if bicarbonate is to be used as a metabolic indicator, it must first be corrected for any change due to altered ventilation. Schwartz provided the most direct method for separating the respiratory and metabolic effect on serum bicarbonate concentrations.[53] He measured the changes in pH and bicarbonate in human volunteers exposed to graded degrees of acute hypo- or hypercapnia, and as well in patients with uncomplicated chronic hypercapnia. Adjustments for chronic hypercapnia include not only the Pco_2 changes as they may affect bicarbonate directly, but also, due to the chronicity of the situation, the renal compensatory mechanism in response to hypercarbia, i.e., newly generated bicarbonate. Renal compensation, as a rule, is insignificant for the first 12 hours after any elevation in Pco_2. Completion of the renal compensatory changes require 3 to 5 days of elevated Pco_2. Therefore, elevations of less than 1 to 2 days follow the rules for *acute* hypercapnic changes on bicarbonate, not chronic hypercapnia.

The following rules can serve as guidelines for separating respiratory and metabolic effects on bicarbonate that CO_2 may induce:

1. For each 10 torr *acute* increase in P_{CO_2}, actual bicarbonate should increase by 1 mEq/liter.
2. For each 10 torr *chronic* increase in P_{CO_2}, actual bicarbonate should increase by 4 mEq/liter.
3. For every 10 torr *acute* decrease in P_{CO_2}, bicarbonate should decrease by 2 mEq/liter.

Thus, these three conditions which have been derived from in vivo determinations in humans through experimental methods can be applied to clinical settings of acid-base disturbances when seen in the I.C.U. patient. They represent in the purest form acute hypercarbia, chronic respiratory acidosis, and acute hyperventilation. For example, if a 70-kg adult is seen in the recovery room or in the I.C.U. immediately after radical gastrectomy and initial blood gases reveal a pH of 7.1, P_{CO_2} of 60, and actual bicarbonate reported as 17 mEq/liter, then acid-base analysis can be made to decide on appropriate therapy. Without pre-existing chronic obstructive pulmonary disease (normal P_{CO_2} before surgery) one may assume that a P_{CO_2} of 60 represents an acute hypercarbic situation. Thus, as P_{CO_2} has increased to 60 torr, bicarbonate concentration would be expected to increase 2 mEq/liter (1 mEq/liter per 10 torr increase in P_{CO_2}). Thus, a corrected bicarbonate would be 15 mEq/liter. If normal bicarbonate is assumed to be 24 mEq/liter, then a deficit of bicarbonate of 9 mEq/liter exists, i.e., a metabolic acidosis in addition to the hypercarbic state. Since the factor 0.4 has been used to estimate the size of the bicarbonate space to be corrected, one may then calculate the total amount of bicarbonate to be administered: 9 mEq/liter $\times$ 0.4 $\times$ 70 = 252 mEq. Standard practice is to give one-half of the total amount to be corrected and remeasure the blood gases within 30 minutes. Thus, 2 amp of bicarbonate could be administered to this patient (132 mEq bicarbonate); this does not preclude administering ventilatory support to correct the postoperative hypoventilation indicated by the P_{CO_2} of 60 torr.

Various fractions of total body weight have been used to estimate the size of the bicarbonate space (0.2 − 0.5). For our clinical practice, the fraction of 0.3 or 0.4 of total body weight can be used as a useful clinical approximation. What is actually done in practice, of course, is to calculate the total deficits on this basis and then give only one-half of the deficit initially. Acid base parameters are then remeasured and the deficit recalculated. Additional therapy is based upon the response to acid-base manipulations and most importantly to the body's physiologic response to the entire resuscitative effort (restoration of intravascular volume, inotropic support, etc.). It is unrealistic to calculate acid-base data as if it exists in vitro since patients respond to total treatment. By using this titration technique for acid base problems in the I.C.U. patient, the necessity to know all about the individual critically ill patient becomes less important since remeasurement, recalculations, and

TABLE 6-14
Acid–Base Disturbances: Observations
and Principles

Carbolic acid ($H_2CO_3 \leftrightharpoons CO_2 + H_2O$) is major acid and under respiratory control
All other acids ("fixed"—because they cannot be eliminated as CO_2 via the lungs)
    are controlled by the kidney
Electrical neutrality must always be preserved
Central nervous system equilibration may lag behind blood changes; thus, control
    stimuli may not seem appropriate to the measured arterial parameters
Chronic disorders must be corrected slowly
Alkalosis, either respiratory or created by metabolic interventions, should be
    avoided
$Paco_2$ reflects respiratory disorders and compensation
True bicarbonate represents the metabolic component and the dissociation equi-
    librium for CO_2; thus, also reflects respiratory function secondarily
In vitro bicarbonate determinations are misleading—apply correction factors
    For each acute 10 torr increase $Paco_2$; add 1 mEq bicarbonate
    For each chronic 10 torr increase in $Paco_2$, add 4 mEq bicarbonate
    For each acute 10 torr decrease in $Paco_2$, subtract 2 mEq bicarbonate

---

alterations in therapy may quickly provide new answers (Table 6-14).

Some technical aspects of blood gas analysis must be taken into account when interpreting acid-base alterations. If the patient's body temperature changes substantially from the normal 37 C, corrections have to be taken into account when blood gas results are reported. Such corrections are best made in the blood gas laboratory *prior to reporting.* All determinations of blood gas are done at 37 C. All samples are, therefore, warmed to 37 C; CO_2 and hydrogen ion concentrations change as temperature changes. The temperature coefficient for pH unit changes are 0.015 pH units per degree Celsius change. If the patient's temperature is less than 37 C, this fraction must be added to the measured pH. Since the Pco_2 coefficient varies with the temperature change, a standard nomogram must be utilized to express corrected Pco_2 as a function of abnormalities in patient's body temperature. Too much heparin may affect the pH of an arterial blood sample. The pH of sodium heparin is approximately 7.0. Likewise, the Pco_2 and Po_2 of heparin approach room air values. We have learned that 0.05 ml sodium heparin (1000 U/ml) will adequately anticoagulate 1 ml of blood; whereas, 0.1 ml will not affect pH, Pco_2, or Po_2 values. The dead space of a 5 ml syringe washed with heparin and then ejected will contain 0.15 to 0.25 ml of heparin. Thus, 2 to 4 ml of blood theoretically contain at least 0.05 ml heparin per ml of blood but no more than 0.1 ml heparin per 1 ml of blood. Preserving anaerobic conditions once the blood gas is drawn is important. Room air has Pco_2 approaching zero and Po_2 of 150 torr. Therefore, air bubbles mixing with a gas sample will result in equilibration between air and

TABLE 6-15

Physiochemical Alterations of Blood Gas Results

Check Your Laboratory System!

Temperature correction (blood gas measured at 37 C)

pH correction

Standard (in vitro) bicarbonate calculations

Heparin induced alterations

Air bubbles—lower P_{CO_2}, may raise P_{O_2}

Calibration range (normally near 150 torr) values above 300 torr may be off by
50 to 100 torr

Hemoglobin concentration

---

blood. Air bubbles may significantly lower P_{CO_2} values and increase P_{O_2} values erroneously.

Thus, technical considerations may affect the values reported, the values delivered, and their interpretation. There can be no greater wish than to insist that the clinicians be cognizant of the possible errors and insure that the blood gas sample of importance can be verified to reflect only the values existing in the patient being treated (Table 6-15).

METABOLIC ACIDOSIS

Acidemia describes an uncompensated metabolic process that results in lowering the arterial pH to less than 7.35. Alveolar hyperventilation usually results as a homeostatic response of the body's attempt to reduce P_{CO_2} and normalize the acidotic pH. The arterial blood pH, however, will usually still be less than 7.40, indicating incomplete compensation. Actual bicarbonate will be less than normal (24 mEq/liter). The typical blood gas pattern one encounters in metabolic acidosis is a pH <7.30; P_{CO_2} <40 torr; and bicarbonate <24 mEq/liter.

One other clinical tool which has been utilized to quantitate diagnosis and express the degree of acidosis has been a determination made from a calculation of the "other" electrolytes, called the anion gap. Serum, sodium, and potassium account for 95 percent (145/155) of all cations present. Chloride and bicarbonate account for only 85 percent (130/155) of extracellular fluid anions. The sum of the cations, therefore, clearly does not equal the sum of the anions; the difference is called the anion gap. All positive changes must be neutralized by equal number of negative charges. Thus, the presence of any anion gap simply means other anions must be present to neutralize the excess cation changes. Ordinarily, these 15 mEq/liter must be accounted for by protein, sulphate, and phosphate.

$$\text{number of cations} = \text{number of anions} + 15$$
$$Na^+ + K^+ = Cl^- + HCO_3^- + 15$$

An elevated anion gap, therefore, is virtually synonymous with the presence of metabolic acidosis. If one adds hydrochloric acid to the extracellular fluid, for each bicarbonate that is bound to hydrogen and eventually excreted as CO_2, the anion gap is not increased because chloride is replaced. Nevertheless, bicarbonate concentration decreases. But if lactic acid, phosphoric acid, or citric acid are added, since they are unmeasured anions, the anion gap will increase. Therefore, if acidosis is present, as determined by blood pH, and if the anion gap is increased, then a finite list of diagnostic possibilities exists. For the I.C.U. patient, this is usually uremia, ketoacidosis, lactic acidosis, or some exogenous toxin such as ethanol or methanol (only applicable to acute admissions from the community).

Anion Gap ≤ 15	Anion Gap > 15
Diarrhea	Ketoacidosis
Pancreatic fistula	Lactic acidosis
Acetazolamide	Uremia
Sulfamylon	Ethanol
Cholestramine	Methanol
HCl	

As a general rule, acid-base balance is maintained until more than 80 percent of renal function is lost. Therefore, uremia acidosis is not seen as a cause of acidosis until the GFR is ≤20 ml/min, i.e., usually associated with a creatinine >4 mg%. On the other hand, if arterial pH indicates acidosis but anion gap is normal, then a different list of possibilities do exist to explain this type of acidosis. Most commonly seen are those associated with bicarbonate loss from diarrhea or pancreatic fistulae. One situation easily excluded is the hyperchloremic acidosis of ureterosigmoidostomy since a normal anion gap is usually present. Certain drugs used in I.C.U. patients can also cause a non-anion gap acidosis, including acetazolamide, sulfamylon, cholestyramine, and hydrochloric acid.

Mixed disorders combining some of these ideologic factors are common in I.C.U. patients although diarrhea and large fistulae losses are typically associated in their pure form with hyperchloremic metabolic acidosis and a decreased actual bicarbonate concentration. If severe extracellular fluid depletion results in true interstitial loss or poor tissue perfusion, then lactate acidosis may be implicated in the acidotic picture. Gastric fluid continuously suctioned through a nasogastric tube, could normalize these acidotic blood values by decreasing chloride and generating bicarbonate in the cells since hydrogen ion is being removed from the body by gastric suction.

Lactic Acidosis For all patients with combined metabolic disturbances, a review of all available data must indicate assessment of the severity, longevity, and the primary metabolic derangements. Azotemia, increased hematocrit, oliguria, low cardiac filling pressures, and low cardiac output all suggest significant volume depletion with cellular hypo-

TABLE 6-16

Metabolic Acidosis

Shock/insufficient resuscitation
Anion gap—diabetic ketoacidosis; lactic acidosis
Uremia; exogenous toxins
Intestinal losses—pancreatic fistula; severe diarrhea
Low flow states—mesenteric ischemia; poor tissue perfusion

---

perfusion as a cause for increased lactic acid production and at least one cause of metabolic acidosis (Table 6-16).

The common thread linking the various presentations of lactic acidosis seems to be the uncoupling of oxidative and phosphorylative processes in the intracellular environment. If not completely uncoupled, these two processes are made clearly less efficient in a wide variety of situations common to I.C.U. patients, such as ethanol intoxication, endotoxin "shock," and tissue hypoxemia. The disorders causing lactic acidosis inhibit oxidative metabolism either by limiting tissue oxygen delivery, or by toxic inhibition of key oxidative enzymes. Blood lactate concentrations, however, are probably not an accurate measure of intracellular lactate. Furthermore, plasma levels of lactic acid reflect a balance between the rate of production of lactic acid in the peripheral tissues and the rate of utilization in the liver. In addition to the overproduction of lactate by the tissue cell mass, some oxidative defects may limit the utilization of lactate by the liver. Anaerobic tissue metabolism produces a lactate ion and a hydrogen ion as end products. When they enter the blood, they exist as lactic acid. Effective clearing of this lactic acid awaits the re-establishment of aerobic metabolism with the subsequent metabolism of lactate primarily in the liver, with CO_2 and water as the ultimate metabolites.

The net rate of production of lactate in all cells is determined by the rate of formation of pyruvate in equilibrium with lactate (Fig. 6-15). In addition, the cytoplasmic redox potential influences the equilibrium between lactate and pyruvate. Formation of pyruvate in turn is determined mainly by factors regulating glycolysis. Normally, lactate concentration in cells and blood is ten times that of pyruvate but the ratio increases when the redox potential of the cells is reduced by hypoxia. Lactate is removed mainly by the liver. The liver converts lactate back to glucose or glycogen or oxidizes it to CO_2. No matter which of these metabolic processes is chosen for metabolism of lactate in the liver, bicarbonate is generated in the process. Since lactate is formed only from pyruvate and consumed only by the reverse reaction, the rate of metabolic removal of lactate depends to a certain extent on the metabolism of pyruvate. Pyruvate is removed by entrance into the mitochondria where it is oxidized or converted to fat, and also by the pyruvate carboxylase reaction which occurs in hepatic and kidney cortex cells, whereby new glucose can be formed from pyruvate. If a block

CORI CYCLE: Salvage mechanism

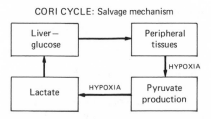

Fig. 6-15. Anaerobic metabolism (cellular hypoxia) produces lactate as an end-product. But lactate produced in peripheral cells may be reconverted into "new" glucose—another form of gluconeogenesis.

in cellular metabolism occurs, which limits the entrance of pyruvate into the Krebs cycle (thus limiting aerobic metabolism) a buildup of pyruvate may be associated with a buildup of lactate (Fig. 6-16). The lactate/pyruvate reactions can be summarized as follows:

$$\text{Pyruvate} + \text{DPNH} + \text{H} \longrightarrow \text{Lactate} + \text{DPN}$$

This reaction requires the presence of lactate dehydrogenase and is reversible.

Thus, the lactate/pyruvate system appears to establish a dynamic equilibrium that is responsive both to oxygen as well as substrate (pyruvate) availability. The metabolic pattern of glucose has been explored as a possible source of lactate accumulation. It is conceivable that when a severely hyperglycemic patient (blood sugar >400 mg%) is given insu-

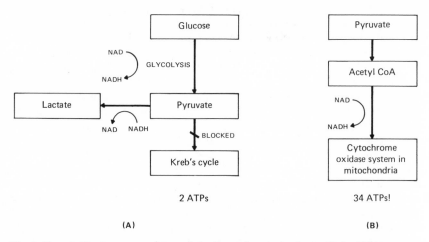

Fig. 6-16. A. During anaerobic metabolism of carbohydrate, little ATP is generated. The reaction cannot proceed to oxidation via the Kreb's cycle; thus lactate accumulates. B. When oxygen is available, the cytochrome oxidase system (Kreb's cycle) functions; this yields an additional 34 moles of ATP for each mole of glucose metabolized.

lin, the cells may be suddenly presented with a large glucose load. At least a temporary increase in lactic acid production would not be unexpected.

Lactic Acidosis in Shock   Shock is probably the most widely recognized cause of lactic acidemia. Lack of oxygen and nutrients being delivered to some or all of the tissue beds results in an increase of the lactate/pyruvate ratio. In fact, the prognostic value of lactate in the shock state has been suggested as a reliable metabolic monitor.[54] Since deficient oxygen delivery is required for lactate build up, defects in either oxygen carrying capacity (arterial content) or cardiac output could result in tissue hypoxia. Likewise, compensation for acute anemias may result in increased cardiac output, therefore still preserving tissue oxidative processes and preventing the accumulation of lactate. In fact, Takaori and Safar infused patients with up to 25 times their blood volume with Ringer's lactate solution.[55] Blood lactate concentration did not rise above base line until the hematocrit had been diluted below 20 percent. Lactic acidosis thus represents a failure of tissue oxygenation—not necessarily related to circulatory homeostasis which is best exemplified by the association of septic shock with high cardiac output and adequate arterial oxygenation.

Concern has been voiced by many clinicians that Ringer's lactate solution may aggravate an existing lactic acidosis when used to treat patients in shock. The use of blood plus Ringer's lactate to treat experimental hemorrhagic shock resulted in more rapid return to normal of blood levels of lactate, excess lactate, and pH than did treatment with the return of shed blood alone.[56] Theoretic objections to the use of lactate-containing solutions for treatment of patients in profound shock include enhancing the in vivo levels of excess lactate attendant upon lactic administration, and lowering blood pH, since the pH of most commerical solutions of Ringer's lactate varies between 6.5 and 6.8. The sodium lactate in Ringer's lactate is not an acid per se and would not be expected to lower the pH. In fact, the sodium lactate has an *alkalinizing* effect after metabolism. Investigation by Carey and associates showed that no difference in measured lactate occurred in the two groups of patients in hemorrhagic shock—one resuscitated with blood plus Ringer's lactate, the other with blood plus normal saline.[57] Subsequent investigation by these same investigators in four major types of shock (hemorrhagic, neurogenic, septic, and cardiogenic) revealed the same effects of Ringer's lactate infusion. The importance of serial determination of lactate as prognostic indicators of survival in shock was examined also by these investigators. The correlation between lactate and excess lactate, and ultimate prognosis was obvious but proved to be of little clinical value in any type of shock they studied. The absolute levels do correlate quite well clinically with depth of shock, but the injuries producing the shock state have a much greater bearing on ultimate survival. Thus, the buffering action of Ringer's lactate is based upon the conversion of lactate ion to carbon dioxide and water with subsequent formation of bicarbonate by the carbonic anhydrase enzymes.

Other Causes of Lactic Acidosis Spontaneous lactic acidosis exists when lactic acidemia occurs prior to the clinical recognition of any underlying disease. Huckabee's definition specifically requires no cardiorespiratory compromise or decreased peripheral perfusion for a diagnosis of spontaneous lactic acidosis.[58] Inability to specifically identify cause of lactic acidosis parallels the very high mortality rates from this primary metabolic disorder. Recently, however, Taradash and Jacobson have reported the successful treatment of patients with primary lactic acidosis utilizing nitroprusside.[59] Such therapy is directed, presumably, at reversing the compartmentalized tissue hypoxia. Although Huckabee's delineation of lactic acidosis as a primary event may be a new disorder, it in fact may be subclinical tissue hypoxia causing an increased production of acid. On the other hand, it may also be a decreased removal of lactate ion by the liver.

Treatment of Metabolic Acidosis The principles and goals for correcting metabolic acidosis due to lactic acidosis can be summarized as follows: (1) diagnose the cause of tissue failure, (2) decrease the lactate concentration, and (3) correct the acidosis. Most of the time these can be accomplished simultaneously by re-establishing aerobic metabolism through hemodynamic resuscitation, with the required addition of bicarbonate only for severe forms of acidosis (pH ≤ 7.2), or in those patients who have some persistent acidosis after hemodynamic resuscitation has been completed. Some patients, on the other hand, produce lactic acid at a rate comparable to or exceeding bicarbonate infusion. Such a metabolic vicious cycle has been associated with an extremely high mortality rate in I.C.U. patients. This event is most commonly seen as an end-stage metabolic marker of death from sepsis or irreversible shock.

Complete correction of metabolic acidosis by the administration of exogenous bicarbonate is not the goal of alkaline therapy. Correction of metabolic acidosis is only a temporary measure to be instituted while the primary cause is corrected. Only correction of the cause can be of any lasting effect. The body tolerates alkalosis (overshoot) much less well than acidosis. Most workers in the area of acid-base metabolism suggest correcting acidosis to only a pH of 7.25 to 7.30. Therefore, even during resuscitation from cardiac arrest, overzealous administration of bicarbonate solution should be and can be averted by obtaining arterial blood samples during resuscitative efforts. The crucial guideline for acid-base correction during resuscitation of cardiac arrest is that death is usually due to hypoxic damage rather than hydrogen ion concentration per se. In fact, most acute metabolic acidosis attendant upon cardiac arrest is due to oxidizable organic acid (lactate). One can minimize any alkaline overshoot by anticipating the conversion of lactate ions to bicarbonate and appropriately limiting bicarbonate replacement to maintain pH 7.30 to 7.35. Complete hemodynamic restoration of aerobic metabolism is associated with metabolizing organically generated anions and the resultant generation of the remaining bicarbonate deficit; the acidosis is, therefore, eliminated with proper systemic therapy. Each mEq/liter of lactate ultimately forms 1 mEq/liter of bicarbonate via aerobic metabolism. Thus, recommended dosages for bicarbonate infusion during CPR should probably not exceed 1 amp (44 mEq) every 3 to 5 minutes. Frequent measurement of arterial blood gases (every 5 to 8 minutes) often reveals that even this dose is excessive. Remember that in low perfusion states, restoration of perfusion is the primary goal and lactic acidosis promptly vanishes when perfusion is re-established.

Acute abrupt interference with gas exchange leads not only to hypoxemia but also to accumulations of CO_2. The compensatory response for acute hypercapnia consists exclusively of tissue buffering which is capable of raising plasma bicarbonate only slightly. Thus, sudden increases in P_{CO_2} to 90 to 100 torr are associated with sudden acidosis, pH 7.05 to 7.1. Prompt increases in alveolar ventilation return P_{CO_2} and pH to normal. The temptation to administer bicarbonate to these patients must be critically appraised; although improvement in the pH may occur, the effect is only evanescent. Furthermore, the cost in terms of sudden volume expansion (1 amp $NaCO_3$ = 300 ml 0.9% NaCl) may be too expensive for the cardiovascular system. Despite these theoretical limitations, in severe bronchial asthma alkalinization seems to be indicated in order to restore bronchomotor responsiveness to epinephrine which can break the vicious cycle. On the other hand, alkali therapy may be life saving when both respiratory and metabolic acidosis can lower pH to dangerous levels.

Sodium-Salt Administration For the support and maintenance of serum bicarbonate levels in chronic mild acidotic states, sodium salts of metabolizable organ acids have been used as an indirect source of bicarbonate. Sodium citrate, lactate, and acetate are most commonly used. These salts are alkalizing only by virtue of their metabolic conversion to bicarbonate and not because of any inherent buffering capacity that they may have. At pH values above those compatible with life, citrate, lactate, and acetate cannot in themselves bind significant amounts of acid. Their chemical reactions proceed as follows:

$$Sodium\ lactate + O_2 \longrightarrow CO_2 + H_2O + NaOH$$

$$CO_2 + H_2O \longrightarrow H_2CO_3$$

$$H_2CO_3 + NaOH \longrightarrow NaHCO_3 + H_2O$$

Sodium lactate and acetate can be useful in situations where calcium and alkali must be mixed in the same solution. Calcium forms an insoluble precipitate with bicarbonate. Sodium bicarbonate is still the most useful alkalizing agent.

Special problems exist which may modify the usual approach to metabolic acidosis. Patients with cardiac or renal failure are prone to volume overload and/or hypernatremia secondary to moderate to large requirements for exogenous sodium bicarbonate. Peritoneal or hemodialysis can provide relief in such situations not only because the organic buffer acetate or lactate when absorbed becomes an immediate source of bicarbonate, but also because dialysis with hypertonic fluids can permit administration of sodium bicarbonate to the extracellular fluid space. Although peritoneal dialysis can lower lactate levels in the blood, many standard peritoneal dialysis solutions contain up to 40 mEq of lactate per liter. In some patients, the solution must be exchanged for an acetate-buffered rather than a lactate-buffered peritoneal dialysate solution.

Therapy of Acidosis with Potassium Deficiency Another problem requiring complex management is the combination of severe acidosis and marked potassium deficiency that can result from massive gastrointestinal losses. In addition, this may also occur in renal tubular acidosis. Correction of acidosis without adequate potassium replacement can lead to severe hypokalemia and profound weakness; on the other hand, administering potassium without correcting the acidosis can lead to marked abrupt increases in serum potassium to dangerous levels long before the total potassium deficit has been corrected. The solution to this problem is careful replacement of *both,* facilitated by separate intravenous lines with extremely frequent monitoring (1 hour or less) of potassium and arterial blood gases along with continuous cardiac rhythm monitoring (Table 6-17).

TABLE 6-17
Metabolic Acidosis—Treatment

Goals
   Diagnose the cause and then correct it!
   Decrease lactate concentration/production
   Correct pH and bicarbonate abnormalities
Calculations
   Assume extracellular space = 30% body weight
   Use actual base deficit (correct if in vitro values reported)
Deficit = 0.3 × BW × base deficit = mEq $NaHCO_3$
Treatment
   Correct by half the calculated value
   Remeasure because:
     Calculations are only a guideline
     Physiologic state is not static; improvement may allow metabolism of lactate; deterioration will be reflected as an inability to correct acidosis (this means that the underlying cause has not been remedied!)

THAM   Although THAM (tris-hydroxy methyl aminomethane) has been used in metabolic acidosis, it offers no advantages over bicarbonate and, in fact, serious side effects detract from its clinical utility. The volumes required plus the fact that it is not directed to reverse the underlying true clinical problem severely limit clinical usefulness if judged by patient survival. THAM will neutralize carbonic acid. It has been suggested to be a better intracellular buffer than exogenously administered bicarbonate; however, objective evidence is lacking.[60]

Summary: Therapy of Metabolic Acidosis   It must be remembered that metabolic acidosis is more a marker of serious cellular metabolic derangement in the critically ill patient than a true cause of any illness; the most important principle is to treat the cause. Severe levels of acidosis, nevertheless, may interfere and compound existing organ dysfunction. As a basis for acid-base therapy, one must remember that most patients in the I.C.U. die with and not because of lactic acidosis. Consequently, all efforts must be directed at uncovering and reversing the underlying cause of the acidosis and reserving alkalinizing therapy only for severe acidosis.

Ketoacidosis   Other than lactate, ketones represent the most important source of fixed acids which may result in severe acid-base derangement. The two major pathways of fatty acid metabolism in the liver are oxidation to carbon dioxide and ketogenesis. Low circulating insulin levels favor mobilizations of fatty acids from adipose tissue to such a great extent that they may overwhelm the liver's ability to oxidize preformed ketones. Ketones, being strong acids, are rapidly buffered by bicarbonate. Therefore, the diagnosis of ketoacidosis is made by noting an anion gap type of acidosis, low bicarbonate and strong serum, and urinary ketones. The two major forms of ketones are acetoacetic acid and β-hydroxybutyric acid (BHB). Tissue hypoxia results in an increase of BHB and a decrease in acetoacetic acid, both being in equilibrium. The standard ketostix, a nitroprusside reaction, does not react with BHB. Therefore, if tissue hypoxia compounds the situation of ketoacidosis, high anion gaps, low bicarbonates, and negative ketostix still do not rule out ketoacidosis. Furthermore, restoration of blood pressure and hemodynamic stability in such patients may result in a paradoxical appearance of biochemical deterioration in face of clinical improvement. A ketone reaction may then become positive as tissue oxidation improves. Continued oxidation of acetoacetic acid reverses this pattern. When normal metabolic pathways are re-established, ketoacids are recycled producing CO_2 and water as metabolites.

METABOLIC ALKALOSIS

Metabolic alkalosis is quite common in critically ill patients but, until recently, has not received the same attention as the more immediately life-threatening derangement—acidosis. Alkalosis can have serious physiologic impacts: increased oxygen consumption, decreased cerebral blood flow, and left shift of the oxyhemoglobin dissociation curve, among others. The immediate compensatory mechanism for metabolic alkalosis is a decrease in ventilation. Theoretically, such hypoventilation, if severe, could result in hypoxemia. Any compensatory decrease in ventilatory response may seriously hinder successful weaning from mechanical ventilation. In addition, the unfavorable leftward shift of the oxyhemoglobin decreases oxygen availability to the tissue. Metabolic alkalosis may also affect CNS function, even producing seizures and coma.

Metabolic alkalosis may be divided into two major categories: those that are salt-responsive (low urine chloride <20 mEq/liter) and those that are salt-resistant (high urine chloride >20 mEq/liter). Under the first category, causes of metabolic alkalosis include large losses of gastric juice, diuretic therapy and compensatory renal conservation of bicarbonate, seen in chronic hypercapnia associated with chronic obstructive pulmonary disease. In the latter salt-resistant group, less common causes, such as hypoaldosteronism and Cushing's syndrome occur. In this latter group, which is rarely seen in I.C.U. patients, the administration of saline is of no value (Table 6-18).

TABLE 6-18
Metabolic Alkalosis

Salt Responsive—all commonly seen in I.C.U. (urine Cl < 20 mEq/liter)
Postresuscitation (lactate + citrate metabolites)
Gastric losses
Diuretic therapy
Chronic hypercapnea
Salt Resistant—rarely seen in I.C.U. (urine Cl > 20 mEq/liter)
Hypoaldosteronism
Cushing's syndrome

Metabolic alkalosis results from any process that tends to elevate plasma bicarbonate. The kidneys normally maintain plasma bicarbonate concentration between 24 and 26 mEq/liter. Acidification of the urine is accomplished by the tubular exchange of the hydrogen ion for sodium ion in tubular fluid. When hydrogen ions are excreted into tubular fluid, sodium and bicarbonate are reabsorbed. Beside the excretion of titratable acid (hydrogen ion), the generation excretion of ammonium salts by the tubular cell serves as another mechanism of acid excretion. Thus, plasma bicarbonate concentration can be maintained in a fairly narrow range coupled with sodium reabsorption and urinary acidification. In addition, another tubular field anion, chloride, may be reabsorbed with sodium to preserve electrical neutrality. If chloride is deficient (hypochloremia) in tubular fluid, only bicarbonate is available for reabsorption with sodium. The tubular extrusion of hydrogen and potassium into tubular fluid is associated with this chloride-deficient state. Furthermore, as serum potassium becomes depleted, intracellular potassium moves out of the cell in exchange for serum hydrogen ions, thus resulting in the accumulation of bicarbonate in the plasma.

Gastric Loss Alkalosis resulting from vomiting or gastric suction, is the most common type of chloride-responsive alkalosis seen in the I.C.U. patient (Fig. 6-17). Gastric chloride loss induces total body chloride depletion as well as active loss of hydrogen ions. This results in a deficiency of an anion suitable for reabsorption with sodium in the proximal renal tubular filtrate. This then blocks the compensatory mechanism usually available to affect the initial gastric loss of hydrogen ions. A greater amount of sodium, therefore, is presented to the distal tubule for exchange with hydrogen and potassium. *One must always remember that the effect of hydrogen excreted into tubular fluid is the same as bicarbonate reabsorption* and that this results in generation of metabolic alkalosis by the kidney. Thus, a continued augmentation of distal tubular hydrogen ion secretion will perpetuate an elevation in extracellular fluid bicarbonate and will also lead to depletion of body potassium. As intracellular potassium depletion occurs, intracellular pH becomes more acid. The kidney responds by conserving potassium and excreting hydrogen ion, and a concomitant generation of a paradoxical aciduria associ-

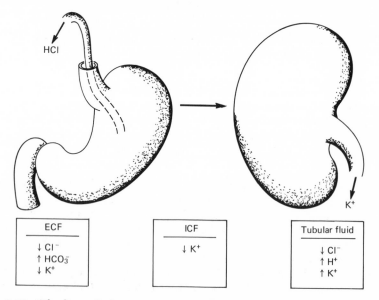

Fig. 6-17. The loss of gastric acid is the most common cause of severe metabolic alkalosis in the I.C.U. Removal of gastric contents from the body results in losses of hydrogen and chloride ions. Combined with the resultant loss of potassium ions through the kidney, a characteristic serum and urine electrolyte profile is created.

ated with metabolic alkalosis. Obviously, the urine of these patients will contain little chloride. When they are given sodium chloride, sodium is again reabsorbed along with chloride in the proximal tubule, ECF is restored in volume and excretion of excess bicarbonate results in correction of the alkalosis.

Although severe renal insufficiency is typically associated with a tendency toward acidosis, metabolic alkalosis develops in the I.C.U. patient in renal failure, due to coincidental large gastric losses. Clearly NaCl infusions in the functionally anephric patient may not be tolerated. On the other hand, this difficult management situation must not be confused with dehydration and consequent azotemia which will respond rapidly to ECF restoration. The overly aggressive use of potent diuretics (furosemide, ethacrynic acid) may lead to prerenal azotemia and an alkalosis created in the volume-deficient state.

Chloride Loss Alkalosis due to chloride depletion, secondary to massive chloride losses via the gastrointestinal tract in patients with adequate renal function, ordinarily responds to extracellular fluid replenishment and chloride replacement as either NaCl or KCl. In renal failure, however, one can use large quantities of neither potassium nor sodium as the chloride vehicle. Various preparations containing hydrochloric acid have been used, including ammonium hydrochloride, arginine hydrochloride, lysine monohydrochloride, but these compounds all deliver an additional nitrogen load and may increase azotemia. In addition, since some element of hepatic dysfunction is frequently coexistent, ammonia infusions are prohibited. In fact, the arginine compound has been removed from the market. Although hypertonic sodium chloride theoretically could be given (if appropriate high ultrafiltration/high flow hemodialysis were also instituted to remove the excess sodium), it seems much simpler to treat this type of alkalosis with the simplest and most direct chloride vehicle which will correct the alkalosis, i.e., hydrochloric acid (Table 6-19).

TABLE 6-19
Metabolic Alkalosis—Rationale for Therapy

Sodium chloride—supplies extracellular fluid, extracellular cation, and chloride for tubular exchange

Potassium chloride—supplies potassium for exchange with hydrogen ion and chloride for bicarbonate exchange

Acetazolamide—carbonic anhydrase inhibitor; results in tubular excretion of bicarbonate

Hydrochloric acid—replaces lost hydrogen and chloride ions, neutralizes excess bicarbonate

Ammonium chloride, lysine monochloride—metabolic processes provide hydrogen ion, chloride ion replaced; rarely useful in I.C.U.

By determining the amount of chloride deficit and the ongoing chloride losses, one may replace such a deficit and losses with 0.1N to 0.2N HCl and D5W solution. This solution contains 100 to 200 mEq of both hydrogen and chloride ions. This must be administered through a large central vein, since peripheral vein HCl infusions may cause tissue necrosis and full thickness skin slough. The pH of the solution is defined as the negative logarithm of the hydrogen ion concentration—in this instance $0.1N = 10^{-1}$ hydrogen ions or a pH of 1. Measuring the electrolyte content of an aliquot of gastric drainage to guide daily chloride replacement may show variations from 50 to 150 mEq/liter. Daily gastric losses can then be titrated with the infusion of 0.1 normal hydrochloric acid. For example, a 60-kg man in acute renal failure has 2000 ml per day of gastric losses, resulting in a serum chloride of 85 mEq/liter; if one assumes a "chloride space" of approximately 30 percent of body weight, then the immediate deficit may be calculated thus:

$$(100 \text{ mEq/liter} - 85 \text{ mEq/liter}) \times 0.3 \times 60 \text{ kg} = 270 \text{ mEq/liter}$$

Thus, a 270 mEq chloride deficit exists. At least 50 percent of the deficit can be safely corrected in 24 hours. If an aliquot of gastric aspirate shows a chloride of 100 mEq/liter, the projected losses over the next 24 hours can be estimated by multiplying 2000 ml $\times$ 100 mEq/liter = 200 mEq. Thus, therapy may be initiated by multiplying 1/2 $\times$ 270 + 200 = 335 mEq chloride which can be administered in a replacement volume calculated to be 2000 ml for gastric loss, 500 ml for net insensible loss, or a maintenance solution of D5W of 2500 ml. Sterile 1.0 normal HCl (150 ml) is added to 850 ml D5W. Two and one-half liters of this 0.15 normal HCl—D5W solution would satisfy the above requirements. When proper chloride balance has been achieved, gastric losses may be replaced ml for ml with 0.1 normal HCl. After correcting the initial alkalosis, the functionally anephric surgical patient can be easily managed if daily sodium and potassium balances are calculated. By adding cimetidine (300 mg every 6 hours I.V.), gastric volume may not be substantially effected but hydrogen ion losses can be significantly decreased.

With adequate renal function, intravenous HCl is not usually required to correct metabolic alkalosis unless the metabolic alkalosis is severe; one should recall that both NaCl and KCl correct alkalosis by suppressing renal acid secretion and increasing renal alkali excretion. These corrective mechanisms when utilized are necessarily slow and more rapid correction can be achieved using simultaneous administration of an HCL infusion. Patients with severe metabolic alkalosis may require large quantities of volume replacement (5 to 7 liters per day) along with KCl replacement in the range of 400 to 600 mEq/day for the first 24 hours. When potassium depletion is also severe, volume expansion with NaCl alone without KCl cannot fully correct the associated alkalosis. Alternately, when chloride deficits are present, hypokalemia and alkalosis cannot be corrected with potassium administration alone;

potassium acetate will fail to correct the abnormalities while potassium chloride will provide the necessary chloride for tubular exchange of bicarbonate.

Similar to metabolic acidosis therapy, the correction of metabolic alkalosis requires the frequent measurement of blood pH and bicarbonate concentration as well as serum potassium in order to document a fall in plasma bicarbonate and a rise in the serum potassium. In addition, when the urine chloride excretion approximates 100 mEq/liter one can fairly well assume that chloride replenishment has been adequate.

With infrequent exceptions, metabolic alkalosis does not seem to result in a compensatory increase in Pco_2 by a reflex decrease in ventilation. Nevertheless, the population at most risk can be found in the I.C.U. In the unconscious, semicomatose, or severely debilitated patient, metabolic alkalosis may precipitate a marked alveolar hypoventilation (Pco_2 = 50 to 60 torr), particularly when bicarbonate concentration is $\geq$ 40 to 45 mEq/liter. If the patient's baseline Pco_2 (COPD) is 50 to 60 torr, then a 10-torr rise due to superimposed metabolic alkalosis can be associated with narcosis.

Hypercapnia   Chronic hypercapnia Pco_2 (70 to 80 torr) is not associated with severe acidosis due to renal compensatory processes of increasing bicarbonate reabsorption. Superimposed acute hypercapnia can develop either when pneumonia or severe respiratory insufficiency supervenes or when oxygen therapy suppresses ventilation in patients whose only respiratory drive is hypoxemia. For severe superimposed infections, antibiotics and assisted ventilation are indicated. Low-flow oxygen therapy and assisted ventilation will correct patients who operate with hypoxic drive. Furthermore, complicating metabolic alkalosis induced by diuretics or vomiting may also impede the ventilatory drive and exacerbate the hypercapnia. In such cases, reduction of plasma bicarbonate to levels appropriate for the patients' usual chronic steady state of CO_2 tension should be achieved by potassium chloride, sodium chloride, or hydrochloric acid administration. Diamox (acetazolamide) can also be employed to enhance bicarbonate excretion. Occasionally, patients will present with Pco_2 55 to 60 torr, bicarbonate 45 to 60 mEq/liter, and pH 7.55 to 7.6; although this pattern is usually seen with chronic respiratory acidosis and superimposed metabolic alkalosis, important exceptions occur. Some patients with these acid-base findings can be shown to have a primary metabolic alkalosis with an unusual degree of respiratory compensation. Distinguishing these disorders involves administering sodium chloride, potassium chloride, or Diamox to correct the alkalosis. If Pco_2 returns to normal after alkalosis is corrected, it can be assumed that the original disturbance was a primary metabolic alkalosis with extreme respiratory compensation (Table 6-20).

Other Manifestations of Alkalosis   The respiratory alkalosis that occurs in association with pulmonary embolism, bacteremia, liver disease, and

TABLE 6-20
Metabolic Alkalosis

Calculation of deficit
  Assume chloride space = 30% body weight
  Assume normal chloride = 100 mEq/liter
  Using measured serum chloride and X, deficit = $(100-X) \times 0.3 \times$ body weight
In mild deficits without continuing losses, use NaCl + KCl; volumes indicated
  by overall fluid, renal, and cardiovascular status
If short term and mild to moderate deficits use acetazolamide 500 mg I.V. q 12
  hr for no longer than 2 days
In severe deficits and/or continued major losses, use 0.1N HCl (100 mEq/liter);
  calculate deficit; replace at 10–15 mEq hr
  Caution: a secure central venous catheter must be used (pH of solution = 1);
    mix 8 ml 12 normal HCl in 1 liter D5W to create approximately 0.1 N HCl
If large gastric losses persist, use cimetidine 300 mg I.V. q 6 hr to reduce gastric
  outpouring of acid which will lessen balance problems

CNS disorders is frequently a therapeutic dilemma. Patients with severe, acute hypocapnia characteristically have only a moderate reduction in plasma bicarbonate and a marked alkalosis. There seems to be little justification for trying to raise CO_2 tensions by giving narcotics or any analgesics to suppress ventilation or acid to lower bicarbonate. There is no evidence that either of these technical manipulations influences morbidity or mortality. The only rational approach is to uncover and correct the underlying cause of hyperventilation.

For the patient with chronic hypercarbia associated with COPD, emphysema, and/or chronic bronchitis, cardiopulmonary reserve is minimal and stress is life threatening. Interpretations of blood gases can be tricky since the patient operates from a different base line; increased Pco_2 and decreased Po_2 are normal. One cannot and should not demand that this patient do better than he was doing prior to the acute problem. The chronically hypercarbic patient may respond to acute stress by increasing alveolar ventilation. This may be difficult to recognize in the arterial blood gas pattern unless the clinical state of the patient was previously documented. Initially, one would interpret such a decrease in Pco_2 and an increase in pH as an uncompensated metabolic alkalosis with hypoxemia. This would be an incorrect interpretation if one did not know the patient "normally" retained CO_2 because of his chronic lung impairment. Likewise, patients with COPD may have superimposed acute ventilatory failure; in these cases, the severity can be judged by assessing the degree of acidemia. In other words, if acute hypercarbia is present with mild degrees of acidemia, one may assume that the baseline state is one of a high Pco_2. If ventilation is needed, the Pco_2 must not be "normalized" ($Pco_2 = 40$ torr), but reduced only enough to restore a normal pH which will reflect the metabolic compensations. A patient who normally has a Pco_2 of 60 to 70 should be ventilated to that "normal" Pco_2 value so as not to disrupt acid-base and electrolyte changes. Maintaining Pco_2 lower than normal will result in acute respiratory alkalosis and consequent increase in the renal excretion of base. Thus, if Pco_2 is abruptly changed from 70 to 40 and the pH changed from 7.4 to 7.55 or above, then the kidney will respond in 24 to 36 hours by readjusting to a true "normal" pH level by excreting bicarbonate.

Also, the COPD patient who requires ventilation support following emergency surgery may acutely alter a "baseline" compensated respiratory acidosis (increased plasma bicarbonate). Lactic acidosis generated during low perfusion states may deplete the bicarbonate buffering capacity. In these patients, regulating mechanical ventilation to maintain Pco_2 at baseline preop values (Pco_2 = 50 to 60) may be associated with moderate severe acidosis (pH 7.20 to 7.30). If pH does not drop below 7.25, allowing hypercarbia (Pco_2 = 50 to 60) to exist will result in renal regeneration of plasma bicarbonate levels which will shift pH to a more normal range (7.35 to 7.45). Once acid-base homeostasis has been reestablished, weaning from mechanical ventilation should be possible.

In addition to the pathophysiologic changes associated with alkalemia affecting central nervous system, cardiovascular, and presumably enzyme function, the weaning period becomes a significant problem since the patient will only be able to generate sufficient minute ventilation to reduce his Pco_2 to a baseline of 70. At this point in time, the Pco_2 of 70 is associated with an acute respiratory acidemia and may be interpreted as an inability to wean.

Furthermore, since many patients with COPD have associated cardiac decompensation, potent "loop" diuretics may be utilized in the initial management. The metabolic effect is to enhance the alkalosis secondary to the action of these loop diuretics resulting in chloride and potassium depletion. This takes approximately 24 hours to develop after use of loop diuretics. Diamox (acetazolamide) can rapidly induce a bicarbonate diuresis in such patients even if they are hyponatremic, leading to a rapid reduction of Pco_2. When diuresis is indicated in these patients, acetazolamide (500 mg) by the I.V. route may provoke a diuresis of bicarbonate-rich urine. The dose may be repeated every 8 to 12 hours, but after 36 to 48 hours most patients become resistant to this diuretic and to its bicarbonate excretion. Acetazolamide is an inhibitor of carbonic anhydrase activity, thereby preventing the generation and tubular secretion of hydrogen ion. In addition to those patients with severe metabolic alkalosis, complicating chronic respiratory disease, this drug may be useful as a diuretic in other common manifestations of metabolic alkalosis seen in the I.C.U. patient. Following resuscitation from hemorrhagic shock with both massive transfusion and Ringer's lactate infusion, the postresuscitation acid-base derangement (if resuscitation has been complete) is usually metabolic alkalosis—primarily due to the citrate of banked blood. If those patients are unable to invoke an effective spontaneous diuresis as an index of normal extracellular fluid resuscitation, diuretics in low doses may assist the mobilization of sequestered fluids and excretion so as to avoid acute volume expansion. Although the potent loop diuretics are most popular, to choose a diuretic which further potentiates metabolic alkalosis does not seem warranted. Consequently, to avoid the alkalosis-induced reflex depression of ventilatory drive, acetazolamide may be utilized, which not only effects a diuretic response but prevents and corrects the excess bicarbonate generated in the extracellular fluid.

Carbenicillin therapy may be associated with an acid-base and metabolic derangement—an increase in anion gap and a large sodium load. Each gram of carbenicillin contains about 5 mEq sodium. Therefore, a standard therapeutic dose for severe septicemia of 30 gm per day is equivalent to 150 mEq sodium load. However, this increased anion gap is due to unmeasured carbenicillin; the anion gap is, therefore, not reflected as acidosis. In fact, metabolic alkalosis with hypokalemia associated with carbenicillin usage is usually noted. The anion of sodium carbenicillin is poorly reabsorbed while sodium is promptly reabsorbed particularly in sodium-added states. Thus, to preserve electrical neutrality within the tubular lumen, potassium and hydrogen are excreted; therefore, hypokalemic metabolic alkalosis results.

SUMMARY OF ACID-BASE DERANGEMENTS

Intracellular metabolism requires a very narrow range of free hydrogen ion concentration (pH) within which enzymatic and biochemical processes may function efficiently and appropriately. Extracellular measurements, while often important, may not reflect the most significant physiologic changes. Significant deviation from these narrow limits are poorly tolerated and may be life threatening. Despite a history of complicated mathematics and confusing terminology, clinical acid-base chemistry can be applied to the care of I.C.U. patients by relying on direct measurements of blood pH and P_{CO_2}. Modern technology in the blood gas laboratory furnishes a calculated actual bicarbonate concentration, which is a far less expensive technique but as accurate as direct measurement.

REFERENCES

1. Moore FD, Olesen KH, McMurray ID et al: The Body Cell Mass and its Supporting Environment. Philadelphia: Saunders, 1963
2. Moore FD, Edelman IS, Olney JM et al: Body sodium and potassium. Metabolism 3:334, 1954
3. Moore FD, Ball MR: The Metabolic Response to Surgery. Springfield, Illinois: Thomas, 1952

4. Trunkey DD, Ulner HMD, Wagner IY et al: The effect of hemorrhagic shock on intracellular muscle action potential in primate. Surgery 74:241, 1973
5. Chaudry IH, Sayeed MM, Baue AE: Effect of hemorrhagic shock on tissue adenine nucleotides in conscious rats. Can J Physiol Pharmacol 52:131, 1974
6. Chaudry IH, Sayeed MM, Baue AE: Insulin resistance in experimental shock: Arch Surg 109:412, 1974
7. Carrico CJ, Canizaro PC, Shires GT: Fluid resuscitation following injury: rationale for the use of balanced salt solutions. Crit Care Med 4:46, 1976
8. McClelland RN, Shires GT, Baxter CR et al: Balanced salt solution in the treatment of hemorrhagic shock. JAMA 199:830, 1967
9. Kirby RR, Civetta JM: The Hyland symposium: "point-counterpoint: factors in pulmonary edema." Crit Care Med 7:83, 1979
10. Lowe RJ, Moss GS, Jilek J et al: Crystalloid versus colloid in the etiology of pulmonary failure after trauma: a randomized trial in man. Surgery 81:676, 1977
11. Zarins CK, Rice CL, Smith DE et al: Role of lymphatics in preventing hypooncotic pulmonary edema. Surg Forum 27:257, 1976
12. Calva E, Mujica A, Bisteni A et al: Oxidative phosphorylation in cardiac infarct: effect of G-I-K solution. Am J Physiol 209:371, 1965
13. Weisul JP, O'Donnel FT, Stone MA et al: Myocardial performance in clinical septic shock. J Surg Res 18:357, 1975
14. Maroko PR, Libley P, Sobel BE et al: Effect of G-I-K infusion on myocardial infarction following experimental coronary artery occlusion. Circulation 45:1160, 1972
15. Civetta JM et al: G-I-K: results of "maximal therapy." Crit Care Med (Abstr) 6:93, 1978
16. Chaudry IH, Sayeed MM, Baue AE: Effect of ATP-MgCl$_2$ administration in shock. Surgery 75:220, 1974
17. Chaudry IH, Sayeed MM, Baue AE: Reversal of insulin resistance by in vivo infusion of ATP in shock. Surg Forum 26:44, 1975
18. McCurdy DK: Hyperosmolar hyperglycemic nonketotic diabetic coma. Med Clin North Am 54:683, 1970
19. Moran WH, Miltenberger FW, Shuayb WA et al: The relationship of ADH secretion to surgical stress. Surgery 65:99, 1964
20. Bartter FC, Schwartz WB: The syndrome of inappropriate secretion of ADH. Am J Med 42:790, 1967
21. Mueller CB, Thomas EJ: Nutritional needs of the normal adult. In Manual of Surgical Nutrition. Committee of Pre and Postoperative Care, American College of Surgeons. Philadelphia: Saunders, 1975, p. 142
22. Wilmore DW, Aulick LH, Pruitt BA: Metabolism during the hypermetabolic phase of thermal injury. Adv Surg 12:193, 1978
23. Becker R, Johnson DW, Woeber KA et al: Depressed serum T$_3$ levels following thermal injury. Fed Proc 35:316, 1976
24. Cahill GF Jr: Starvation in man. N Engl J Med 282:668, 1970
25. Long CL, Spencer JL, Kinney JM et al: Carbohydrate metabolism in man: effect of elective operations and major injury. J Appl Physiol 31:110, 1971
26. Kinney JM, Duke JH Jr, Long CL et al: Tissue fuel and weight loss after injury. J Clin Pathol (Suppl) 4:65, 1978
27. Blackburn GL, Maini BS, Pierce EC: Nutrition in the critically ill patient. Anesthesiology 47:181, 1977

28. Pietsch JB, Meakins JL, MacLean LD: Delayed hypersensitivity response: application in clinical surgery. Surgery 82:349, 1977

29. Meakins JL, McLean APH et al: Delayed hypersensitivity and neutrophil chemotaxis: effect of trauma. J Trauma 18:240, 1978

30. Woolfson AMJ, Heatley RV, Allison SP: Insulin to inhibit protein catabolism after injury. N Engl J Med 300:14, 1979

31. Fischer JE, Funovics JM, Aguirre A et al: The role of plasma amino acids in hepatic encephalopathy. Surgery 78:276, 1975

32. Fischer JE, Rosen HM, Ebeid AM et al: The effect of normalization of plasma amino acids on hepatic encephalopathy in man. Surgery 80:77, 1976

33. Freund H, Yoshimura N, Lunetta L et al: The role of the branched-chain amino acids in decreasing muscle catabolism in vivo. Surgery 83:611, 1978

34. Dobbie RP, Hoffmeister JA: Continuous pump-tube enteric hyperalimentation. Surg Gynecol Obstet 143:273, 1976

35. Gamble JL: Physiologic information gained from studies on the life-raft ration. Harvey Lect 42:247, 1947

36. Blackburn GL, Flatt JP, Clowes GHA et al: Peripheral intravenous feeding with isotonic amino acid solutions. Am J Surg 125:447, 1973

37. Wolfe BM, Culebras JM, Tweedle D et al: Effect of glucose on the nitrogen-sparing effect of amino acids given intravenously. Surg Forum 27:39, 1976

38. Touloukian RJ, Downing SE: Cholestasis associated with long-term parenteral hyperalimentation. Arch Surg 106:58, 1973

39. Kinney JM: Energy requirements of the surgical patient. In Manual of Surgical Nutrition. Committee on Pre and Postoperative Care, American College of Surgeons. Philadelphia: Saunders, 1975, p. 223

40. Anderson GH, Patel DG, Jeejeebhoy KN: Design and evaluation by nitrogen balance and blood aminograms of an amino acid mixture for total parenteral nutrition of adults with gastrointestinal disease. J Clin Invest 53:904, 1974

41. Abel RM, Beck CH Jr, Abbott WM et al: Improved survival from acute renal failure following treatment with intravenous essential L-amino acids and glucose, N Engl J Med 288:695, 1973

42. Baldessarini RJ, Fischer JE: Serotonin metabolism in rat brain after surgical diversion of the portal venous circulation. Nature [New Biol] 254:25, 1973

43. Long JM, Wilmore DW, Mason AD et al: The effect of carbohydrate and fat intake on nitrogen excretion during total intravenous feedings. Ann Surg 185:417, 1977

44. Jarstrand C, Berghem L, Lahnborg G: Human granulocyte and R-E system function during intralipid infusion. J Parent Ent Nutrit 2:633, 1978

45. Page M, Alberti KG et al: Treatment of diabetic coma with continuous low-dose infusion of insulin. Br Med J 2:687, 1974

46. Fischer JE: Total parenteral nutrition. Boston: Little, Brown, 1976

47. Travis SF, Sugarman HJ et al: Alteration of red-cell glycolytic intermediates and oxygen transport as a consequence of hypophosphatemia in patients receiving intravenous hyperalimentation. N Engl J Med 285:763, 1971

48. Kinney JM, Askanazi J, Gump FE et al: Use of the ventilatory equivalent to separate hypermetabolism from increased dead space ventilation in the injured or septic patient. Presented at American Association Surgery of Trauma, Lake Tahoe, Nevada, September, 1978

49. Allinson R: Plasma trace elements during total parenteral nutrition. J Parent Ent Nutrit 2:35, 1978

50. Ryan JA, Abel RM, Abbott WM et al: Catheter complications in total parenteral nutrition. N Engl J Med 290:757, 1974

51. Sanderson I, Deitel M: Intravenous hyperalimentation without sepsis. Surg Gynecol Obstet 136:577, 1973
52. Mitchell JH, Wildenthal K, Johnson RL: The effects of acid-base disturbances on cardiovascular and pulmonary function. Kidney Int 1:375, 1972
53. Brackett NC, Cohen JJ, Schwartz WB: Carbon dioxide titration curve of normal man. N Engl J Med 272:6, 1965
54. Broder G, Weil MH: Excess lactate: an index of reversibility of shock in human patients. Science 143:1457, 1964
55. Takaori M, Safar P: Treatment of massive hemorrhage with colloids and crystalloid solutions. JAMA 199:297, 1967
56. Shires GT, Coln D, Carrico J et al: Fluid therapy in hemorrhagic shock. Arch Surg 88:688, 1964
57. Carey LC, Lowery BD, Cloutier CT: Hemorrhagic shock. Curr Probl Surg, January 1971, p. 48
58. Huckabee WE: Lactic acidosis. Am J Cardiol 12:663, 1963
59. Taradash MR, Jacobson LB: Vasodilator therapy of idiopathic lactic acidosis. N Engl J Med 293:468, 1975
60. Bleich HL, Schwartz WB: Tris buffer (THAM). N Engl J Med 274:782, 1966

INDEX